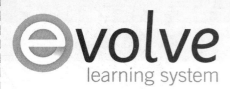

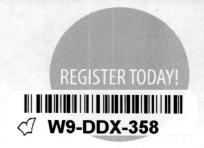
To access your Student Resources, visit the web address below:

http://evolve.elsevier.com/Sorrentino/essentials/

Evolve Student Learning Resources for *Workbook and Competency Evaluation Review for Mosby's Essentials for Nursing Assistants,* Fourth Edition offers the following features:

- **Video Clips**

  Demonstrate important steps in procedures included in the textbook

- **Audio Glossary**

  Provides definitions of all key terms in addition to audio pronunciations for selected key terms

- **Useful Spanish Vocabulary and Phrases**

  Includes helpful translations of common healthcare terms and phrases

- **Skills Evaluation**

  Reviews procedures that may be covered on competency evaluations

- **Checklists**

  Allow for instructor and self-evaluation

- **Body Spectrum**

  Provides interactive review of Anatomy and Physiology content

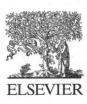

ELSEVIER

Workbook and Competency Evaluation Review for

Mosby's Essentials for
Nursing Assistants

FOURTH EDITION

BERNIE GOREK, BS, MA

Gerontology Consultant
New England, North Dakota

Competency Evaluation Review by
LEIGHANN N. REMMERT, BSN, RN

Clinical Instructor, Capital Area School of Practical Nursing
Springfield, Illinois

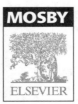

MOSBY
ELSEVIER

3251 Riverport Lane
Maryland Heights, Missouri 63043

WORKBOOK AND COMPETENCY EVALUATION REVIEW FOR
MOSBY'S ESSENTIALS FOR NURSING ASSISTANTS

ISBN: 978-0-323-06874-1

Notices

The content and procedures in this book are based on information currently available. They were reviewed by instructors and practicing professionals in various regions of the United States. However, agency policies and procedures may vary from the information and procedures in this book. In addition, research and new information may require changes in standards and practices.

Standards and guidelines from the Centers for Disease Control and Prevention (CDC) and the Occupational Safety and Health Administration (OSHA) may change as new information becomes available. Other federal and state agencies also may issue new standards and guidelines. So may accrediting agencies and national organizations.

You are responsible for following the policies and procedures of your employer and the most current standards, practices, and guidelines as they relate to the safety of your work.

To the fullest extent of the law, neither the Publisher nor the authors or editors, assume any liability for any injury and/or damage to persons or property as a matter of products liability, negligence or otherwise, or from any use or operation of any methods, products, instructions, or ideas contained in the material herein.

ISBN: 978-0-323-06874-1

Executive Editor: Susan R. Epstein
Senior Developmental Editor: Maria Broeker
Publishing Services Manager: Jeff Patterson
Project Manager: Tracey Schriefer
Designer: Jessica Williams

Printed in the United States of America

Last digit is the print number: 9 8 7 6 5

Working together to grow
libraries in developing countries

www.elsevier.com | www.bookaid.org | www.sabre.org

ELSEVIER   BOOK AID International   Sabre Foundation

To my husband, Tom.
Thank you for your assistance, your support,
your humor, and your love.

Preface

This workbook is written to be used with *Mosby's Essentials for Nursing Assistants*, fourth edition by Sheila A. Sorrentino, Leighann N. Remmert, and Bernie Gorek. Any reference to the "textbook" in this workbook refers to *Mosby's Essentials for Nursing Assistants*, fourth edition.

This workbook is designed to help you apply what you have learned in each chapter. You are encouraged to use this workbook as a study guide. Various types of study questions (matching, fill in the blanks, and multiple choice) and learning exercises are included in each chapter to help you understand and apply the information in the textbook.

Case studies are provided for each chapter. They will help you think about what you have learned and apply your knowledge in practical situations. Likewise, the **Additional Learning Activities** encourage discussion and practical application of the information presented in each chapter. These activities are meant to challenge you and add to the learning experience.

Procedure checklists are provided that correspond with the procedures in *Mosby's Essentials for Nursing Assistants*, fourth edition. NNAAP™ skills are identified. These checklists are intended to help you become confident and skilled when performing procedures that affect the quality of care you provide.

The answers to the workbook questions are provided in the *TEACH Instructor Resources and Program Guide*, which accompanies the textbook. Your instructor will provide answers as needed.

The **Competency Evaluation Review** includes a general review section and two practice exams with answers to help you prepare for the written certification exam. It also features a skills review guide that helps you practice procedures required for certification.

Nursing assistants are important members of the health and nursing teams. Completing the exercises in this workbook will increase your knowledge, skills, and confidence. The goal is to prepare you to provide the best possible care and to help you develop pride in the important work you do.

1 INTRODUCTION TO HOSPITALS AND NURSING CENTERS

STUDY QUESTIONS

Matching

Match each term with the correct definition.

1. _____ A nurse who has completed a 1-year nursing program and has passed a licensing test

2. _____ A long-term care center that provides complex care for severe health problems

3. _____ The many health care workers whose skills and knowledge focus on the person's total care

4. _____ Provides a room, meals, laundry, and supervision

5. _____ A person who has passed a nursing assistant training and competency evaluation program; performs delegated nursing tasks under the supervision of a licensed nurse

6. _____ A long-term care center that provides health care services to persons who need regular or continuous care

7. _____ An agency or program for persons who are dying

8. _____ Those who provide nursing care; RNs, LPNs/LVNs, and nursing assistants

9. _____ A federal law requiring that nursing centers provide care in a manner and in a setting that maintains or improves each person's quality of life, health, and safety

10. _____ Complex medical care or rehabilitation when hospital care is no longer needed

11. _____ A nurse who has completed a 2-, 3-, or 4-year nursing program and has passed a licensing test

12. _____ Provides housing, personal care, support services, health care, and social activities in a home-like setting to persons needing help with daily activities

A. Board and care home
B. Health care team (interdisciplinary health team)
C. Omnibus Budget Reconciliation Act of 1987 (OBRA)
D. Licensed practical nurse (LPN)
E. Registered nurse (RN)
F. Nursing center (nursing facility, nursing home)
G. Nursing team
H. Nursing assistant
I. Skilled nursing facility (SNF)
J. Subacute care
K. Assisted living residence (ALR)
L. Hospice

Fill in the Blanks

13. Hospitals and long-term care centers provide

    health care services. _____ is the focus of care.

14. Define the following terms:

    A. Acute illness _____

    _____

    _____

    B. Chronic illness _____

    _____

    _____

    C. Terminal illness _____

    _____

    _____

15. Persons who live in long-term care centers are

    called _____.

16. _____

_____ is a document that explains the person's rights and expectations during hospital stays.

17. Long-term care centers are designed to meet the needs of persons who cannot care for themselves at home, but do not need hospital care. Describe the following types of persons cared for in long-term care centers:

A. Confused and disoriented persons _____

_____

_____

_____

B. Short-term residents _____

_____

_____

_____

C. Persons needing respite care _____

_____

_____

_____

D. Mentally ill persons _____

_____

_____

_____

18. Disabilities occurring before 22 years of age are

called _____.

19. An Alzheimer's unit is designed for _____

_____

_____

20. A hospital has a governing body called the

_____.

21. In nursing centers, department directors report

to _____.

22. The goal of the health team is to _____

_____.

23. You are concerned about the care a team member is providing a patient. Which health team

member should you tell? _____

_____

24. Which health team member is responsible for the entire nursing staff and the care given?

_____

_____

25. Nursing education staff are responsible for:

A. _____

B. _____

C. _____

D. _____

E. _____

F. _____

26. Describe primary nursing. _____

_____

_____

_____

_____

27. _____ is a federal health insurance program for persons 65 years of age or older.

28. A nursing center resident is not able to exercise her rights. Who can do so for her?

_____

_____

29. Nursing centers must inform residents of their rights.

A. When are residents informed of their rights?

_____

_____

_____

B. How are residents informed of their rights?

_____

_____

_____

30. A resident tells you he will not take his walk this morning. What should you do?

_____

_____

31. Residents have the right to be free from abuse. This includes _____

   _____

   _____ .

32. Involuntary seclusion involves:

   A. _____

   _____

   _____

   B. _____

   _____

   _____

   C. _____

   _____

   _____

33. A doctor's order is needed for restraint use. Restraints are not used:

   A. For _____

   B. To _____

34. Nursing center activity programs must promote

   _____

   _____

   _____ .

35. Health care agency standards are set by

   _____

   _____

   _____ .

36. Write the meanings of the following abbreviations:

   A. LPN _____

   B. ALR _____

   C. RN _____

   D. OBRA _____

   E. SNF _____

   F. DON _____

   G. LVN _____

   H. DRG _____

   I. RUG _____

   J. CMG _____

   K. OT _____

   L. HMO _____

   M. PT _____

37. A patient is having difficulty swallowing. Which health team member evaluates swallowing

   disorders? _____

38. A resident cannot hold on to his fork when he tries to eat. Which health team member evaluates the problem and designs eating utensils to help the person eat independently?

   _____

Multiple Choice
Circle the **BEST** Answer

39. An ombudsman is
   A. A nursing center administrator
   B. Someone who promotes the interests of another person
   C. Someone who assists the medical director
   D. A health care agency's legal advisor

40. Team nursing
   A. Focuses on tasks and jobs
   B. Involves a team of nursing staff led by an RN
   C. Involves a primary nurse who is responsible for the resident's total care
   D. Involves a case manager coordinating the person's care

41. Which is a health care payment program sponsored by the federal government and operated by the states?
   A. Private insurance
   B. Medicaid
   C. Medicare
   D. Prospective payment

42. This prospective payment system is for SNF payments.
   A. Diagnosis-related groups (DRGs)
   B. Resource utilization groups (RUGs)
   C. Case mix groups (CMGs)
   D. Private insurance

43. Managed care
   A. Is a health insurance plan sponsored by the federal government
   B. Is a nursing care pattern
   C. Deals with health care delivery and payment
   D. Is required by OBRA

44. Nursing center residents have the right to information. This includes the following *except* the right to
    A. See all of his or her records
    B. Be fully informed of his or her total condition
    C. Information about his or her doctor
    D. Information about his or her roommate
45. If a person does not give consent or refuses treatment, it cannot be given.
    A. True
    B. False
46. A resident received a letter from her daughter. You know that the person cannot read. You can open the letter without the person's consent.
    A. True
    B. False
47. Which action promotes courteous and dignified care?
    A. Styling the person's hair the way you like it
    B. Rearranging pictures in the person's room
    C. Allowing the person to choose what clothing to wear
    D. Doing everything for the person
48. Which action does *not* promote the person's privacy?
    A. Draping the person properly during care procedures
    B. Knocking on the door before entering the person's room
    C. Closing the bathroom door when the person uses the bathroom
    D. Providing care with the room door open
49. Which statement about restraints is *correct?*
    A. Restraints are always used when patients and residents are confused.
    B. To keep them safe, all older patients and residents are restrained at night.
    C. Restraints are always used for persons at risk for falling.
    D. A doctor's order is needed for restraint use.
50. Which is *not* part of your role in the survey process?
    A. Reviewing staffing patterns
    B. Providing quality care
    C. Helping keep the agency clean
    D. Following agency procedures

CROSSWORD

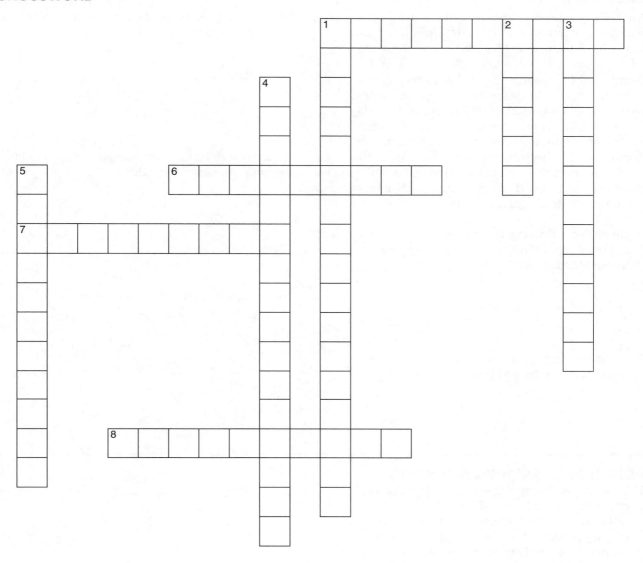

Across

1. Fills drug orders written by doctors; monitors and evaluates drug actions and interactions
6. Diagnoses and treats diseases and injuries
7. Assesses and plans for nutritional needs
8. Prevents, diagnoses, and treats foot disorders

Down

1. Assists persons with musculo-skeletal problems; focuses on restoring function and preventing disability
2. Assists with spiritual needs
3. Deals with social, emotional, and environmental issues affecting illness and recovery
4. Performs delegated nursing tasks under the supervision of a licensed nurse
5. Tests hearing; prescribes hearing aids; works with persons who are hard-of-hearing

CASE STUDY

Mr. George Jansen is a 66-year-old man who had surgery to repair a fractured right hip. His wife died 2 years ago. His son lives in the same city. The son is married and has a 16-year-old daughter. Mr. Jansen's son and daughter-in-law work full time. Mr. Jansen lives alone and works part time as a school janitor. This is his third day in the hospital. It is his second day after surgery. He has Medicare Part A and Part B. Mr. Jansen's doctor told him this morning that he is ready for discharge from the hospital. However, he will need more rehabilitation. The case manager is helping Mr. Jansen with discharge plans.

Answer the following questions:

1. Is Mr. Jansen's condition acute, chronic, or terminal? Explain.

2. What care and services might Mr. Jansen need when he is discharged from the hospital?

3. Which health team members might be involved in Mr. Jansen's care?

4. Which health care agencies might be involved in meeting Mr. Jansen's needs?

5. How might Mr. Jansen pay for his care?

ADDITIONAL LEARNING ACTIVITIES

1. Look in the yellow pages of the telephone book or search for the information online. List the hospitals, nursing centers, and assisted living residences (ALRs) in your community. If the services provided are identified, list them.

2. Collect brochures from the hospitals, nursing centers, and ALRs in your community. Compare the content.
   A. What services are provided?

B. Are hospice services available?

C. Are Alzheimer's disease and dementia care available?

D. What other information about the hospital, nursing center, and ALR is provided?

3. Look at your health insurance policy.
   A. Do you know which services are covered and which are not?

   B. Does your policy limit where you can go for health care? Explain.

4. Read the section in this chapter about "resident rights" under OBRA.
   A. Explain why these rights are important to you.

   B. Explain how you might react if one or more of your rights were limited or taken away.

2 THE NURSING ASSISTANT

STUDY QUESTIONS

Matching
Match each term with the correct definition.

1. _____ Laws dealing with relationships between people

2. _____ Laws concerned with offenses against the public and society in general

3. _____ Injuring a person's name and reputation by making false statements to a third person

4. _____ To authorize another person to perform a nursing task in a certain situation

5. _____ The intentional mistreatment or harm of another person

6. _____ Saying or doing something to trick, fool, or deceive a person

7. _____ Unlawful restraint or restriction of a person's freedom of movement

8. _____ Violating a person's right not to have his or her name, photo, or private affairs exposed or made public without giving consent

9. _____ An unintentional wrong in which a person did not act in a reasonable and careful manner and a person or the person's property was harmed

10. _____ A document that describes what the agency expects you to do

A. Delegate
B. Negligence
C. Job description
D. Fraud
E. Civil law
F. False imprisonment
G. Abuse
H. Criminal law
I. Invasion of privacy
J. Defamation

Fill in the Blanks

11. In order to protect patients and residents from harm, you need to know:

    A. _____

    B. _____

    C. _____

    D. _____

12. The Omnibus Budget Reconciliation Act of 1987 (OBRA) requires each state to have a nursing

    assistant _____

    _____.

    It must be successfully completed by nursing

    assistants working in _____

    _____

    _____.

13. List the three main content areas included in the National Nurse Aide Assessment Program's (NNAAP™) Written Examination.

    A. _____

    B. _____

    C. _____

14. The _____ is an official listing of persons who have successfully completed a nursing assistant training and competency evaluation program.

15. What information about each nursing assistant is contained in the nursing assistant registry?

    A. _____

    _____

    B. _____

    _____

C. _____

_____

D. _____

_____

E. _____

_____

F. _____

_____

G. _____

_____

16. Agencies must provide educational programs for nursing assistants. They must also evaluate their work. What is the purpose of these requirements? _____

_____

_____

17. To protect persons from harm, you must understand:

A. _____

B. _____

C. _____

18. Before you perform a nursing task you must make sure that:

A. _____

_____

B. _____

_____

C. _____

_____

D. _____

_____

19. The _____

tells you what the agency expects you to do.

20. Do not take a job that requires you to:

A. _____

_____

B. _____

_____

21. List 8 role limits for nursing assistants (things you should never do).

A. _____

_____

B. _____

_____

C. _____

_____

D. _____

_____

E. _____

_____

F. _____

_____

G. _____

_____

H. _____

_____

22. RNs can delegate nursing tasks to _____

_____

_____.

23. Delegation decisions must result in _____

_____.

24. List the 4 steps of delegation described by the National Council of State Boards of Nursing (NCSBN).

A. _____

B. _____

C. _____

D. _____

25. During the communication step, the nurse must provide clear and complete directions about the following:

A. _____

B. _____

C. _____

D. _____

E. _____

F. _____

26. After completing a delegated task, you must

_____

_____

27. The NCSBN's *Five Rights of Delegation* is another way to view the delegation process. List the *Five Rights of Delegation*.

A. _____

B. _____

C. _____

D. _____

E. _____

28. An _____ behaves and acts in the right way. He or she does not cause a person harm.

29. Ethical behavior involves not being

_____ or

_____

30. You discuss with a patient the problems you are having disciplining your teenager. This is

_____

31. False imprisonment involves:

A. _____

B. _____

C. _____

32. The Health Insurance Portability and Accountability Act of 1996 (HIPAA) protects the privacy and security of a person's health information. Protected health information refers to:

A. _____

B. _____

_____

33. Failure to comply with HIPAA rules can result in

_____

_____

34. You are admitting a person to the hospital. You tell the person that you are a nurse. This is

_____

35. Consent is informed when _____

_____

_____

36. A patient is unconscious. The doctor orders intravenous therapy and oxygen. How is legal consent for these treatments obtained?

_____

_____

37. List three ways in which a person may give consent.

A. _____

B. _____

C. _____

38. Abuse is a crime. Abuse has one or more of the following elements:

A. _____

B. _____

C. _____

D. _____

E. _____

39. A nursing center resident is allowed to lie in bed in the same position all day. The person's son finds her bed wet with urine when he visits. The person is crying. The staff is guilty of

_____

40. You see a resident's daughter slap him. This is

_____

41. Involuntary seclusion is _____

_____

_____

42. A person refuses to take needed drugs and does not keep doctors' appointments. The person has poor nutrition and poor hygiene and refuses help from others. This is

_____

43. OBRA does not allow agencies to employ

persons who _____

_____

_____

44. Write the meanings of the following abbreviations:

A. HIPAA _____

_____

B. OBRA _____

_____

C. NATCEP _____

_____

D. NCSBN_____

_____

E. CNA _____

_____

Multiple Choice
Circle the **BEST** Answer

45. OBRA requires each state to have a nursing assistant training program. How many hours of instruction does OBRA require?
    A. 16
    B. 40
    C. 50
    D. 75
46. To successfully complete the competency evaluation, how many attempts does OBRA allow you?
    A. Only one attempt
    B. At least two attempts
    C. At least three attempts
    D. At least four attempts
47. The nursing assistant registry is
    A. A skills evaluation
    B. A list of rules and responsibilities for nursing assistants
    C. An official listing of persons who have successfully completed a nursing assistant training and competency evaluation program
    D. A procedure book
48. Retraining and a new competency evaluation program are required
    A. For nursing assistants who have not worked for 24 months
    B. Whenever a nursing assistant changes jobs
    C. If a nursing assistant has a poor performance review
    D. Whenever a nursing assistant is accused of abuse
49. Nursing assistants
    A. Function under the supervision of licensed nurses
    B. Decide what should or should not be done for a person

C. Supervise other nursing assistants
D. Take telephone orders from the doctor

50. The nurse asks you to perform a task that is not in your job description. You should
    A. Perform the task after the nurse shows you how
    B. Refuse to perform the task and explain why
    C. Ask a co-worker to assist you with the task
    D. Report the nurse to the administrator
51. The nurse asks you to apply an ankle brace to a patient's right ankle. You do not understand the directions. What should you do?
    A. Ask the patient to tell you how to apply the brace.
    B. Ask the nursing assistant who cared for the patient yesterday to show you how to apply the brace.
    C. Ask another nursing assistant to apply the brace.
    D. Explain to the nurse that you do not understand the instructions.
52. You agree to perform a task. You must do the following *except*
    A. Complete the task safely
    B. Ask for help when you are unsure
    C. Report what you did and your observations to the nurse
    D. Delegate the task to another nursing assistant if you are busy
53. You can refuse to perform a delegated task for the following reasons *except*
    A. The task is not in your job description
    B. You do not know how to use the equipment
    C. You do not want to perform the task because it is unpleasant
    D. The nurse's directions are unclear
54. Nursing assistants *do not* delegate.
    A. True
    B. False
55. Which is *not* a code of conduct for nursing assistants?
    A. Respect each person as an individual.
    B. Carry out the directions and instructions of the nurse if you have time.
    C. Be loyal to your employer and co-workers.
    D. Keep the person's information confidential.
56. As a nursing assistant, you help patients, residents, and families. That which separates helpful behaviors from those that are not helpful is
    A. A nursing task
    B. Protected health information
    C. Professional boundary
    D. Ethics

57. Which action is *not* good work ethics?
    A. Completing tasks safely
    B. Providing for privacy when performing care measures
    C. Performing a task that is not in your job description
    D. Asking the nurse to explain instructions if you do not understand
58. Which action protects a person's right to privacy?
    A. Opening the person's mail without consent
    B. Listening to a resident's phone conversation with his daughter
    C. Discussing a patient's treatment with his roommate
    D. Asking visitors to leave the room when care is given
59. An RN asks you to perform a task beyond the legal limits of your role. You agree to perform the task. Harm is caused. Who is responsible?
    A. You and the RN
    B. Only the RN
    C. Only you
    D. The entire nursing team
60. Sometimes refusing to follow the nurse's directions is your right and duty.
    A. True
    B. False

61. Two nursing assistants are making fun of the way a resident walks. This is
    A. Sexual abuse
    B. Verbal abuse
    C. Neglect
    D. Physical abuse
62. A resident's granddaughter takes money from the resident's purse while she is asleep. This is
    A. Involuntary seclusion
    B. Mental abuse
    C. Financial exploitation
    D. Verbal abuse
63. You suspect a person you are caring for is being abused. You must
    A. Report your observations to the nurse
    B. Call the police
    C. Tell a co-worker
    D. Tell the person's doctor
64. Threatening a person with punishment is
    A. Physical abuse
    B. Neglect
    C. Emotional abuse
    D. Involuntary seclusion
65. Which is *not* a sign of elder abuse?
    A. Complaints of stiff and painful joints
    B. Weight loss
    C. Bleeding and bruising in the genital area
    D. Frequent injuries

CROSSWORD

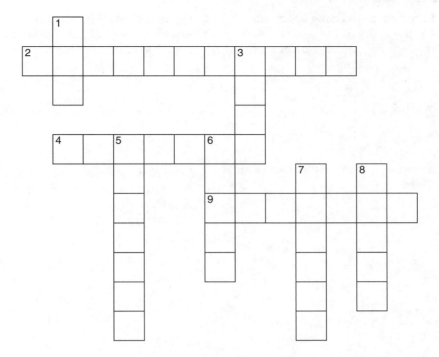

Across
2. Negligence by a professional person
4. Intentionally attempting or threatening to touch a person's body without the person's consent
9. Touching a person's body without his or her consent

Down
1. A rule of conduct made by a government body
3. A wrong committed against a person or the person's property
5. Making false statements orally
6. Making false statements in print, writing, or through pictures or drawings
7. Knowledge of what is right conduct and wrong conduct
8. An act that violates a criminal law

CASE STUDY

Miss Mary Adams is a 52-year-old woman. She was admitted to the hospital 2 days ago with nausea, vomiting, and complaints of abdominal pain. The nurse tells you in report that Miss Adams is very anxious. She also has some demanding behaviors. Miss Adams has had her signal light on three times in the past 30 minutes. While walking by her room, you overhear a co-worker talking to Miss Adams in a loud voice. The co-worker tells Miss Adams, "I can't keep coming in here to straighten your linens. I am very busy. If you keep using your signal light, I will take it away. I need to spend my time with patients who really need me."

Answer the following questions:
1. Is your co-worker's behavior toward Miss Adams a form of abuse? Explain.

2. What is your responsibility in this situation?

3. Whom should you notify about what you heard?

ADDITIONAL LEARNING ACTIVITIES

1. Read the code of conduct for nursing assistants. (Box 2-6 on p. 24 in the textbook)
   A. List ways you might apply this code in a job setting.

   B. Discuss the importance of this code with your classmates.

2. If you are asked to perform a task that you feel is unsafe, how might you handle the request?
   A. What could you say?

   B. To whom will you talk to about your concerns?

3. List any job functions that you are opposed to doing for moral or religious reasons.
   A. How will you advise your employer of your concerns?

3 WORK ETHICS

STUDY QUESTIONS

Matching

Match each term with the correct definition.

1. _____ Trusting others with personal and private information

2. _____ The most important thing at the time

3. _____ To spread rumors or talk about the private matters of others

4. _____ To trouble, torment, offend, or worry a person by one's behavior or comments

5. _____ Staff members work together as a group; each person does his or her part to provide safe and effective care

6. _____ Behavior in the workplace

A. Gossip
B. Harassment
C. Confidentiality
D. Teamwork
E. Work ethics
F. Priority

Fill in the Blanks

7. Professionalism involves _____

_____

_____.

8. Work ethics involves:

A. _____

B. _____

C. _____

D. _____

9. To function at your best, you need good

_____ and

_____ health.

10. For good nutrition, you need _____

_____.

11. Regular exercise is needed for _____

_____

_____.

12. If you smoke, you must practice hand washing and good personal hygiene because

_____

_____

_____.

13. You must never report to work under the influence of alcohol or drugs because

_____

_____

_____

_____.

14. Why should you keep your fingernails short, and neatly shaped? _____

_____

15. You should not wear perfume, cologne, or after-shave lotion to work because _____

_____

_____.

16. List 8 ways to find out about agencies and jobs.

    A. _____

    B. _____

    C. _____

    D. _____

    E. _____

    F. _____

    G. _____

    H. _____

17. Employers want to hire people who:

    A. _____

    B. _____

    C. _____

    D. _____

    E. _____

18. Explain why it is important for you to be at work on time and when scheduled. _____

    _____

    _____

    _____

19. Define the following qualities and traits for good work ethics:

    A. Caring _____

    _____

    _____

    B. Empathetic _____

    _____

    _____

    C. Honest _____

    _____

    _____

20. You are completing a job application. It is important to follow directions because

    _____

    _____

21. You are completing a job application. A question on the application does not apply to you. What should you do? _____

    _____

    _____

22. When completing a job application, you will be asked to supply references. How many references should you be prepared to supply?

    _____ What information about each reference should you be prepared to give? _____

    _____

    _____

23. Lying on a job application is _____.

24. You are reviewing the job description during your job interview. You should advise the interviewer of any functions you cannot perform because of _____

    _____.

25. List 3 things you need to do when you accept a job.

    A. _____

    _____

    B. _____

    _____

    C. _____

    _____

26. What can you expect to occur during an agency's new employee orientation program?

    A. _____

    B. _____

    C. _____

27. Some agencies have preceptor programs. A preceptor is _____

    _____.

28. _____ and _____ are common reasons for losing a job.

29. To eavesdrop means to _____

_____ .

30. You are scheduled to return from your meal break at 12 noon. Explain why it is important to return from your meal break on time.

_____

_____

_____

31. _____ ,

_____ ,

_____ , and

_____

help you decide what to do and when.

32. Priorities change as _____ change.

33. _____ is the response or change in the body caused by any emotional, physical, social, or economic factor.

34. Sexual harassment involves _____

_____

_____ .

35. You are resigning from a job. You should include the following in your notice:

    A. _____

    B. _____

    C. _____

Multiple Choice
Circle the **BEST** Answer

36. To look professional, do the following *except*
    A. Wear a clean uniform daily
    B. Wear a lot of jewelry
    C. Wear your name badge or photo ID
    D. Wear a wristwatch with a second hand

37. You are getting ready for a job interview. You should do the following *except*
    A. Bathe, brush your teeth, and wash your hair
    B. Make sure your hands and fingernails are clean
    C. Make sure your shoes are clean and in good repair
    D. Wear clean jeans and a T-shirt

38. Being on time for a job interview shows that you are
    A. Courteous
    B. Anxious
    C. Helpful
    D. Dependable

39. When you arrive for a job interview, you should
    A. Tell the receptionist your name and why you are there
    B. Spend time visiting with the receptionist until it is time for your interview
    C. Ask the receptionist how long you will have to wait
    D. Ask the receptionist questions about the job

40. You want to make a good impression for a job interview. Which is *correct?*
    A. Stand until asked to take a seat.
    B. Look down or away from the interviewer when answering questions.
    C. Give short "yes" or "no" answers.
    D. Give long answers and explanations to all questions.

41. You can ask questions at the end of the interview. Which is *not* a good question?
    A. What is the greatest challenge of this job?
    B. What are the uniform requirements?
    C. Can I have four days off next month?
    D. How will my performance be evaluated?

42. How soon after a job interview should you send a thank-you note?
    A. Within 24 hours
    B. Within 3 days
    C. Within one week
    D. Whenever you have time

43. You are always willing to help and work with others. You are being
    A. Cheerful
    B. Respectful
    C. Cooperative
    D. Enthusiastic

44. Knowing your own feelings, strengths, and weaknesses is the quality of
    A. Cooperation
    B. Self-awareness
    C. Caring
    D. Courtesy

45. You have just completed a 2-week preceptor program. You are still not comfortable with some of your job duties. What should you do?
    A. Resign from your job.
    B. Discuss your concerns with the administrator.
    C. Do the best you can.
    D. Ask for more orientation time.

46. Proper speech and language at work involves
    A. Speaking clearly
    B. Shouting to be heard
    C. Using abusive language when needed
    D. Arguing with the person when you know you are right
47. Which of these statements reflects a negative attitude?
    A. "Can I help you?"
    B. "Please show me how this works."
    C. "I can't, I'm too busy."
    D. "Thank you for your help."
48. You can share information about a resident with
    A. The resident's family
    B. The nurse supervising your work
    C. Your co-worker during lunch
    D. Your family and friends
49. Which action will keep personal matters out of the workplace?
    A. Letting family and friends visit you on the unit
    B. Using an agency copy machine to copy recipes for a co-worker
    C. Taking agency pens and pencils home
    D. Making personal phone calls during meals and breaks
50. Setting priorities involves the following *except* deciding
    A. Which person has the greatest needs
    B. What tasks need to be done at a set time
    C. What tasks you enjoy doing most
    D. How much help you need to complete a task
51. Stress in your personal life affects your work.
    A. True
    B. False
52. To reduce stress, do the following *except*
    A. Give yourself praise
    B. Get enough rest and sleep
    C. Spend time with unhappy people
    D. Laugh with others
53. Harassment is *not* legal in the workplace.
    A. True
    B. False
54. Harassment involves only sexual behavior.
    A. True
    B. False
55. Victims of sexual harassment are always women.
    A. True
    B. False
56. You feel that you are being harassed at work. Which is *correct*?
    A. Tell your co-workers.
    B. Ignore it. You do not want to cause trouble.
    C. Ask your family and friends for advice.
    D. Report it to your supervisor and the human resource officer.
57. Common reasons for losing a job include the following *except*
    A. Poor attendance
    B. Falsifying a record
    C. Having, using, or distributing drugs in the work setting
    D. Politely refusing to perform a task you were not trained to do
58. You can lose your job for failing to maintain patient confidentiality.
    A. True
    B. False

4 COMMUNICATING WITH THE HEALTH TEAM

STUDY QUESTIONS

Matching

Match each term with the correct definition.

1. _____ The exchange of information
2. _____ A type of card file that summarizes the person's drugs, treatments, diagnoses, care measures, equipment, and special needs
3. _____ The identification of a disease or condition by a doctor
4. _____ A written or electronic account of a person's condition and response to treatment and care
5. _____ A written guide about the person's care
6. _____ Describes a health problem that can be treated by nursing measures
7. _____ An action or measure taken by the nursing team to help the person reach a goal
8. _____ A written guide required by OBRA giving direction for the resident's care
9. _____ A word element placed before a root; it changes the meaning of a word
10. _____ The oral account of care and observations
11. _____ A word element placed after a root to change the meaning of the word
12. _____ A part of a word

A. Medical diagnosis
B. Prefix
C. Medical record
D. Kardex
E. Communication
F. Nursing intervention
G. Nursing diagnosis
H. Suffix
I. Reporting
J. Word element
K. Comprehensive care plan
L. Nursing care plan

Fill in the Blanks

13. Health team members share information about:

   A. _____

   B. _____

   C. _____

14. Agency policies about medical records address:

   A. _____

   B. _____

   C. _____

   D. _____

   E. _____

   F. _____

15. If you have access to the medical record you

   must _____

   _____.

16. Which medical record forms relate to your work?

   A. _____

   B. _____

   C. _____

   D. _____

   E. _____

17. The _____ is completed when the person is admitted to the agency. It has the person's identifying information.

18. The graphic sheet is used to record _____ _____ _____.

19. In long-term care, summaries of care describe _____ _____.

20. List the 5 steps of the nursing process in the correct order.

    A. _____

    B. _____

    C. _____

    D. _____

    E. _____

21. You collect the following data about a patient. Identify the subjective data with an "s" and the objective data with an "o."

    A. _____ pain

    B. _____ nausea

    C. _____ vomiting

    D. _____ dizziness

    E. _____ clear yellow urine

    F. _____ warm moist skin

    G. _____ numbness

    H. _____ pulse rate of 80 beats per minute

22. _____ are what is most important for the person.

23. Goals are aimed at _____ _____ _____.

24. Describe the purpose of the nursing care plan.

    _____

    _____

    _____

    _____

25. The comprehensive care plan identifies:

    A. _____

    B. _____

    C. _____

    D. _____

26. The nurse uses an _____ to communicate delegated measures and tasks to you.

27. You do not understand a task on your assignment sheet. What should you do?

    _____

    _____

    _____

    _____

28. List and define the two types of resident care conferences required by OBRA.

    A. _____

    _____

    _____

    _____

    B. _____

    _____

    _____

    _____

29. Anyone who reads your charting should know:

    A. _____

    B. _____

    C. _____

30. Convert the following times from standard clock time to 24-hour clock time:

    A. 6:15 PM _____

    B. 8:00 AM _____

    C. 2:30 PM _____

    D. 5:02 PM _____

    E. 10:55 AM _____

    F. 1:29 PM _____

    G. 1:33 AM _____

    H. 9:00 PM _____

31. Convert the following times from 24-hour clock time to standard clock time:

    A. 1600 _____

    B. 0945 _____

    C. 1115 _____

    D. 2120 _____

    E. 1705 _____

32. List the word elements (parts of words).

    A. _____

    B. _____

    C. _____

33. Medical terms are formed by combining word elements. When translating medical terms, begin with the _____ .

34. Define the following directional terms:

    A. Anterior (ventral) _____

    B. Distal _____

    C. Lateral _____

    D. Medial _____

    E. Posterior (dorsal) _____

    F. Proximal _____

35. You are recording care given. You are unsure of an abbreviation. What should you do?

    _____

36. Computer systems _____,

    _____,

    _____,

    _____,

    and _____

    information. The right to _____ must be protected.

37. When speaking on the phone, you give much information by:

    A. _____

    B. _____

    C. _____

38. List the information you need to write when taking a phone message.

    A. _____

    B. _____

C. _____

39. List the steps for transferring a phone call.

    A. _____

    B. _____

    C. _____

40. The problem-solving process involves these steps:

    A. _____

    B. _____

    C. _____

    D. _____

    E. _____

    F. _____

41. _____ and _____ help prevent and resolve conflicts.

42. Write the meanings of the following abbreviations:

    A. ADL _____

    B. ePHI _____

    C. MDS _____

Multiple Choice

Circle the **BEST** Answer

43. For good communication, do the following *except*
    A. Use familiar words
    B. Be brief and concise
    C. Give un-needed information
    D. Give information in a logical and orderly manner

44. Which team members have access to a person's medical record?
    A. The person's family members
    B. Staff members involved in the person's care
    C. Laundry staff
    D. All dietary staff

45. All nursing interventions need a doctor's order.
    A. True
    B. False

46. Care is given during this step of the nursing process.
    A. Assessment
    B. Planning
    C. Implementation
    D. Evaluation

47. Nursing assistants have a key role in the nursing process.
    A. True
    B. False
48. Which statement about resident care conferences is *correct?*
    A. Family members are not allowed to attend.
    B. The resident is required to attend.
    C. Residents may refuse suggestions made by the health team.
    D. Residents attend only if invited by the doctor.
49. You are reporting resident care. Which is *incorrect?*
    A. Report your observations to the nurse.
    B. Report the care that was given by a co-worker.
    C. Reports must be prompt, thorough, and accurate.
    D. Report immediately any changes from normal.
50. When recording do the following *except*
    A. Use ink
    B. Use only agency-approved abbreviations
    C. Use correct spelling and grammar
    D. Use correcting fluid if you make a mistake
51. When recording, do the following
    A. Erase errors
    B. Skip lines
    C. Record your judgments
    D. Make sure writing is readable and neat
52. When using electronic charting, which action is *incorrect?*
    A. Using another person's username
    B. Checking the time your entry is made
    C. Checking for accuracy
    D. Saving your entry
53. Intake and output are recorded on the
    A. Graphic sheet
    B. Kardex
    C. Admission sheet
    D. Nursing care plan
54. Which is a nursing diagnosis?
    A. Breast cancer
    B. Pneumonia
    C. Bowel incontinence
    D. Diabetes
55. Priorities and goals are set. Which step in the nursing process is this?
    A. Assessment
    B. Planning
    C. Implementation
    D. Evaluation
56. Which prefix means "away from"?
    A. ab
    B. anti
    C. dis
    D. epi
57. Which root means "head"?
    A. broncho
    B. cephal(o)
    C. hema
    D. nephr(o)
58. The suffix "algia" means
    A. Cell
    B. Tumor
    C. Disease
    D. Pain
59. What does the medical term "gastritis" mean?
    A. Difficulty urinating
    B. Nerve pain
    C. Inflammation of the stomach
    D. Excision of the ovary
60. Which medical term means study of the skin?
    A. Glossitis
    B. Dermatology
    C. Neuralgia
    D. Bacteriogenic
61. You are using a computer to record care given. Which action will *not* protect the person's privacy?
    A. Preventing others from seeing what is on the screen
    B. Logging off after making an entry
    C. Not leaving printouts where others can read them
    D. Using e-mail to report confidential information
62. Which is *not* a guideline for answering phones?
    A. Give a courteous greeting.
    B. Cover the receiver with your hand when not speaking to the caller.
    C. Return to a caller on hold within 30 seconds.
    D. Do not give confidential information to any caller.
63. Conflict can arise on the job over work schedules, absences, and amount and quality of work performed. Which action will *not* help resolve conflict?
    A. Asking your supervisor to meet with you
    B. Discussing the problem with co-workers during lunch break
    C. Giving facts and specific examples
    D. Identifying ways to solve the problem
64. Your co-worker frequently does not clean the tub after use. You should
    A. Ask your supervisor for some time to talk privately so you can explain the problem
    B. Confront your co-worker in the hallway
    C. Tell the nurse you will not work with the person
    D. Make sure all team members know how lazy the person is

CROSSWORD

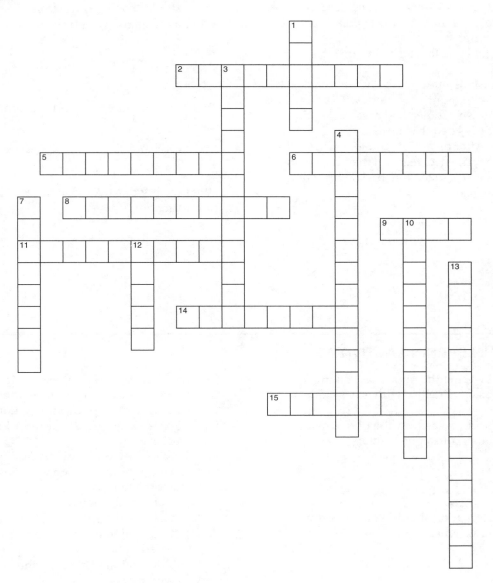

Across

2. Involves measuring if the goals in the planning step of the nursing process were met
5. Data (information) that are seen, heard, felt, or smelled
6. Subjective data
8. Data (things) a person tells you about that you cannot observe through your senses
9. The word element, which contains the basic meaning of the word
11. Involves collecting information about the person
14. A clash between opposing interests or ideas
15. The written account of care and observations

Down

1. Another term for the medical record
3. A shortened form of a word or phrase
4. Carrying out or performing the nursing measures in the care plan
7. Setting priorities and goals
10. Using the senses of sight, hearing, touch, and smell to collect information
12. Objective data
13. The method nurses use to plan and deliver nursing care

CASE STUDY

Mr. Juan Gomez is a 75-year-old resident of Valley View Nursing Center. You have been assigned his care this morning.

Mr. Gomez told you that he had a bowel movement at 0500 (5:00 AM).

You helped Mr. Gomez get ready for breakfast by assisting him with mouth care and with washing his face and hands. Mr. Gomez had breakfast sitting in the chair beside his bed. He ate everything on his breakfast tray. After breakfast, you took Mr. Gomez for a walk. He walked 20 feet and then complained of being tired. You assisted him back to his room and helped him into bed.

Answer the following questions:

1. What information would you report and record?

2. To whom should you report the information?

3. What form would you use to record each piece of information?

ADDITIONAL LEARNING ACTIVITIES

1. Practice answering the phone and taking a written message. Practice with a classmate or friend.
   A. How would you answer the phone in a professional, courteous manner?

   B. What information should you write down when taking a message?

   C. What steps would you take before putting a person on hold?

2. Practice your observation, recording, and reporting skills. Ask a classmate or member of your family to help. Use Box 4-1 on p. 51 in the textbook as a guide for recording your observations.
   A. Talk to the person for about 5 minutes. Use a note pad to write down your observations. Include the following:
      (1) Color and length of hair
      (2) Color of eyes
      (3) Description of any jewelry the person is wearing
      (4) Description of clothing the person is wearing
      (5) Any special features (birth marks, scars, and so on)
      (6) Any information the person gave you about himself or herself
   B. Use your notes to give a verbal report.
   C. Discuss the accuracy of your observations.

3. Read the following vignette involving conflict in the workplace. Then answer the questions at the end of the vignette.

You are assigned to care for Mrs. Amy Martin. When you return from your lunch break, Mrs. Martin's signal light is on. When you answer her signal light, Mrs. Martin tells you that her light has been on for 25 minutes. Mrs. Martin also tells you that another nursing assistant walked in to her room and told her that she would have to wait until her nursing assistant returned from lunch.

    A. How might you feel?

    B. What would you say to Mrs. Martin?

    C. With whom would you discuss the situation?

    D. Where would you discuss the situation?

    E. What steps would you take to solve the problem?

4. Make flash cards of the prefixes, root words, and suffixes in Chapter 4. Write the meaning of each on the back of each flash card. Use the flash cards to help you study and learn medical terms. Work alone, with a classmate, or with a friend.

5 UNDERSTANDING THE PERSON

STUDY QUESTIONS

Matching
Match each term with the correct definition.

1. _____ Relate to love, closeness, and affection

2. _____ Experiencing one's potential

3. _____ To think well of oneself and to see oneself as useful and having value

4. _____ To focus on verbal and nonverbal communication; using sight, hearing, touch, and smell

A. Self-esteem
B. Love and belonging needs
C. Listening
D. Self-actualization

Fill in the Blanks

5. The _____ or _____ is the most important person in the agency.

6. The whole person has _____, _____, _____, and _____ parts.

7. Define a need. _____ _____ _____

8. List the basic needs for life as described by Abraham Maslow (from the lowest level to the highest level).

   A. _____
   B. _____
   C. _____
   D. _____
   E. _____

9. Persons in hospitals and nursing centers feel safer and more secure if they know what will happen. For every task the person should know:

   A. _____
   B. _____
   C. _____
   D. _____

10. A person's culture influences health _____ and _____.

11. Where will you find information about the person's cultural and religious practices?

    _____

12. Religion relates to _____.

13. List 5 causes of anger.

    A. _____
    B. _____
    C. _____
    D. _____
    E. _____

14. List 6 nonverbal signs of anger.

    A. _____
    B. _____
    C. _____
    D. _____
    E. _____
    F. _____

15. Causes of demanding behavior include:

    A. _____
    B. _____
    C. _____
    D. _____

16. A nursing center resident has difficulty hearing. The person also has poor vision. The nurse tells you to write messages to communicate. When writing messages you need to:

    A. _____

    B. _____

    C. _____

17. _____ communication

    does not use words.

18. The meaning of touch depends on _____,

    _____,

    _____, and

    _____.

19. You may use touch to communicate. Touch

    should be _____, not _____,

    _____, or _____.

20. Body language sends messages through

    _____

    _____

21. Listening requires that you care and have interest. You need to follow these guidelines:

    A. _____

    B. _____

    C. _____

    D. _____

    E. _____

22. Giving opinions is a communication barrier.

    Opinions involve _____

    _____

    _____.

23. Failure to listen is a communication barrier

    because _____

    _____

    _____

24. How might illness and disability affect

    communication? _____

    _____

    _____

25. A patient has visitors. You need to give care. What should you do?

    _____

    _____

    _____

    _____

    _____

Multiple Choice

Circle the **BEST** Answer

26. Communication that uses written or spoken words is
    A. Holism
    B. Verbal communication
    C. Body language
    D. A direct question

27. Which action shows respect for the whole person?
    A. Addressing the person using his or her title
    B. Addressing the person using his or her first name
    C. Calling an older person Grandma or Grandpa
    D. Calling a person Honey or Sweetheart

28. Which needs are the most important for survival?
    A. Self-esteem
    B. Safety and security
    C. Physical
    D. Love and belonging

29. Which needs relate to feeling safe from harm, danger, and fear?
    A. Physical
    B. Safety and security
    C. Love and belonging
    D. Self-esteem

30. A nursing center resident needs assistance with walking. She wants to attend church services in the center's chapel. Which is *correct*?
    A. Assist her to attend church services.
    B. Tell her family about her request.
    C. Tell her that you are too busy.
    D. Ask the nurse what to do.

31. A nursing center resident stays in his room most of the day. He does not attend activities. He does not talk to his family when they visit. This behavior is
    A. Self-centered behavior
    B. Demanding behavior
    C. Withdrawal
    D. Anger

32. Inappropriate sexual behavior is always on purpose.
    A. True
    B. False

33. A person with aggressive behavior
    A. Is critical of others
    B. May swear, bite, hit, pinch, scratch, or kick
    C. Has little or no contact with others
    D. Has dementia

34. You are giving a patient a complete bed bath. She complains about how you are giving the bath. She also tells you that her breakfast was terrible. She tells you, "Nobody knows what they are doing and nobody cares about me." Which action is *not* helpful?
    A. Explaining that you are giving her bath in the right way and you do know what you are doing
    B. Listening and using silence; letting her express her feelings
    C. Staying calm and professional
    D. Discussing the situation with the nurse

35. Which action will *not* promote effective communication?
    A. Respecting the person's religion and culture
    B. Giving the person time to process information
    C. Telling the person that you are repeating information
    D. Asking questions to see if the person understood you

36. Which is *correct*, when using verbal communication?
    A. Look away from the person.
    B. Speak clearly, slowly, and distinctly.
    C. Use slang or vulgar words.
    D. Shout to be heard.

37. A person for whom you are caring cannot speak or read. How should you communicate with the person?
    A. Use gestures.
    B. Use nods and blinks.
    C. Follow the care plan.
    D. Use touch.

38. Nonverbal messages more truly reflect a person's feelings than words do.
    A. True
    B. False

39. You must never control your body language.
    A. True
    B. False

40. Which communication method focuses on certain information?
    A. Listening
    B. Open-ended questions
    C. Clarifying
    D. Direct questions

41. Using silence shows the person that
    A. You are uncomfortable
    B. You care and respect the person's feelings
    C. You are being rude
    D. You are not listening

42. Which is *not* a communication barrier?
    A. Using touch
    B. Giving opinions
    C. Pat answers
    D. Changing the subject

43. When communicating with foreign-speaking persons, which is *not* helpful?
    A. Speaking loudly
    B. Speaking distinctly
    C. Keeping messages short and simple
    D. Using gestures and pictures

44. You ask a person, "How do you feel about being here?" Which communication method have you used?
    A. A direct question
    B. Clarifying
    C. Silence
    D. An open-ended question

45. A person may acquire a disability any time from birth through old age.
    A. True
    B. False

46. This means being unable to respond to verbal stimuli.
    A. Comatose
    B. Disability
    C. Nonverbal
    D. Holism

47. A patient for whom you are caring is comatose. When giving care do the following *except*
    A. Explain care measures step-by-step as you do them
    B. Tell the person when you are finishing care
    C. Avoid touching the person when possible
    D. Tell the person when you are leaving the room

48. The presence or absence of family or friends affects the person's quality of life.
    A. True
    B. False
49. You give visitors support by answering their questions about the person's condition.
    A. True
    B. False
50. You observe that a patient's visitor is upsetting him. Which action is *correct*?
    A. Ask the visitor to leave.
    B. Report your observation to the nurse.
    C. Ask the person if you can help.
    D. Do nothing. It is none of your business.

51. Often the person who is comatose can hear and can feel touch and pain.
    A. True
    B. False
52. Which is ethical behavior?
    A. Insulting a person's health care beliefs
    B. Arguing with a person about religious beliefs
    C. Trying to force your views on another person
    D. Respecting a person's cultural practices

CROSSWORD

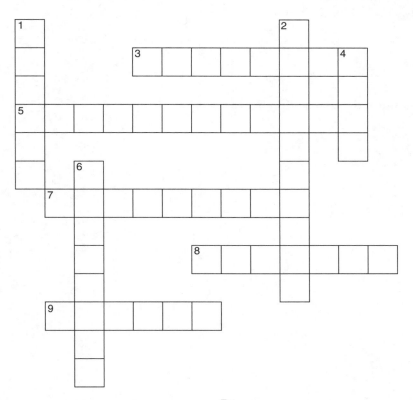

Across

3. Spiritual beliefs, needs, and practices
5. Messages sent through facial expressions, gestures, posture, hand and body movements, gait, eye contact, and appearance
7. Communication that does not use words
8. The characteristics of a group of people passed from one generation to the next
9. A concept that considers the whole person; the whole person has physical, social, psychological, and spiritual parts that are woven together and cannot be separated

Down

1. Communication that uses written or spoken words
2. Any lost, absent, or impaired physical or mental function
4. Something necessary or desired for maintaining life and mental well-being
6. Being unable to respond to verbal stimuli

CASE STUDY

Mrs. Sarah Stein was admitted to Pine Crest Nursing Center today. She is an 80-year-old widow of Jewish religion. She came to America from Germany with her parents when she was 12 years old. She speaks German and English fluently. She was a college professor and taught at the local university for 20 years. She was married for 55 years. Her husband died 2 years ago. Mrs. Stein has difficulty hearing and wears eyeglasses. She walks with a cane. Before coming to Pine Crest Nursing Center, she lived with her married daughter for 2 years. Her daughter felt it was no longer safe for her mother to live with her because she was alone most of the day. Mrs. Stein has fallen twice during the past month and has lost 5 pounds.

Answer the following questions:

1. What characteristics make Mrs. Stein unique?

2. How might her culture and religion affect her care plan?

3. How might the RN use the nursing process to help the nursing team meet Mrs. Stein's needs?

4. What feelings might Mrs. Stein have about moving to Pine Crest Nursing Center?
   A. What measures might help her adjust?

5. What needs might Mrs. Stein's daughter have?
   A. What measures might help her adjust?

ADDITIONAL LEARNING ACTIVITIES

1. Review the Caring About Culture boxes in Chapter 5 in the textbook.

    A. List some ways that knowing about a person's cultural and religious practices might help you give better care.

    B. Do you have cultural and/or religious beliefs that are important to you? Explain.

    (1) How do these beliefs influence your health practices?

2. Observe the nonverbal communication during social contacts with family and friends.

    A. Are you aware of your nonverbal communication? Explain.

    B. How do others communicate with you using nonverbal communication?

    C. Do you ever receive mixed messages from a person's verbal and nonverbal communication? Explain.

6 BODY STRUCTURE AND FUNCTION

STUDY QUESTIONS

Matching

Match each term with the correct definition.

1. _____ The basic unit of body structure

2. _____ The skin

3. _____ The point where two or more bones meet

4. _____ Consists of the brain and spinal cord

5. _____ The substance in red blood cells that carries oxygen and gives blood its color

6. _____ The uniting of the sperm and ovum into one cell

A. The integumentary system
B. The central nervous system
C. Cell
D. A joint
E. Fertilization
F. Hemoglobin

Matching (Immune System)

The following terms relate to the immune system. Match each term with the correct definition.

7. _____ The body's reaction to a certain threat

8. _____ Normal body substances that are involved in destroying abnormal or unwanted substances

9. _____ Substances that can cause an immune response

10. _____ White blood cells that digest and destroy microorganisms and other unwanted substances

11. _____ White blood cells that produce antibodies

12. _____ The body's reaction to anything it does not recognize as a normal body substance

13. _____ Cells that destroy invading cells

14. _____ Cells that cause the production of antibodies that circulate in the plasma

A. B lymphocytes (B cells)
B. Antigens
C. Specific immunity
D. Nonspecific immunity
E. Antibodies
F. T lymphocytes (T cells)
G. Phagocytes
H. Lymphocytes

Fill in the Blanks

15. Explain why you need to know the body's normal structure and function. _____
_____
_____
_____
_____

16. List and describe the basic structures of the cell.

A. _____
B. _____
C. _____
D. _____

17. Chromosomes are _____
_____

18. Cells reproduce by _____.
    This process is called _____.

19. _____ tissue covers internal and external body surfaces.

20. _____ tissue stretches and contracts to let the body move.

21. What is the function of nerve tissue? _____
    _____
    _____

22. The largest system is the _____
    _____

23. _____ gives the skin its color.

24. _____,
    _____,
    _____,
    and _____ are skin appendages.

25. List three functions of the musculo-skeletal system.
    A. _____
    B. _____
    C. _____

26. Name the types of bones and their function.
    A. _____
    _____
    B. _____
    _____
    C. _____
    _____
    D. _____
    _____

27. A membrane called _____ covers bones.

28. _____ acts as a lubricant so the joint can move smoothly.

29. Describe the movement of each type of joint.
    A. Ball-and-socket _____
    _____
    B. Hinge _____
    _____
    C. Pivot _____
    _____

30. _____ muscles can be consciously controlled.

31. List the 3 functions of muscles.
    A. _____
    B. _____
    C. _____

32. Strong, tough connective tissues called _____ connect muscles to bones.

33. The _____ controls, directs, and coordinates body functions.

34. Name and describe the two main divisions of the nervous system.
    A. _____
    _____
    _____
    B. _____
    _____
    _____

35. The 3 main parts of the brain are:
    A. _____
    B. _____
    C. _____

36. The outside of the cerebrum is called the _____.
    It controls _____
    _____.

37. The brainstem contains the _____,

_____,

and _____.

38. The _____

lies within the spinal column. It contains
pathways that conduct messages to and from the
brain.

39. What is the function of the cerebrospinal fluid?

_____

_____

_____

40. The peripheral nervous system has 12 pairs of

_____

and 31 pairs of _____.

41. Some peripheral nerves form the _____

_____

This system controls _____

_____

42. The autonomic nervous system is divided into

the _____ and the

_____.

43. Name the 5 senses.

A. _____

B. _____

C. _____

D. _____

E. _____

44. Where are touch receptors located?

_____

45. The _____ gives

the eye its color.

46. _____

varies with the amount of light entering the eye.

47. The ear functions in _____

and _____.

48. The circulatory system is made up of the

_____,

_____,

and _____.

49. List 4 functions of the circulatory system.

A. _____

_____

_____

B. _____

_____

_____

C. _____

_____

D. _____

_____

50. The blood consists of _____

_____.

51. _____ are needed for blood

clotting.

52. The _____ is the thick,

muscular part of the heart.

53. Name and describe the two phases of heart
action.

A. _____

_____

_____

B. _____

_____

_____

54. The 3 groups of blood vessels are:

A. _____

B. _____

C. _____

102. Where does digestion begin?
    A. In the esophagus
    B. In the stomach
    C. In the large intestine
    D. In the mouth
103. In the stomach, food is mixed and churned with gastric juices to form a semi-liquid substance called
    A. Chyme
    B. Bile
    C. Peristalsis
    D. Saliva
104. The basic working unit of the kidney is the
    A. Glomerulus
    B. Nephron
    C. Renal pelvis
    D. Ureter
105. Urine is stored in the
    A. Bladder
    B. Kidney
    C. Nephron
    D. Urethra
106. Male sex cells are called
    A. Semen
    B. Prostate
    C. Sperm
    D. Testosterone
107. The female sex cell is called a/an
    A. Progesterone
    B. Cervix
    C. Ovum
    D. Vagina

108. The male hormone is
    A. Estrogen
    B. Progesterone
    C. Sperm
    D. Testosterone
109. The tissue lining the uterus is the
    A. Menstruation
    B. Cervix
    C. Fundus
    D. Endometrium
110. Female external genitalia are called the
    A. Labia
    B. Hymen
    C. Uterus
    D. Vulva
111. Which gland is called the "master gland"?
    A. Pituitary
    B. Thyroid
    C. Adrenal
    D. Parathyroid
112. Insulin is secreted by the
    A. Thyroid
    B. Pancreas
    C. Gonads
    D. Pituitary
113. If there is too little insulin, sugar cannot enter the cells. Excess amounts of sugar build up in the blood. This condition is called
    A. Blood sugar
    B. Glucocorticoid
    C. Diabetes
    D. Epinephrine

Labeling

114. Label the 3 types of joints.

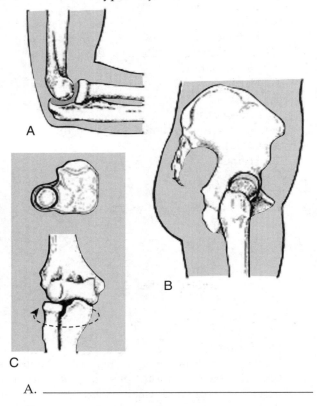

115. Label the major parts of the central nervous system.

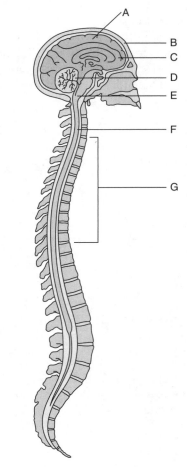

A. _____

B. _____

C. _____

A. _____

B. _____

C. _____

D. _____

E. _____

F. _____

G. _____

116. Label the structures of the heart.

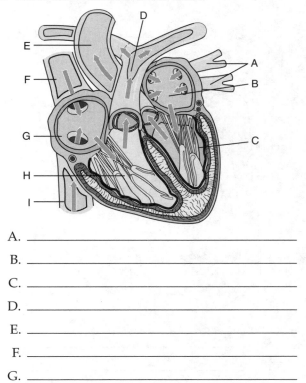

A. _____
B. _____
C. _____
D. _____
E. _____
F. _____
G. _____
H. _____
I. _____

117. Label the structures of the male reproductive system.

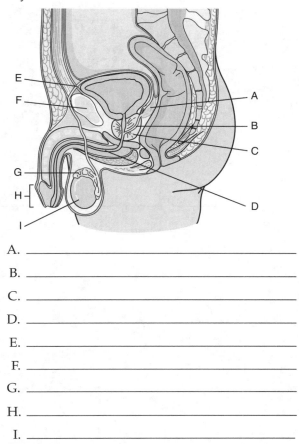

A. _____
B. _____
C. _____
D. _____
E. _____
F. _____
G. _____
H. _____
I. _____

118. Label the structures of the female external genitalia.

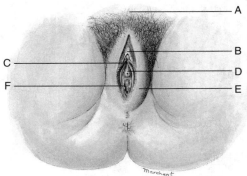

A. _____

B. _____

C. _____

D. _____

E. _____

F. _____

119. Label the glands of the endocrine system.

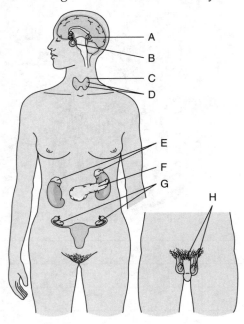

A. _____

B. _____

C. _____

D. _____

E. _____

F. _____

G. _____

H. _____

CROSSWORD

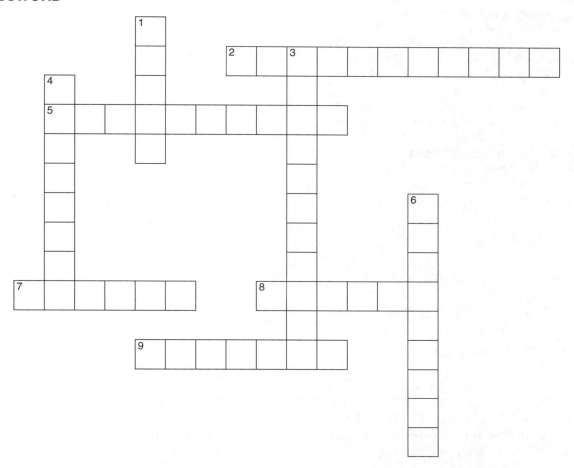

Across

2. Involuntary muscle contractions in the digestive system that move food through the alimentary caral

5. The burning of food for heat and energy by the cells

7. Organs that work together to perform special functions

8. A groups of cells with similar functions

9. A chemical substance secreted by the endocrine glands into the bloodstream

Down

1. Groups of tissues with the same function

3. The process of supplying the cells with oxygen and removing carbon dioxide from them

4. Protection against a disease or condition; the person will not get or be affected by the disease

6. The process of physically and chemically breaking down food so that it can be absorbed for use by the cells

CASE STUDY

This chapter provides the student with a basic knowledge of body structure and function. The body is made up of systems. The systems are related to and depend on each other for proper function and survival. Injury or disease of one part affects the whole body.

Basic knowledge of the body's structure and function should result in safe and dignified care.

Answer the following questions:
1. How might a basic knowledge of body structure and function help you:
   A. Meet the person's physical needs?

   B. Meet the person's safety and security needs?

   C. Understand the reasons for the care you give?

   D. Treat the person and the person's body with dignity and respect?

   E. Make accurate observations about the person?

ADDITIONAL LEARNING ACTIVITIES

1. List and define the three layers of connective tissue that line the brain and spinal cord. (See p. 83 in the textbook.)

2. Describe how the sympathetic nervous system and the parasympathetic nervous system balance each other. (See p. 83 in the textbook.)

3. Explain how the eye uses light to see. (See p. 84 in the textbook.)

4. Outline how the blood flows through the circulatory system. (See p. 86 in the textbook.)

5. Outline the process of respiration. (See pp. 86-87 in the textbook.)

6. Outline the process of digestion. (See pp. 87-88 in the textbook.)

7. Explain how urine is formed and how it passes through the urinary system. (See pp. 88-89 in the textbook.)

8. Outline the process of menstruation. (See pp. 90-91 in the textbook.)

9. Outline the process of fertilization. (See p. 91 in the textbook.)

10. If available in your school or class site, use anatomical models to practice identifying body structures. Also, practice locating the body structures on your own body.

7 CARE OF THE OLDER PERSON

STUDY QUESTIONS

Matching
Match each term with the correct definition.

1. _____ Difficulty swallowing

2. _____ Difficult, labored, or painful breathing

3. _____ The care of aging people

4. _____ The study of the aging process

5. _____ Between 75 and 84 years of age

6. _____ The time when menstruation stops and menstrual cycles end

7. _____ 85 years of age and older

8. _____ Between 65 and 74 years of age

9. _____ The physical, emotional, social, cultural, and spiritual factors that affect a person's feelings and attitudes about his or her sex

A. Menopause
B. Old-old
C. Young-old
D. Dysphagia
E. Geriatrics
F. Sexuality
G. Dyspnea
H. Old
I. Gerontology

Fill in the Blanks

10. With aging, normal changes occur in body _____ and _____.

These changes increase the risk for _____,

_____,

and _____.

11. Growth is _____ _____ _____.

12. Development relates to _____ _____ _____.

13. Growth and development occur in a _____,

_____,

and_____.

14. A development task is _____

_____

_____.

15. List 5 social changes that occur with aging.

A. _____

B. _____

C. _____

D. _____

E. _____

16. When a person's partner dies, the person loses

a _____,

_____,

_____,

and _____.

17. List 6 age related changes in the musculo-skeletal system.

A. _____

B. _____

C. _____

D. _____

E. _____

F. _____

18. List 3 measures that help prevent bone loss and loss of muscle strength.

    A. _____

    B. _____

    C. _____

19. _____,

    _____, and

    _____

    help prevent respiratory complications from bedrest.

20. Persons with _____, or

    _____,

    often need foods providing soft bulk such as whole grains and cooked fruits and vegetables.

21. List 4 age related changes in the digestive system.

    A. _____

    B. _____

    C. _____

    D. _____

22. As a result of age related changes in the digestive system, _____,
    foods are hard to chew and irritate the intestines.

23. List 4 age related changes in the male reproductive system.

    A. _____

    B. _____

    C. _____

    D. _____

24. Nursing centers are options for _____

    _____.

25. The person needing nursing center care may suffer some or all of the following losses. Loss of:

    A. _____

    B. _____

    C. _____

D. _____

E. _____

26. The losses listed in the previous question may

    cause the person to feel _____,

    _____,

    and _____.

27. Frequency of sexual activity decreases for many men and women. Reasons for this include:

    A. _____

    B. _____

    C. _____

    D. _____

    E. _____

28. You are giving a male resident a bed bath. You notice that he is becoming aroused. What actions

    should you take? _____

    _____

    _____

    _____

29. A nursing center provides a temporary or permanent residence for some persons. The

    setting must be _____

    _____

    _____.

30. An _____
    is someone who supports or promotes the needs and interests of another person.

31. List 6 functions of a long-term care ombudsman.

    A. _____

    B. _____

    C. _____

    D. _____

    E. _____

    F. _____

32. Ombudsman services are useful when:

    A. _____

    _____

    B. _____

    _____

33. Nursing center residents have the right to voice

_____ and

_____.

Multiple Choice
Circle the **BEST** Answer

34. Which is *not* a developmental task of infancy?
    A. Tolerating separation from parents or primary caregivers
    B. Learning to walk
    C. Learning to eat solid foods
    D. Beginning to have emotional relationships with parents, brothers, and sisters

35. Which is a developmental task of adolescence?
    A. Learning basic reading, writing, and arithmetic skills
    B. Learning how to study
    C. Becoming independent from parents and adults
    D. Selecting a partner

36. Adjusting to decreased strength and loss of health is a developmental task of
    A. Adolescence
    B. Young adulthood
    C. Middle adulthood
    D. Late adulthood

37. Which statement about retirement is *correct*?
    A. All people enjoy retirement.
    B. Retirement usually means increased income.
    C. All people retire because they want to.
    D. Some people retire because of poor health or disability.

38. Most older people have regular contact with family and friends.
    A. True
    B. False

39. Some children care for older parents. Which statement is *incorrect*?
    A. This helps some older persons feel secure.
    B. Tensions may occur.
    C. Some older persons lose dignity and self-respect.
    D. This is always a good arrangement for the parent and the child.

40. Changes in the integumentary system include the following *except*
    A. The skin loses its elasticity
    B. The skin loses its fatty tissue layer
    C. Oil and sweat secretion increases
    D. The skin has fewer nerve endings

41. Changes in the skin occur with aging. Care measures include the following *except*
    A. Using mild soaps or soap substitutes
    B. A daily bath
    C. Using lotions, oils, and creams to prevent drying
    D. Protecting the person from drafts

42. A resident complains of cold feet. Which care measure is *correct*?
    A. Soaking the person's feet in very warm water
    B. Providing the person with socks
    C. Giving the person a bath
    D. Providing the person with a heating pad

43. Age related changes in the musculo-skeletal system cause bones to break easily. Which measure is *not* helpful?
    A. Turning and moving the person gently
    B. Helping the person to get out of bed
    C. Helping the person to walk
    D. Keeping the person in bed as much as possible

44. Which is *not* a result of age related nervous system changes?
    A. More sleep is needed.
    B. Blood flow to the brain is decreased.
    C. Reflexes slow.
    D. Memory is shorter.

45. Painful injuries or diseases may go unnoticed by an older person because
    A. Older persons are confused
    B. Hearing and vision losses occur
    C. Touch and sensitivity to pain and pressure are reduced
    D. Activity is decreased

46. Changes in the circulatory system result in
    A. Loss of appetite
    B. Poor circulation in many parts of the body
    C. Decreased ability to sleep
    D. Agitation and restlessness

47. A patient has severe circulatory changes. You know that
    A. Bedrest is needed
    B. Everything must be done for the person
    C. Personal care items are kept nearby
    D. The person is encouraged to walk long distances

48. Which measure does *not* promote normal breathing?
    A. Placing heavy bed linens over the person's chest
    B. Assisting with turning, repositioning, and deep breathing
    C. Positioning the person in semi-Fowler's position
    D. Encouraging the person to be as active as possible

49. Which is *not* a result of age related changes in the digestive system?
    A. Improved taste and smell
    B. Flatulence and constipation
    C. Indigestion
    D. Swallowing problems

50. Changes in the urinary system result in
    A. Less concentrated urine
    B. Urinary frequency and urgency
    C. Decreased risk for urinary tract infections
    D. Blood in the urine
51. Which measure will help reduce the need to urinate during the night?
    A. Limiting fluid intake to 1000 mL daily
    B. Taking all fluids before 1300 (1:00 PM)
    C. Drinking only water after 12:00 noon
    D. Taking most fluids before 1700 (5:00 PM)
52. Older persons are at risk for urinary tract infection.
    A. True
    B. False
53. Which is *not* an age related change in the female reproductive system?
    A. Orgasm is less intense.
    B. Vaginal walls become thinner and drier.
    C. The ovaries and uterus increase in size.
    D. External genitalia shrink and lose elastic tissue.
54. Which measure can help a nursing center resident cope with loneliness?
    A. Telling the person not to worry
    B. Ignoring the person's feelings
    C. Feeling sorry for the person
    D. Visiting with the person a few times during your shift
55. Mr. and Mrs. Adams have been married for 52 years. They no longer have sexual intercourse. Which statement is *correct?*
    A. They are too old for sexual intercourse.
    B. They have lost sexual needs and desires.
    C. They can express closeness and intimacy in other ways.
    D. They no longer love one another.
56. A resident makes sexual advances toward you. Which action is *correct?*
    A. Refusing to care for the person
    B. Telling the person's family
    C. Discussing the matter with the nurse
    D. Ignoring the matter
57. Very few older persons are healthy and live in their own homes.
    A. True
    B. False
58. Love, affection, and intimacy are needed throughout life.
    A. True
    B. False

59. Married couples living in nursing centers are allowed to share the same room.
    A. True
    B. False
60. Ms. Irma Adams and Mr. John Moore are nursing center residents. You see them kissing in Mr. Moore's private room. What should you do?
    A. Tell the nurse at once.
    B. Close the door for privacy.
    C. Escort Ms. Adams to her room.
    D. Discuss what you saw with co-workers in the lunchroom.
61. Which measure promotes sexuality?
    A. Letting the person practice grooming routines
    B. Choosing clothing for the person
    C. Judging the person's sexual relationships
    D. Entering the person's room without knocking
62. Sexually aggressive behaviors are always intentional.
    A. True
    B. False
63. A person you are caring for touches you in a sexual way. Which action is *incorrect?*
    A. Asking the person not to touch you and stating the places you were touched
    B. Telling the person that the behavior makes you uncomfortable
    C. Discussing the matter with the nurse
    D. Telling the person that you will report the behavior to the ombudsman
64. A resident wishes to voice a grievance about his roommate. The resident wants to talk to an ombudsman. Which statement is *incorrect?*
    A. The person has the right to voice his grievance.
    B. The person must discuss his concerns with the nurse.
    C. The center must post the names, addresses, and phone numbers of local and state ombudsmen.
    D. You must know the center's policies for contacting an ombudsman.
65. You may be involved in a survey process. Which action is *incorrect?*
    A. Making sure each person's room is neat and clean
    B. Sharing your complaints about your work schedule with members of the survey team
    C. Protecting each person's rights
    D. Placing soiled linens in designated areas

CASE STUDY

Mrs. June Chaney and Mr. Warren Anderson live at Green Acres Nursing Center. They have both been widowed for several years. Since moving to Green Acres, they have developed a relationship. They attend the same activities, eat at the same table in the dinning room, and sit side by side in the recreation room. They are frequently seen holding hands and kissing. Sometimes they are together in Mrs. Chaney's room with the door closed. Mr. Anderson's son tells you that he is not happy about the relationship and wants you to keep his father and Mrs. Chaney apart.

Answer the following questions:

1. How are Mr. Anderson and Mrs. Chaney expressing their sexuality?

2. Should Mr. Anderson and Mrs. Chaney be allowed to continue their relationship? Explain your answer.

3. How might you address the concerns expressed by Mr. Anderson's son?

ADDITIONAL LEARNING ACTIVITIES

1. Ask an older relative, friend, or neighbor if you can interview him or her. Ask the person:
   A. What physical, social, and emotional changes he or she has experienced over the past 10 to 20 years?
   B. What support systems have helped the person adjust to the changes?
   C. What brings meaning and quality to the person's life?

2. Read about the changes that occur as people age. Think about how these changes might affect you and your life-style as you age.
   A. Do you have fears or concerns? Explain.

   B. How might you adjust to the changes?

   C. What can you do now to slow or decrease the effects of aging?

D. Which people and what possessions might you have the most difficulty giving up? Explain.

3. List some ways you can help persons you care for express their sexuality.

4. You may have to deal with persons who are sexually aggressive toward you.
   A. How do you feel about this?

   B. How might you handle these uncomfortable situations?

8 PROMOTING SAFETY

STUDY QUESTIONS
Matching

Match each term with the correct definition.

1. _____ A sudden catastrophic event in which many people are injured and killed, and property is destroyed

2. _____ A state of being unaware of one's surroundings and being unable to react or respond to people, places, or things

3. _____ The loss of cognitive and social function caused by changes in the brain

4. _____ Any chemical in the workplace that can cause harm

5. _____ Violent acts directed toward persons at work or while on duty

6. _____ When breathing stops from the lack of oxygen

A. Dementia
B. Suffocation
C. Workplace violence
D. Disaster
E. Hazardous substance
F. Coma

Fill in the Blanks

7. Where will you find the safety measures needed

    by the person? _____

    _____

    _____

8. List 8 factors that increase the risk of accidents and injuries.

    A. _____

    B. _____

    C. _____

    D. _____

    E. _____

    F. _____

    G. _____

    H. _____

9. List 6 drug side effects that increase a person's risk for accidents and injuries.

    A. _____

    B. _____

    C. _____

    D. _____

    E. _____

    F. _____

10. Cognitive function involves:

    A. _____

    B. _____

    C. _____

    D. _____

    E. _____

    F. _____

11. To identify the person before giving care, use the

    _____.

12. Explain why calling the person by name is *not* a safe way to identify the person.

    _____

    _____

    _____

13. When checking the ID bracelet with the assignment sheet, you need to carefully check the person's full name because _____

_____

_____.

14. An alert and oriented nursing center resident chooses not to wear an ID bracelet. What is the correct procedure for identifying the person before giving care? _____

_____

15. You notice that a patient's ID bracelet is too tight. What should you do? _____

_____

16. List 4 common causes of burns.

A. _____

B. _____

C. _____

D. _____

17. List 6 common causes of suffocation.

A. _____

B. _____

C. _____

D. _____

E. _____

F. _____

18. _____ is when the heart stops suddenly and without warning.

19. The most common cause of choking is _____

_____.

20. With _____,
you should stay with the person and encourage the person to keep coughing to expel the object.

21. _____ is often called the "universal sign of choking."

22. Describe the signs and symptoms of severe airway obstruction. _____

_____

_____

_____

_____

_____

23. _____ are used to relieve severe airway obstruction.

24. When is equipment unsafe?

A. _____

B. _____

C. _____

25. Frayed cords and over-loaded electrical outlets can cause _____,

_____,

and _____.

26. List 7 warning signs of a faulty electrical item.

A. _____

B. _____

C. _____

D. _____

E. _____

F. _____

G. _____

27. Where should you connect bed power cords?

_____

_____

28. Explain why you should turn off equipment before unplugging it. _____

_____

_____

29. How many workers are needed to safely transfer a person to a stretcher? _____

30. When can you leave a person on a stretcher alone? _____

31. Exposure to hazardous substances can occur in the workplace. List 7 hazardous substances found in health care agencies.

    A. _____

    B. _____

    C. _____

    D. _____

    E. _____

    F. _____

    G. _____

32. Every hazardous substance has a material safety data sheet (MSDS). You need to check the MSDS before:

    A. _____

    B. _____

    C. _____

33. List the 3 things needed for a fire.

    A. _____

    B. _____

    C. _____

34. The word RACE will help you remember what to do first if a fire occurs. What do the letters R-A-C-E stand for?

    A. R _____

    B. A _____

    C. C _____

    D. E _____

35. You answer the phone at the nurses' station. The caller tells you that there is a bomb in the hospital. What should you do? _____

    _____

    _____

36. Explain why nurses and nursing assistants are at risk for workplace violence. _____

    _____

    _____

37. _____ involves identifying and controlling risks and safety hazards affecting the agency.

38. The intent of risk management is to:

    A. _____

    B. _____

    C. _____

    D. _____

39. Errors in care must be reported at once. Errors in care include:

    A. _____

    B. _____

    C. _____

40. Write the meaning for the following abbreviations:

    A. AED _____

    B. CPR _____

    C. FBAO _____

    D. MSDS _____

Multiple Choice
Circle the **BEST** Answer

41. Cognitive relates to
    A. Dementia
    B. Impaired hearing
    C. Knowledge
    D. Balance and coordination

42. Loss of muscle function, loss of sensation, or loss of both muscle function and sensation is
    A. Dementia
    B. Paralysis
    C. Coma
    D. Suffocation

43. When identifying the person, which is *incorrect?*
    A. Use at least one identifier.
    B. Compare identifying information on the assignment sheet with that on the ID bracelet.
    C. Call the person by name when you check the ID bracelet.
    D. Carefully check all the information.

44. Safety measures to prevent burns include the following *except*
    A. Do not allow smoking in bed
    B. Do not allow smoking near oxygen equipment
    C. Measure bath water temperature before the person gets into the tub
    D. Turn on hot water first, then cold water

45. To prevent poisoning, do the following
    A. Remove all personal care items from the person's room
    B. Inspect the person's drawers every shift
    C. Follow agency policy for storing personal care items
    D. Remind patients and residents not to drink shampoo, mouthwash, or lotion
46. Which measure helps prevent suffocation?
    A. Leaving a person alone in the bathtub
    B. Giving small amounts of oral foods and fluids to persons with feeding tubes
    C. Using bed rails for all patients and residents
    D. Reporting loose teeth or dentures to the nurse
47. This method is used to relieve choking in the very obese and in pregnant women.
    A. The Heimlich maneuver
    B. Chest thrusts
    C. Back blows
    D. Abdominal thrusts
48. Which action will *not* help prevent equipment accidents?
    A. Inspecting power cords for damage
    B. Using two-pronged plugs on all electrical devices
    C. Keeping electrical items away from water
    D. Turning off equipment before unplugging it
49. Which measure promotes wheelchair safety?
    A. Make sure the casters point toward the back of the chair.
    B. Position the person's feet on the footplates.
    C. Pull the chair backward when transporting the person.
    D. Have the person stand on the footplates when transferring from the wheelchair.
50. A resident needs to be transferred to another room on a stretcher. Which action will *not* promote stretcher safety?
    A. Locking the stretcher wheels before transferring the person to the stretcher
    B. Fastening the safety straps when the person is properly positioned on the stretcher
    C. Raising the side rails and keeping them up during transport
    D. Moving the stretcher head first
51. You find a bottle of liquid in the tub room without a label. Which action is *correct*?
    A. Open the bottle to see what is inside.
    B. Leave the bottle and get the nurse.
    C. Take the bottle to the nurse and explain the problem.
    D. Ask a co-worker what is in the bottle.

52. When must you check material safety data sheets (MSDSs)?
    A. Before using a hazardous substance
    B. Before cleaning up a leak or spill
    C. Before disposing of a hazardous substance
    D. All of the above are correct
53. Which is *not* a fire prevention measure?
    A. Following safety measures for oxygen use
    B. Supervising persons who smoke
    C. Emptying ashtrays into metal wastebaskets lined with plastic bags
    D. Storing flammable liquids in their original containers
54. The first thing you must do when a fire occurs is to
    A. Pull the fire alarm
    B. Rescue persons in immediate danger
    C. Get the fire extinguisher
    D. Turn off electrical equipment
55. Do *not* use elevators if there is a fire.
    A. True
    B. False
56. A patient is receiving oxygen therapy. Which is *incorrect*?
    A. A "NO SMOKING" sign is placed on the person's door and near his bed.
    B. Smoking materials are kept in the person's bedside stand.
    C. The person and his visitors are reminded not to smoke in the person's room.
    D. Materials that ignite easily are removed from the person's room.
57. Special safety measures are practiced where oxygen is used and stored.
    A. True
    B. False
58. You are caring for a person who becomes agitated and aggressive. Which measure promotes safety?
    A. Using touch to calm the person
    B. Keeping your hands free
    C. Telling the person to calm down
    D. Standing close to the person
59. Which measure will help keep a patient's personal belongings safe?
    A. Sending all personal belongings home with the family
    B. Completing a personal belongings list
    C. Locking all personal belongings in the safe
    D. Keeping all personal belongings in the person's closet
60. In nursing centers, shoes and clothing are labeled with the person's name.
    A. True
    B. False

61. Accidents and errors in care are reported only if someone is injured.
    A. True
    B. False
62. You promote safety by doing as much for the person as possible.
    A. True
    B. False
63. This is any event that has harmed or could harm a patient, resident, visitor, or staff member.
    A. Hazard
    B. Disaster
    C. Risk factor
    D. Incident
64. You notice that a light bulb has burned out in a resident's bathroom. Which action is *correct?*
    A. Get a new light bulb and change the light bulb.
    B. Do nothing. Assume the nurse already knows about the problem.
    C. Tell the resident to be extra careful when using the bathroom.
    D. Follow agency policy for reporting such problems.
65. You forgot to give a resident a bath. Which is *correct?*
    A. You can give the bath tomorrow.
    B. Tell the next shift to give the bath.
    C. You must tell the nurse.
    D. No one was harmed. It is not important.

CASE STUDY

Mr. John Wilson is 80 years old. He is a resident at Pine View Nursing Center. He is recovering from surgery to repair a fractured right leg. He is learning to use a walker. He is receiving oxygen for a chronic lung disease. He wears eyeglasses and has very poor vision without his glasses. Mr. Wilson has smoked a pack of cigarettes a day for the past 60 years. He is alert and oriented and able to make his needs known.

Answer the following questions:

1. What accident risk factors does Mr. Wilson have?

2. What types of accidents or injuries is Mr. Wilson at risk for?

3. What nursing measures might help decrease Mr. Wilson's risks for accidents and injury?

4. What is your role in providing a safe setting for Mr. Wilson?

ADDITIONAL LEARNING ACTIVITIES

1. Carefully review the safety measures to prevent burns, poisoning, and suffocation.
   A. List the safety measures you practice in your home related to each.
   B. List the safety measures you practice in your workplace related to each.

C. Do you have a fire safety plan in your home? Explain.

D. If you do not already have one, develop an evacuation plan for your home. Make sure that there are at least two possible exits from each room. Schedule regular fire drills with your family.

2. Make a list of emergency phone numbers (Poison Control, Police, Ambulance, Hospital, and Doctor). Keep the list by each phone in your home. Make sure all family members know where the list is.

3. Carefully review the procedure for relieving choking—adult or child (over 1 year of age).
   A. Under the supervision of a qualified instructor practice the procedure. Use the procedure checklist on p. 193 as a guide.

4. Carefully review the procedure for using a fire extinguisher.
   A. Under the supervision of your instructor, practice the procedure. Use the procedure checklist on p. 195 as a guide.

9 PREVENTING FALLS

STUDY QUESTIONS
Fill in the Blanks

1. At what time of the day do most falls occur?

   _____

   _____

2. Explain why falls are more likely to occur during

   shift changes. _____

   _____

   _____

3. List 5 bathroom and shower/tub room safety
   measures to prevent falls.

   A. _____

   _____

   B. _____

   _____

   C. _____

   _____

   D. _____

   _____

   E. _____

   _____

4. Explain why wheeled equipment is pulled, not

   pushed, through doorways. _____

   _____

   _____

5. Why should you do a safety check of the

   person's room after visitors leave? _____

   _____

   _____

6. A resident's care plan states that he needs bed
   rails. When must his bed rails be up?

   _____

   _____

7. Bed rails cannot be used unless _____

   _____.

   They must be _____

   _____.

8. How will you know which patients or residents

   use bed rails? _____

   _____

   _____

   _____

9. If the person uses bed rails, you need to:

   A. _____

   _____

   B. _____

   _____

   C. _____

   _____

10. A patient does not use bed rails. How will you
    promote the person's safety when giving care?

    _____

    _____

    _____

11. What is the purpose of hand rails in hallways

    and stairways? _____

    _____

    _____

12. What is the purpose of grab bars in bathrooms

    and showers/tub rooms? _____

    _____

13. Bed wheels have locks to prevent the bed from moving. You need to lock bed wheels when:

   A. _____

   B. _____

14. To use a transfer belt safely, follow _____
   _____.

15. While assisting a person with ambulation, the person starts to fall. Explain why you should ease the person to the floor (do not try to prevent the fall). _____
   _____
   _____
   _____

16. You and a co-worker need to move a patient from the bed to a stretcher. Which measures will increase the person's comfort? _____
   _____
   _____
   _____
   _____
   _____

Multiple Choice
Circle the **BEST** Answer

17. A history of falls increases the risk of falling again.
   A. True
   B. False
18. Persons older than 65 years are at risk for falling.
   A. True
   B. False
19. Which is a factor increasing the risk of falls?
   A. Wearing eyeglasses
   B. Wearing hearing aids
   C. Living in one's own home
   D. Foot problems
20. A patient is incontinent of urine. The person is at increased risk of falling.
   A. True
   B. False
21. Which is *not* a safety measure to prevent falls?
   A. The bed is kept in the highest horizontal position.
   B. Furniture is placed for easy movement.
   C. Bed wheels are locked for transfers.
   D. Crutches, canes, and walkers have non-skid tips.

22. Which statement about bed rails is *incorrect?*
   A. Bed rails are considered restraints.
   B. Bed rails are necessary for all nursing center residents.
   C. A person can get trapped or entangled in bed rails.
   D. The person or legal representative must give consent for raised bed rails.
23. A patient uses bed rails. You promote the person's comfort by
   A. Making sure needed items are within reach
   B. Keeping the bed in the highest horizontal position
   C. Raising both bed rails when giving care
   D. Leaving the person alone when the bed is raised
24. Bed wheels must be locked at all times except when moving the bed.
   A. True
   B. False
25. A transfer belt is unsafe for persons with certain conditions involving the chest or abdomen.
   A. True
   B. False
26. Transfer belts are always applied over clothing.
   A. True
   B. False
27. You are applying a transfer belt on a woman. Which is *incorrect?*
   A. Apply the belt around the woman's waist over clothing.
   B. You should be able to slide your open, flat hand under the belt.
   C. Make sure the woman's breasts are not caught under the belt.
   D. Secure the buckle over the woman's spine.
28. A person starts to fall while you are assisting her with ambulation. You ease the person to the floor. The person is confused and tries to get up. You should force the person to remain on the floor until the nurse arrives.
   A. True
   B. False
29. You must complete an incident report after a patient or resident falls.
   A. True
   B. False
30. Which is *not* a safety measure to prevent falls?
   A. Meeting fluid needs
   B. Placing bed rails on all beds
   C. Wiping up spills at once
   D. Responding to alarms at once

CASE STUDY

Miss Lynn Adams is a new nursing center resident. She is 86 years old. Miss Adams wears eyeglasses and a hearing aid in her right ear. She has arthritis and high blood pressure. In report, the nurse tells you that Miss Adams has been a little confused since admission to the nursing center 2 days ago.

Answer the following questions:

1. What factors increase Miss Adams' risk for falling?

2. What safety measures might help prevent Miss Adams from falling?

ADDITIONAL LEARNING ACTIVITIES

1. Review the safety measures to prevent falls in Box 9-2 on p. 122 in the textbook.
   A. List the safety measures you practice in your home.

   B. List the safety measures you practice in your workplace.

2. Review the procedures for:
   A. Applying a transfer/gait belt
   B. Helping the falling person
   C. Under the supervision of your instructor, practice each procedure. Use the procedure checklists on pp. 196 and 197 as a guide.

STUDY QUESTIONS

Matching

Match each term with the correct definition.

1. _____ Any action that punishes or penalizes a person

2. _____ An indication or characteristic of a physical or psychological condition

3. _____ Any change in place or position for the body or any part of the body that the person is physically able to control

4. _____ Any drug that is used for discipline or convenience and not required to treat medical symptoms

A. Freedom of movement
B. Medical symptom
C. Chemical restraint
D. Discipline

Fill in the Blanks

5. _____ have rules for using restraints. Like the Omnibus Budget Reconciliation Act of 1987 (OBRA), these rules protect _____.

6. Restraints may only be used to _____ _____ or _____ _____.

7. List 7 risks of restraint use.

   A. _____
   B. _____
   C. _____
   D. _____
   E. _____
   F. _____
   G. _____

8. Restraints cannot be used for staff convenience. Convenience is any action that:

   A. _____
   B. _____
   C. _____

9. The nurse restrains a resident to the chair in the person's room so he can make rounds without being interrupted. This action is _____ _____.

10. According to the Centers for Medicare & Medicaid Services (CMS), physical restraints include these points:

    A. _____ _____
    B. _____ _____
    C. _____ _____
    D. _____ _____

11. Drugs cannot be used if they _____ _____.

12. List 6 mental effects of restraint use.

    A. _____
    B. _____
    C. _____
    D. _____
    E. _____
    F. _____

13. List 6 legal aspects of restraint use.

   A. _____

   _____

   B. _____

   _____

   C. _____

   _____

   D. _____

   _____

   E. _____

   _____

   F. _____

   _____

14. A resident's doctor writes an order for a restraint. What information does the doctor's order include?

   A. _____

   B. _____

   C. _____

   D. _____

15. The nurse tells you to apply a wrist restraint to a patient's right wrist. You do not understand why the restraint is being used. What should you do?

   Explain. _____

   _____

   _____

   _____

16. Explain why you should never secure restraints to the bed rails. _____

   _____

   _____

   _____

17. You apply a belt restraint to a resident in a wheelchair. What information must you report to the nurse?

   A. _____

   B. _____

   C. _____

   D. _____

   E. _____

   F. _____

   G. _____

   H. _____

   I. _____

   J. _____

   K. _____

   L. _____

18. You are applying a belt restraint to a patient. The person is confused and resists your efforts. What should you do? _____

   _____

   _____

   _____

19. Before you apply any restraint, what information do you need from the nurse and the care plan?

   A. _____

   B. _____

   C. _____

   D. _____

   E. _____

   F. _____

   G. _____

   H. _____

   I. _____

   J. _____

   K. _____

   L. _____

   M. _____

   N. _____

20. A patient has a wrist restraint on his right wrist. You are checking the circulation in the person's right wrist. What signs and symptoms must you report to the nurse at once?

   A. _____

   _____

   B. _____

   _____

   C. _____

   _____

   D. _____

   _____

21. Why are persons restrained in the supine position monitored constantly? _____

_____

_____

22. One of your patients has a wrist restraint. Why should you keep a scissors in your pocket?

_____

_____

_____

23. What is the purpose of bed rail covers and gap protectors? _____

_____

_____

24. When applying a restraint to a person's chest, you must _____

_____

_____

_____.

25. Criss-crossing vest restraints in back can cause

_____.

26. You must remove a restraint at least every 2 hours. What care measures do you need to perform before you re-apply the restraint?

A. _____

B. _____

C. _____

D. _____

E. _____

F. _____

G. _____

27. Remove easily means _____

_____

_____

_____

28. Write the meaning of the following abbreviations:

A. CMS _____

B. FDA _____

C. TJC _____

Multiple Choice
Circle the **BEST** Answer

29. Knowing and treating the cause of certain behaviors can prevent restraint use.
    A. True
    B. False
30. Physical restraints
    A. Restrict freedom of movement or normal access to one's body
    B. Must be used to control a person's behavior
    C. Are effective in preventing falls
    D. Should never be used
31. Which is a physical restraint?
    A. The person is moved closer to the nurses' station.
    B. The person is taken to a supervised activity.
    C. The person wears padded hip protectors under his or her clothing.
    D. The person's chair is placed so close to the wall that the person cannot move.
32. The most serious risk from restraints is
    A. Loss of dignity
    B. Fractured hip
    C. Increased agitation
    D. Death from strangulation
33. Which is *not* a restraint alternative?
    A. An exercise program is provided.
    B. A floor cushion is placed next to the person's bed.
    C. The person's bed sheets are tucked in so tightly that the person cannot move.
    D. Extra time is spent with the restless person.
34. Which of the following measures is a restraint alternative?
    A. The person is kept in his or her room with the door closed.
    B. The person is allowed to wander in a safe area.
    C. The person's wheelchair is placed tight against a table. The wheelchair wheels are locked.
    D. Bed rails are used to keep the person in bed.
35. Restraints cannot be used without consent.
    A. True
    B. False
36. A resident is confused. The person cannot give informed consent for restraint use. Who does so for the person?
    A. The doctor
    B. The RN
    C. The agency's administrator
    D. The person's legal representative

37. You may need to apply restraints or care for persons who are restrained. Which action is *unsafe?*
    A. Using the restraint noted in the person's care plan
    B. Using only restraints that have manufacturer instructions and warning labels
    C. Using a restraint to position a person on the toilet
    D. Padding bony areas and skin
38. For safe use of restraints
    A. Keep bed rails down when using vest, jacket, or belt restraints
    B. Position the person in the supine position when using vest, belt, or jacket restraints
    C. Tie restraints according to agency policy
    D. Secure restraints to the bed rail
39. A belt restraint is used to restrain a person on the toilet.
    A. True
    B. False
40. Back cushions are used when a person is restrained in a chair.
    A. True
    B. False
41. How often do you need to check the person's circulation if mitt, wrist, or ankle restraints are used?
    A. At least every 15 minutes
    B. At least every 30 minutes
    C. Every hour
    D. Every 2 hours

42. Restraints can increase confusion and agitation.
    A. True
    B. False
43. Which restraints limit arm movement?
    A. Mitt restraints
    B. Wrist restraints
    C. Belt restraints
    D. Vest restraints
44. Which type of restraint is the *most* restrictive?
    A. A mitt restraint
    B. A wrist restraint
    C. A belt restraint
    D. A vest restraint
45. You are applying a wrist restraint. The person is in bed. Where should you tie the straps?
    A. To the head board
    B. To the bed rail out of the person's reach
    C. To the footboard
    D. To the moveable part of the bed frame out of the person's reach

CASE STUDY

Mr. Howard Hein is a 76-year-old man in the hospital. He is recovering from abdominal surgery. Mr. Hein has a large abdominal dressing. He is receiving intravenous (IV) therapy (receiving nutrition and medications through a catheter in his vein). The (IV) catheter is in his left arm. He receives pain medication every 4 hours.

Mr. Hein is very restless and moves around a lot in bed. He is agitated at times. He has removed his abdominal dressing and has pulled the IV catheter from his arm. The RN has scheduled an emergency care planning conference.

Mr. Hein has a daughter, a son, and two adult grandchildren who visit daily. The daughter and son will be attending the care planning conference.

Answer the following questions:

1. What safety risk factors does Mr. Hein have?

2. What behaviors does Mr. Hein have that interfere with his treatment?

3. What are possible causes for Mr. Hein's behaviors?

4. What restraint alternatives might the health team try?

5. Before the doctor orders a restraint, what must he or she do?

6. If a restraint is ordered:
   A. What are the risk factors?

   B. What safety measures must be followed?

   C. What must be reported and recorded about the restraint?

   D. How will you provide for Mr. Hein's basic needs?

   E. How will you provide for Mr. Hein's quality of life?

ADDITIONAL LEARNING ACTIVITIES

1. You are caring for a person who is restrained. List some things you can do to protect the person's quality of life. Discuss how you would want to be treated.

2. Under the supervision of your instructor, practice with a classmate the procedure for applying restraints.
   A. Use the procedure checklist on p. 198. Remember that restraints can cause serious injury and even death. They must always be applied correctly.
3. Under the supervision of your instructor, allow a classmate to practice applying restraints to you. Discuss how it feels to be restrained. Answer these questions.
   A. Did you feel safe? Explain.

   B. Did you feel comfortable? Explain.

   C. Did you feel in control? Explain.

4. Imagine that you are in a nursing center or hospital. You are having a lot of pain. You do not know the staff. The medication you are taking makes you drowsy. You are not sure what day it is. You have an IV in your right arm and a tube in your nose. You are frightened.
   A. What behaviors might you have?

   B. What could be some reasons for your behaviors?

   C. Might the staff believe that you are confused? Explain.

   D. Would you feel safer and less fearful if you were restrained?

   E. What measures might make you feel safe and less fearful?

11 PREVENTING INFECTION

STUDY QUESTIONS

Matching

Match each term with the correct definition.

1. _____ Items contaminated with blood, body fluids, secretions, or excretions

2. _____ A disease caused by pathogens that spread easily; a contagious disease

3. _____ The process of destroying pathogens

4. _____ A human or animal that is a reservoir for microbes but does not have signs and symptoms of infection

5. _____ The process of destroying all microbes

6. _____ Practices used to remove or destroy pathogens and to prevent their spread from one person or place to another person or place; clean technique

7. _____ A microbe that does not usually cause an infection

8. _____ A small living plant or animal seen only with a microscope

A. Carrier
B. Microorganism (a microbe)
C. Sterilization
D. Biohazardous waste
E. Medical asepsis
F. Disinfection
G. Non-pathogen
H. Communicable disease

Fill in the Blanks

9. Where are microbes found? _____

10. Microbes need a _____ to live and grow.

11. _____ organisms can resist the effects of antibiotics.

12. A _____ is in a body part. A _____ involves the whole body.

13. The chain of infection is a process. Describe the process.

_____

_____

_____

_____

_____

_____

14. List the portals of exit and the portals of entry used by pathogens to leave and enter the body.

A. _____

B. _____

C. _____

D. _____

E. _____

F. _____

15. The _____ system protects the body from disease and infection.

16. In medical asepsis, an item or area is _____ when it is free of pathogens.

17. A resident with dementia does not understand aseptic practices. When do you need to assist the person with hand washing?

A. _____

B. _____

C. _____

D. _____

18. Explain why hand lotions or hand creams are applied to the hands after practicing hand hygiene.

_____

_____

_____

19. Germicides are _____

_____

_____.

20. List 3 aseptic measures that help protect the susceptible host.

A. _____

_____

_____

B. _____

_____

C. _____

_____

_____

21. _____ are used to keep pathogens within a certain area. The _____ _____ is followed.

22. Isolation precautions are based on _____

_____

_____.

23. If a person requires isolation precautions, you need to do the following:

A. _____

B. _____

C. _____

24. _____ are used for all persons whenever care is given.

25. Standard Precautions prevent the spread of infection from:

A. _____

B. _____

C. _____

D. _____

26. The personal protective equipment needed for Standard Precautions depends on:

A. _____

_____

_____

B. _____

_____

_____

27. _____ are always worn when gowns are worn.

28. List the 3 types of Transmission-Based Precautions.

A. _____

B. _____

C. _____

29. To provide care for a patient, the nurse tells you that you need to wear gloves, a mask, goggles, and a gown. List the order in which you should apply this attire.

A. _____

B. _____

C. _____

D. _____

30. Wear gloves whenever contact with _____,

_____,

_____,

_____,

_____, and

_____ is likely.

31. You notice an itchy rash on your hands after you remove your gloves. What should you do?

_____

32. Some patients and residents are allergic to latex. Where will you find this information?

_____

33. Which part of a mask is contaminated?

_____

34. You need to wear a mask to provide care. When should you practice hand hygiene? _____

_____

35. Which parts of goggles and face shields are considered clean?

_____

_____

36. Explain how contaminated items are removed from the person's room. _____

_____

_____

37. Double-bagging of items is *not* needed unless

_____

_____.

38. Masks, gowns, goggles, and face shields can change how you look. This can cause fear and agitation in some persons. Before putting on personal protective equipment (PPE), you need to do the following:

A. _____

B. _____

39. _____
protects against exposure to the human immunodeficiency virus (HIV) and the hepatitis B virus (HBV).

40. Bloodborne pathogens are spread to others by

_____ and

_____.

41. Immunity means _____

_____

_____.

42. You need to discard contaminated needles and sharp instruments in containers that are

_____,

_____, and

_____.

These containers are color-coded in _____

and have the _____ symbol.

43. List the times you need to decontaminate work surfaces.

A. _____

B. _____

C. _____

D. _____

44. What should you use to clean up broken glass?

_____

_____

45. An exposure incident is _____

_____

_____.

46. Parenteral means _____

_____

_____.

47. The source individual is _____

_____

_____.

48. The Centers for Disease Control and Prevention (CDC) serves to _____

_____

_____

49. Write the meaning of the following abbreviations:

A. AIIR _____

B. HAI _____

C. MRSA _____

D. OPIM _____

E. TB _____

F. VRE _____

G. OSHA _____

Multiple Choice

Circle the **BEST** Answer

50. Microbes are destroyed by
    A. Water
    B. A warm environment
    C. A dark environment
    D. Heat and light
51. A carrier can pass a pathogen to others.
    A. True
    B. False
52. Healthcare-associated infections (HAIs) are prevented by the following *except*
    A. Medical asepsis
    B. The immune system
    C. Standard Precautions
    D. The Bloodborne Pathogen Standard
53. Which of the following is *not* a sign or symptom of infection?
    A. Fever
    B. Increased appetite
    C. Pain and tenderness
    D. Redness and swelling
54. The most important measure to prevent the spread of infection is
    A. Sterilization of equipment
    B. Hand hygiene
    C. Surgical asepsis
    D. Isolation precautions
55. An alcohol-based hand rub can be used to decontaminate your hands
    A. When they are visibly dirty or soiled with blood, body fluids, secretions, or excretions
    B. Before eating
    C. After using the restroom
    D. After removing gloves
56. Which is *not* a rule for hand washing with soap and water?
    A. Wash your hands under warm running water.
    B. Stand away from the sink.
    C. Keep your hands and forearms higher than your elbows.
    D. Rub your palms together to work up a good lather.
57. Single use equipment items are discarded after use.
    A. True
    B. False
58. When cleaning equipment, do the following *except*
    A. Wear personal protective equipment
    B. Rinse the item in hot water first
    C. Wash the item with soap and hot water
    D. Scrub thoroughly using a brush if necessary

59. Disposable gloves are worn when using chemical disinfectants.
    A. True
    B. False
60. All non-pathogens and pathogens are destroyed by
    A. Disinfection
    B. Cleaning
    C. Sterilization
    D. Hand hygiene
61. Which aseptic measure controls reservoirs?
    A. Washing the overbed table with soap and water before placing a meal tray on it
    B. Wearing personal protective equipment as needed
    C. Holding soiled linens away from your uniform
    D. Providing good skin care
62. Which aseptic measure controls a portal of entry?
    A. Cleaning away from your body
    B. Providing perineal care after bowel elimination
    C. Emptying urinals promptly
    D. Cleaning and disinfecting the shower after use
63. Which is an aseptic practice?
    A. Taking equipment from one person's room to another
    B. Holding equipment and linen close to your uniform
    C. Covering your nose and mouth when coughing or sneezing
    D. Shaking linen to remove wrinkles
64. You help prevent the spread of infection by
    A. Cleaning toward your body
    B. Using leak-proof plastic bags for soiled linens
    C. Holding equipment and linens against your uniform
    D. Cleaning from the dirtiest area to the cleanest area
65. Which is *not* a rule for isolation precautions?
    A. Collect all needed items before entering the room.
    B. Use paper towels to handle contaminated items.
    C. Do not touch any clean area or object if your hands are contaminated.
    D. Wear gloves to turn faucets on and off.

66. Which statement about wearing gloves is *correct?*
    A. Gloves are easier to put on when hands are wet.
    B. Remove a torn glove when you complete the task.
    C. The same pair of gloves are worn for persons in the same room.
    D. Change gloves when moving from a contaminated body site to a clean body site.

67. Gloves are removed so the inside part is on the outside. The inside is clean.
    A. True
    B. False

68. Which statement is *correct?*
    A. A gown must completely cover you from your neck to your knees.
    B. The gown opens in the front.
    C. Gowns are used more than once.
    D. Gowns are clean on the outside.

69. A wet or moist mask is contaminated.
    A. True
    B. False

70. The Bloodborne Pathogen Standard is a regulation of
    A. OBRA
    B. Medicare
    C. OSHA
    D. Medicaid

71. Hepatitis B is spread by
    A. The fecal-oral route
    B. Blood and sexual contact
    C. Contaminated water
    D. Coughing and sneezing

72. Which statement about the hepatitis B vaccine is *incorrect?*
    A. You can receive the vaccination within 10 working days of being hired.
    B. You can refuse the vaccination.
    C. If you refuse the vaccination, you can have it at a later time.
    D. You pay for the vaccination.

73. Which work practice is required by OSHA?
    A. Store food and drinks where blood or OPIM are kept.
    B. Practice hand hygiene before removing gloves.
    C. Wash hands as soon as possible after skin contact with blood or OPIM.
    D. Recap and remove needles by hand.

74. Which is *not* a safety measure for using PPE?
    A. Remove PPE when a garment becomes contaminated.
    B. Wash and decontaminate disposable gloves for re-use.
    C. Place used PPE in marked areas or containers.
    D. Wear gloves when you expect contact with blood or OPIM.

75. OSHA requires the following measures for contaminated laundry *except*
    A. Handle it as little as possible
    B. Wear gloves or other needed OPIM
    C. Bag contaminated laundry in the dirty utility room
    D. Place wet, contaminated laundry in leak-proof containers before transport

76. When do you need to report an exposure incident?
    A. At once
    B. At the end of your shift
    C. Only if you request blood testing
    D. When you have time

77. The Centers for Disease Control and Prevention is
    A. A state agency
    B. An OBRA agency
    C. A federal agency
    D. A survey team

78. Persons requiring isolation precautions may feel lonely. You can help the person by doing the following *except*
    A. Encouraging family to stay away to prevent the spread of microbes
    B. Providing hobby materials if possible
    C. Organizing your work so you can stay to visit with the person
    D. Saying "Hello" from the doorway often

79. Your co-worker's patient requires droplet precautions. Your co-worker asks you to help answer the signal lights of her other patients while she is in the person's room. You should
    A. Do so willingly and pleasantly
    B. Tell your co-worker that you have your own work to do
    C. Report your co-worker's behavior to the nurse
    D. Ignore the request and complete your own assignment

CROSSWORD

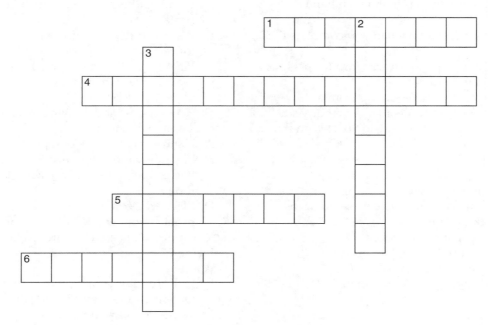

Across
1. Being free of disease-producing microbes
4. The process of becoming unclean
5. The absence of all microbes
6. A microorganism

Down
2. A microbe that is harmful and can cause an infection
3. A disease state resulting from the invasion and growth of microbes in the body

---

CASE STUDY

Miss Joan McMillan is a 50-year-old patient. She was admitted to the hospital with severe acute respiratory syndrome (SARS). She is in an airborne infection isolation room (AIIR). She is on airborne precautions. Miss McMillan is hard-of-hearing. She has difficulty seeing without her eyeglasses. She has very few visitors. She lives in her own home in a small rural town about 50 miles from the hospital.

Answer the following questions:
1. What precautions are required when providing care for Miss McMillan?

2. What guidelines will you follow if you need to transport Miss McMillan to another area of the hospital for tests?

3. What measures might help prevent the person from feeling lonely?

ADDITIONAL LEARNING ACTIVITIES

1. List the measures you practice in your personal life to prevent infection.

2. List the special care needs of the person requiring isolation precautions. Describe how you can help meet the person's needs.

3. View the CD Companion: Skills to help you learn and practice the Hand Washing procedure.

4. Review the procedures described in Chapter 11. Using the procedure checklists provided on pp. 202-205:
   A. Practice the procedures for hand washing, removing gloves, donning and removing a gown, and donning and removing a mask.
   B. Observe a classmate performing the procedures.

12 BODY MECHANICS

STUDY QUESTIONS

Matching
Match each term with the correct definition.

1. _____ The back-lying or supine position
2. _____ The way the head, trunk, arms, and legs are aligned with one another
3. _____ Using the body in an efficient and careful way
4. _____ A semi-sitting position; the head of the bed is raised between 45 and 60 degrees
5. _____ The side-lying position
6. _____ The area on which an object rests
7. _____ The amount of effort needed to perform a task
8. _____ Body alignment
9. _____ Lying on the abdomen with the head turned to one side
10. _____ The lateral position
11. _____ A left side-lying position in which the upper leg is sharply flexed so it is not on the lower leg and the lower arm is behind the person
12. _____ The science of designing a job to fit the worker

A. Body mechanics
B. Force
C. Base of support
D. Sims' position
E. Body alignment
F. Dorsal recumbent position
G. Fowler's position
H. Posture
I. Side-lying position
J. Ergonomics
K. Prone position
L. Lateral position

Fill in the Blanks

13. _____, _____, and _____ can result from improper use and positioning of the body during activity or rest.

14. _____ lets the body move and function with strength and efficiency.

15. Your strongest and largest muscles are in the _____, _____, _____, and _____.

16. For good body mechanics, you need to _____ _____ to lift a heavy object.

17. For good body mechanics, hold items _____ to your body and base of support.

18. The goal of ergonomics is to _____ _____ _____.

19. Work-related musculo-skeletal disorders (MSDs) are _____ _____ _____ _____.

20. Early signs and symptoms of MSDs include

_____

_____

_____ .

21. Describe these risk factors for MSDs in nursing team members:

    A. Repeating action _____

    _____

    _____

    B. Awkward postures _____

    _____

    _____

22. Signs and symptoms of back injury include:

    A. _____

    B. _____

    C. _____

23. _____ are serious threats from lying or sitting too long in one place.

24. A contracture is _____

    _____

    _____ .

25. _____

    _____

    help prevent contractures.

26. You are positioning a person in Fowler's position. For good alignment, you need to:

    A. _____

    B. _____

    C. _____

27. You have positioned a person in the prone position. Where should you place small pillows?

    _____

    _____

28. You are positioning a person in a chair. For good alignment you need to:

    A. _____

    _____

B. _____

_____

_____

C. _____

_____

_____

Multiple Choice

Circle the **BEST** Answer

29. Which is *not* involved in good body mechanics?
    A. Keep objects close to your body when you lift, move, or carry them.
    B. Push, slide, or pull heavy objects.
    C. Work with sudden motions.
    D. Turn your whole body when changing the direction of your movement.

30. To pick up a box using good body mechanics, which is *correct?*
    A. Use the muscles of the lower back.
    B. Bend your hips and knees.
    C. Hold the box away from your body.
    D. Stand with your feet very close together.

31. After helping move a patient up in bed, you feel pain in your lower back. When should you report this?
    A. As soon as possible
    B. Only if the pain gets worse
    C. Before your next scheduled break
    D. At the end of your shift

32. Which is *not* a rule for body mechanics?
    A. Use an upright working posture.
    B. Bend your back, not your legs.
    C. Keep objects close to your body when you lift, move, or carry them.
    D. Avoid unnecessary bending and reaching.

33. Regular position changes and good alignment promote the following *except*
    A. Comfort and well-being
    B. Breathing
    C. Circulation
    D. Contractures and pressure ulcers

34. Whether in bed or in a chair, the person is repositioned
    A. Every hour
    B. At least every 2 hours
    C. At least every 4 hours
    D. Every shift and when the person requests

35. Which will *not* promote comfort and safety when moving the person?
    A. Providing for privacy
    B. Telling the person what you are going to do before and during the procedure
    C. Moving the person with quick, firm movements
    D. Using pillows as directed by the nurse for support and alignment
36. Before repositioning the person, you need the following information from the nurse and the care plan *except*
    A. How to use body mechanics
    B. How many staff members need to help you
    C. What assist devices to use
    D. What observations to report and record
37. A person is positioned in a chair. If restraints are used, a pillow must be used behind the person's back.
    A. True
    B. False

38. Which action promotes the person's independence?
    A. Positioning the person's wheelchair so the person can see outside
    B. Letting the person stay in the same position for up to 4 hours
    C. Letting the person help as much as safely possible
    D. Arranging the person's room for your convenience
39. Transferring and positioning a person should be done by one worker whenever possible.
    A. True
    B. False

Labeling
Label each position.

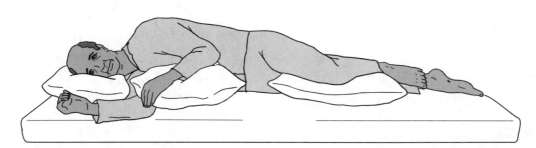

40. _____

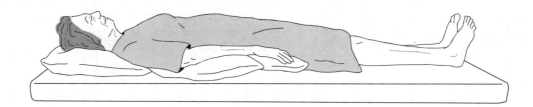

41. _____

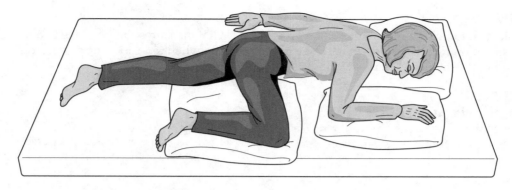

42. _____

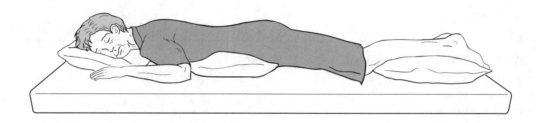

43. _____

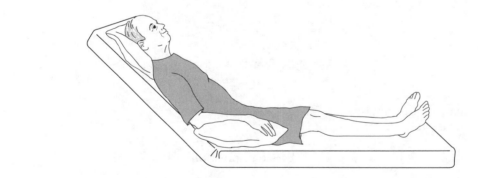

44. _____

CASE STUDY

The nurse asks you to assist a resident to move up in bed. The person is an 85-year-old woman. She is weak. You know that the person has osteoporosis and arthritis.

Answer the following questions:

1. What information do you need from the nurse and the care plan before you assist the person to turn in bed?

2. What measures can you take to avoid causing pain when repositioning the person?

3. How can you ensure that the person is comfortable after you have moved her up in bed?

ADDITIONAL LEARNING ACTIVITIES

1. Review the rules for body mechanics.
   A. Do you practice these rules in your daily activities? Explain.

   B. Do you practice these rules in your work activities? Explain.

   C. Are there ways you can change how you move and work to decrease your risk for injury?

   B. Supine position

   C. Lateral position

   D. Sims' position

   E. Chair position

2. List the measures needed for good alignment for each of the following positions (see pp. 177-179 in the textbook):
   A. Fowler's position

3. Practice proper positioning (Fowler's, supine, prone, lateral, and Sims') with a classmate or family member. Use pillows to promote comfort and body alignment. Assume each position yourself.

13 SAFELY HANDLING, MOVING, AND TRANSFERRING THE PERSON

STUDY QUESTIONS

Matching
Match each term with the correct definition.

1. _____ Sitting on the side of the bed

2. _____ The rubbing of one surface against another

3. _____ Moving the person from one place to another

4. _____ Turning the person as a unit, in alignment, with one motion

5. _____ When skin sticks to a surface while muscles slide in the direction the body is moving

A. Transfer
B. Logrolling
C. Dangling
D. Shearing
E. Friction

Fill in the Blanks

6. When performing a procedure, you must give step-by-step directions. When giving directions, you need to:

   A. _____

   B. _____

   C. _____

   D. _____

   E. _____

7. To promote mental comfort when handling, moving, or transferring a person, you must always:

   A. _____

   _____

   _____

   B. _____

   _____

   _____

8. You are getting ready to move a person up in bed. The person can be without a pillow. Why should you place the pillow upright against the

   headboard? _____

   _____

   _____

9. To safely handle, move, and transfer the person, the nurse and health team determine:

   A. _____

   B. _____

   C. _____

   D. _____

10. These measures reduce friction and shearing:

    A. _____

    B. _____

11. Explain how you would move or transfer each of the following persons:

    A. A male resident with a dependence level of

    Code 4: Total dependence _____

    _____

    _____

    _____

    B. A female resident with a dependence level of

    Code 2: Limited assistance _____

    _____

    _____

    _____

12. After moving a person up in bed, what observations do you need to report and record?

    A. _____

    B. _____

    C. _____

    D. _____

    E. _____

13. It is best to have help and to use an assist device when moving persons up in bed. You can perform this procedure alone *only if:*

    A. _____

    B. _____

    C. _____

    D. _____

    E. _____

    F. _____

    G. _____

14. Explain why assist devices are used to move persons up in bed. _____

    _____

    _____

    _____

15. Some incontinence products are used as assist devices. For use as assist devices, incontinence products must:

    A. _____

    B. _____

    C. _____

16. You are moving a patient up in bed using an assist device. How should you stand?

    _____

    _____

    _____

17. Explain why you need to move the person to the side of the bed before turning him or her.

    _____

    _____

    _____

18. You are moving a person to the side of the bed. You need to use a mechanical lift or assist device method following OSHA guidelines and for the following persons:

    A. _____

    B. _____

    C. _____

19. You will move a resident in segments. Which part of the person's body do you need to move first? _____

20. What information do you need from the nurse and the care plan before turning a person?

    A. _____

    B. _____

    C. _____

    D. _____

    E. _____

    F. _____

    G. _____

    H. _____

    I. _____

    J. _____

    K. _____

21. To safely turn a person, do the following:

    A. _____

    B. _____

    C. _____

22. Logrolling is used to turn the following persons:

    A. _____

    B. _____

    C. _____

    D. _____

23. You are assisting a patient to dangle. The person complains of feeling dizzy. What should you do?

    _____

24. You are assisting a patient to dangle. After the person is in the sitting position, you need to check the person's condition by:

    A. _____

    B. _____

    C. _____

    D. _____

25. To transfer a person means _____

    _____

    _____.

26. Explain why you need to know about areas of weakness before you transfer a person.

    _____

    _____

    _____

    _____

27. After transferring a person, what observations do you need to report and record?

    A. _____

    B. _____

    C. _____

    D. _____

    E. _____

    F. _____

28. The person wears _____ footwear for transfers.

29. Transfer belts are used to:

    A. _____

    B. _____

30. A person's left side is weak. When transferring the person, which side moves first?

    _____

    _____

31. You are transferring a person from the chair to the bed. The number of staff members needed for a transfer depends on the person's

    _____,

    _____,

    and _____.

32. You are preparing to transfer a resident from the wheelchair to bed. The person's left side is her weak side. How will you position the wheelchair for the transfer? _____

    _____

    _____

33. The nurse tells you to transfer a resident using a mechanical lift. You have not used the lift before. What should you do?

    _____

    _____

    _____

34. How will you promote the person's mental comfort when using a mechanical lift to transfer him or her? _____

    _____

    _____

35. How is the wheelchair positioned for wheelchair to toilet transfers? _____

    _____

    _____

    _____

    _____

36. List 4 measures to promote pride and independence while handling, moving, and transferring a person.

    A. _____

    B. _____

    C. _____

    D. _____

Multiple choice
Circle the **BEST** Answer

37. You need to reposition an older person in bed. Which will *not* help prevent injuries?
    A. Following the rules for body mechanics
    B. Trying to move the person by yourself
    C. Keeping the person in good alignment
    D. Making sure the person's face is not obstructed by a pillow or other device

38. A person with dementia resists your efforts to transfer her from the bed to the chair. Which will *not* prevent work-related injuries?
    A. Proceeding quickly and forcefully
    B. Using a calm and pleasant voice
    C. Diverting the person's attention
    D. Getting a co-worker to help you

39. Before handling, moving, or transferring a person, you need the following information from the nurse and the care plan *except*
    A. The person's height and weight
    B. The person's dependence level
    C. If the person has a weak side
    D. The person's age

40. A lift sheet is used to move a person up in bed. Which is *incorrect?*
    A. Two workers are needed.
    B. Shearing and friction are reduced.
    C. Place the sheet under the person from her waist to her knees.
    D. Roll the sides of the lift sheet up close to the person.

41. You need to move a person in segments. Which helps protect you from injury?
    A. Move the person toward you.
    B. Move the person away from you.
    C. Use a mechanical lift.
    D. Have two co-workers help you.

42. A slide board is used to move a person up in bed. The device is removed after the person is moved.
    A. True
    B. False

43. Two or three staff members are needed to logroll a person.
    A. True
    B. False

44. A 90-year-old resident has arthritis. Before turning the person, you need to move her to the side of bed. You need to move her in segments.
    A. True
    B. False

45. You are helping a patient to dangle. Which is *incorrect?*
    A. Provide support if necessary.
    B. Ask the person how she feels.
    C. Check the person's pulse and respirations.
    D. Leave the person alone if she tells you she is OK.

46. When preparing to dangle a person, the head of the bed should be
    A. As flat as possible
    B. Slightly raised
    C. Raised to a sitting position
    D. In the position the person prefers

47. You are transferring a person from the bed to the chair. Which is *correct?*
    A. The person wears non-skid footwear.
    B. The person is helped out of bed on her weak side.
    C. The bed is kept in the high position.
    D. The person places her arms around your neck.

48. You are assisting a patient transfer from the bed to the wheelchair. You must do the following *except*
    A. Lock wheelchair wheels
    B. Make sure wheelchair footplates are down
    C. Remove or swing the front rigging out of the way
    D. Lower the bed to its lowest position

49. Which statement about mechanical lifts is *incorrect?*
    A. Persons who cannot help themselves are transferred with mechanical lifts.
    B. The slings, straps, hooks, and chains must be in good repair.
    C. The person's weight must not exceed the lift's capacity.
    D. If you know how to use one type of lift, you know how to use all types.

50. You are using a mechanical lift to transfer a resident. You should instruct the person to hold on to the swivel bar.
    A. True
    B. False

51. Before transferring a person to the toilet, you need to
    A. Practice hand hygiene
    B. Remove the elevated toilet seat
    C. Check the towel bar to make sure it is secure
    D. Have the person wear warm slippers

52. To safely reposition a person in the wheelchair, you need to do the following *except*
    A. Follow the nurse's directions and the care plan
    B. Explain the procedure to the person
    C. Lock the wheelchair wheels
    D. Pull the person from behind the wheelchair
53. You are repositioning a patient in the wheelchair. The person is able to assist. Which is *correct?*
    A. Stand behind the person.
    B. Ask the person to place his folded hands in his lap.
    C. Position the person's feet on the footplates.
    D. Lock the wheelchair wheels.

54. Which action promotes the person's independence?
    A. Focusing on the person's disabilities
    B. Letting the person stay in the same position for up to 4 hours
    C. Letting the person help as much as safely possible
    D. Positioning the person's wheelchair farther away from the bed than necessary

CASE STUDY

You are caring for an 82-year-old resident living at Pine View Nursing Center. The person is 5 feet and 11 inches tall and weighs 190 pounds. The person cannot walk. He uses a wheelchair. He cannot stand without assistance. He is able to bear some weight on his legs to assist with transfers from his bed to the wheelchair and from the wheelchair onto the toilet. The person's right side is his strong side. He needs help to change positions when in bed.

1. For what skin problems is the person at risk?

2. How can you protect the person from friction and shearing during transfers and when turning and moving him in bed?

3. When assisting the person with transfers, which side will you move first?

4. How often do you need to help with repositioning?

ADDITIONAL LEARNING ACTIVITIES

1. View the CD Companion: Skills to help you learn and practice the following procedures:
   A. Turning and Positioning the Person
   B. Transferring the Person to a Chair or Wheelchair

2. Review the procedures described in Chapter 13.
   A. Under the supervision of your instructor, practice each procedure.
      (1) Use the procedure checklists provided on pp. 206-226.
      (2) Take your turn being the patient or resident.

(3) Discuss the experience with your classmates and instructor. Answer these questions.
    A. Were your safety needs met?

    B. Were your comfort needs met?

14 ASSISTING WITH COMFORT

STUDY QUESTIONS

Matching

Match each term with the correct definition.

1. _____ Having the means to be completely free from public view while in bed

2. _____ A chronic condition in which the person cannot sleep or stay asleep all night

3. _____ The amount and quality of sleep are decreased

4. _____ The head of the bed is raised 30 degrees; or the head of the bed is raised 30 degrees and the knee portion is raised 15 degrees

5. _____ The sleeping person leaves the bed and walks about

6. _____ The head of the bed is lowered and the foot of the bed is raised

7. _____ A semi-sitting position; the head of the bed is raised 60 to 90 degrees

8. _____ The head of the bed is raised and the foot of the bed is lowered

9. _____ A semi-sitting position; the head of the bed is raised between 45 and 60 degrees

10. _____ To ache, hurt, or be sore

A. Reverse Trendelenburg's position
B. Insomnia
C. Pain
D. Full visual privacy
E. Sleep deprivation
F. Sleep-walking
G. Semi-Fowler's position
H. Fowler's position
I. Trendelenburg's position
J. High-Fowler's position

Fill in the Blanks

11. _____ is a state of well-being.

12. The person's unit is _____

_____

_____.

This area is _____.

13. To protect older and ill persons from cool areas and drafts, you need to:

A. _____

B. _____

C. _____

D. _____

E. _____

F. _____

14. Smoking causes odors. If you smoke you need to:

A. _____

B. _____

C. _____

15. Common health care sounds may disturb patients or residents. List 4 ways to help decrease noise.

A. _____

B. _____

C. _____

D. _____

16. Explain how lighting is adjusted in dementia care units. _____

_____

_____

_____

17. Explain why hospital beds are raised horizontally to give care. _____

_____

_____

18. A resident has a manual bed. Explain why it is important to keep the cranks down when not in use. _____

_____

_____

19. Bed wheels must be locked when you:

A. _____

B. _____

20. List the 6 basic bed positions.

A. _____

B. _____

C. _____

D. _____

E. _____

F. _____

21. List the parts of the hospital bed system.

A. _____

B. _____

C. _____

D. _____

E. _____

22. Hospital bed systems have seven entrapment zones. Entrapment means _____

_____

_____

_____

23. Persons at greatest risk for entrapment include persons who:

A. _____

B. _____

C. _____

D. _____

E. _____

F. _____

G. _____

H. _____

24. The overbed table is used for _____

_____

_____

_____

25. Explain the purpose of raised toilet seats.

_____

_____

_____

26. Beds are made in the following ways.

A. A _____ bed is not in use. Top linens are not folded back.

B. An _____ bed is in use. Top linens are fan-folded back.

C. An _____ bed is made with the person in it.

D. A _____ bed is made to transfer a person from a stretcher.

27. Place clean linens on a _____.

28. When are wet, damp, or soiled linens changed?

_____

29. What is the purpose of a cotton drawsheet?

_____

_____

_____

30. Before making a bed, what information do you need from the nurse and the care plan?

   A. _____

   B. _____

   C. _____

   D. _____

   E. _____

   F. _____

   G. _____

   H. _____

31. Why is it important to follow Standard Precautions and the Bloodborne Pathogen Standard when removing linen from the person's bed? _____
_____
_____

32. After making a bed, you must _____
_____
_____
_____.

33. You are putting the top sheet on a closed bed. The hem stitching should face
_____.

34. Describe how you should place the pillow on the person's bed. _____
_____
_____

35. A closed bed becomes an open bed by _____
_____
_____.

36. A surgical bed also is called _____
_____
_____.

37. A patient received a strong pain-relief drug. You must practice these safety measures:

   A. _____

   B. _____

   C. _____

   D. _____

38. A patient received a pain-relief drug. How long do you need to wait before giving care?
_____

39. List 9 factors affecting pain.

   A. _____

   B. _____

   C. _____

   D. _____

   E. _____

   F. _____

   G. _____

   H. _____

   I. _____

40. List 6 factors that affect the amount and quality of sleep.

   A. _____

   B. _____

   C. _____

   D. _____

   E. _____

   F. _____

41. Sleep disorders involve _____
_____
_____.

42. List 3 things you can do to help reduce noise in patient and resident areas?

   A. _____

   B. _____

   C. _____

43. You answer a signal light for a patient assigned to your co-worker. You do not know the person. What can you do to promote safe and quality care? _____
_____
_____
_____
_____
_____

Multiple Choice
Circle the **BEST** Answer

44. To maintain the person's unit, you need to
    A. Adjust the temperature so it is comfortable for you
    B. Arrange personal items the way you prefer
    C. Keep the signal light within the person's reach at all times
    D. Empty the person's wastebasket weekly

45. You are assisting a patient with a bath. You notice many small scraps of paper with notes on them lying on the person's bedside stand. You can throw them in the trash to keep the unit neat and clean.
    A. True
    B. False

46. Which room temperature range is usually comfortable for most healthy people?
    A. 65° F to 68° F
    B. 68° F to 74° F
    C. 72° F to 82° F
    D. 82° F to 90° F

47. Which action will *not* help reduce odors?
    A. Dispose of incontinence products at the end of your shift.
    B. Check incontinent persons often.
    C. Keep laundry containers closed.
    D. Provide good hygiene.

48. To reduce odors, you need to
    A. Change wet or soiled linens every 4 hours
    B. Empty, clean, and disinfect bedpans promptly
    C. Use a room deodorizer every 4 hours
    D. Dispose of ostomy products at the end of your shift

49. A person has dementia. Which statement is *incorrect?*
    A. The person may not understand the meaning of sounds.
    B. The person may have extreme reactions to sounds.
    C. The person's reaction to sound is less severe at night.
    D. A strange room can make the person's reaction to sounds worse.

50. Good lighting is needed for safety and comfort. Which is *correct?*
    A. Provide bright light to help the person relax.
    B. Provide dim lighting during the night.
    C. Adjust lighting the way visitors request.
    D. Keep light controls within the person's reach.

51. Which bed positions require a doctor's order?
    A. Flat and Fowler's
    B. Fowler's and semi-Fowler's
    C. Semi-Fowler's and reverse Trendelenburg's
    D. Trendelenburg's and reverse Trendelenburg's

52. A resident tells you that he does not like his mattress because it is too hard. What should you do?
    A. Tell the person that it is the only mattress available.
    B. Call maintenance and ask for a new mattress.
    C. Tell the nurse about the person's complaint.
    D. Ask the person's family to bring a more comfortable mattress.

53. Which item *cannot* be placed on the overbed table?
    A. A bedpan
    B. The water pitcher
    C. A box of tissues
    D. A book

54. Where should you store the person's bedpan and toilet paper?
    A. On the overbed table
    B. On the lower shelf in the bedside stand
    C. In the person's closet
    D. In the person's bathroom

55. Each person's unit must have at least one chair. The chair must
    A. Be a reclining chair
    B. Be a straight back chair
    C. Not move or tip during transfers
    D. Be provided by the person or family

56. The privacy curtain must be pulled completely around the person's bed
    A. Always when giving care
    B. Only when the person's roommate is present
    C. Only when the room door is open
    D. Only if the person requests it to be

57. Persons who are confused do not need signal lights.
    A. True
    B. False

58. For the person's safety, you must
    A. Keep the signal light within the person's reach
    B. Place the signal light on the person's weak side
    C. Remind the person to signal only in emergencies
    D. Take the signal light away from a person if he or she uses it too often

59. OBRA requires closet space for each nursing center resident.
    A. True
    B. False

60. To keep beds neat and clean, you need to
    A. Straighten linens whenever loose or wrinkled and at bedtime
    B. Check for and remove food and crumbs once each shift
    C. Straighten linens whenever they become wet, soiled, or damp
    D. Change all linens daily
61. This type of bed is made for persons who are out of bed for a short time.
    A. A closed bed
    B. An occupied bed
    C. An open bed
    D. A surgical bed
62. You are making a closed bed for a new resident. Which piece of linen is placed on the bed first?
    A. Bottom sheet
    B. Cotton drawsheet
    C. Mattress pad
    D. Pillow case
63. This type of bed is made after a person is discharged.
    A. An open bed
    B. A closed bed
    C. An occupied bed
    D. A surgical bed
64. You are making an occupied bed. Which is *incorrect?*
    A. Keep the bed in the lowest position.
    B. If the person uses bed rails, the far bed rail is up.
    C. Keep the person in good alignment.
    D. After making the bed, lock the bed wheels.
65. You have finished making a surgical bed for a resident arriving by stretcher. After making the bed, you should leave the bed in its highest position.
    A. True
    B. False
66. Wear gloves when removing linen from the person's bed.
    A. True
    B. False
67. Which is a rule for bed making?
    A. Shake linens to remove wrinkles.
    B. Hold linens against your uniform.
    C. Place dirty linen on the floor.
    D. Follow the rules of medical asepsis.
68. You brought an extra pillow case into a patient's room. What should you do?
    A. Take it back to the linen closet.
    B. Put it in the dirty laundry.
    C. Use it for another patient.
    D. Put it in the patient's closet.
69. Which statement about pain is *incorrect?*
    A. Pain can cause anxiety.
    B. Pain seems worse when a person is tired.
    C. Dealing with pain is often easier when family and friends offer support.
    D. Pain affects all persons in the same way.
70. Changes in usual behavior may signal pain in persons with dementia.
    A. True
    B. False
71. Which occurs during sleep?
    A. Stress and tension increase.
    B. The body uses more energy than when awake.
    C. Tissue healing and repair occur.
    D. Body functions speed up.
72. Sleep problems are *uncommon* in persons with Alzheimer's disease and other dementias.
    A. True
    B. False
73. Which of these measures will *not* promote sleep?
    A. Giving a back massage
    B. Reducing noise
    C. Keeping the room cool and well lighted
    D. Positioning the person in good alignment
74. A resident asks for a bedtime snack. Which will *not* help promote sleep?
    A. Coffee and a brownie
    B. Milk
    C. Toast
    D. Crackers and milk

CASE STUDY

Ms. Angela Lopez and Ms. Lois Green share a room at Pine View Nursing Center.

Ms. Lopez has the bed by the window. She likes to sleep with the window open. She likes the privacy curtain between her bed and Ms. Green's bed open so she can see out the door. Family and friends visit Ms. Lopez often. They often bring her ethnic foods. She sometimes hides food in her drawers and closet.

Ms. Green is a very private person. She chills easily. She likes to go to bed early. Listening to opera music helps her fall asleep. Ms. Green has many figurines, which she likes to display in a cabinet she brought from home. She worries about them getting broken. She also brought her own reclining chair from home.

Answer the following questions:

1. What challenges does the interdisciplinary health team have in meeting the needs of each resident?

2. How can the rights of each resident be promoted?

3. How can the interdisciplinary health team promote each person's comfort and quality of life?

ADDITIONAL LEARNING ACTIVITIES

1. Discuss the importance of personal space in your daily life. Answer the following questions.
   A. How would you feel about sharing a room with another person?

   B. How would you decide what items to take with you and what items to leave behind?

2. Make a list of factors that affect your ability to sleep. Answer the following questions.
   A. What temperatures are most comfortable for you? How do you adapt to changes in temperature?

   B. Are there certain odors that prevent sleep? How do you control the odors in your environment?

C. How do noises and sounds affect your ability to sleep? What sounds keep you awake? Are there sounds that help you relax?

D. How do you control the light in your environment to help you sleep?

E. Do you have certain rituals that help you sleep? Explain.

F. How might you use what you know about your personal comfort needs to help you provide better care?

3. How much sleep do you need to feel rested?
   A. How does lack of sleep affect your daily activities?

4. Practice gathering linen in the correct order for bedmaking. List the correct order on an index card. Carry the card with you until you have the order memorized.

5. View the CD Companion: Skills to help you learn and practice the Making an Occupied Bed procedure.

6. Practice the procedures in Chapter 14. Use the procedure checklists provided on pp. 227-233.

7. Observe classmates performing the procedures in Chapter 14. Use the procedure checklists provided on pp. 227-233.

15 ASSISTING WITH HYGIENE

STUDY QUESTIONS

Matching

Match each term with the correct definition.

1. _____ Routine care given before breakfast

2. _____ Routine hygiene done after lunch and before the evening meal

3. _____ Breathing fluid, food, vomitus, or an object into the lungs

4. _____ Care given at bedtime

5. _____ Mouth care

6. _____ Cleaning the genital and anal areas

7. _____ Care given after breakfast

A. Morning care
B. Oral hygiene
C. Evening care (PM care)
D. Early morning care (AM care)
E. Afternoon care
F. Aspiration
G. Perineal care (peri-care)

Fill in the Blanks

8. The _____ is the body's first line of defense against disease.

9. Intact skin prevents _____ from entering the body.

10. You will assist patients and residents with personal hygiene. You need to protect the person's right

    to _____

    and _____.

11. Oral hygiene does the following:

    A. _____

    B. _____

    C. _____

    D. _____

    E. _____

12. A patient has his own teeth. You assist the person with oral hygiene. What observations do you need to report and record?

    A. _____

    B. _____

    C. _____

    D. _____

    E. _____

13. Explain why you need to follow Standard Precautions and the Bloodborne Pathogen Standard when giving oral hygiene.

    _____

    _____

    _____

    _____

14. Many people brush their own teeth. You may have to brush the teeth of persons who:

    A. _____

    B. _____

    C. _____

15. Explain why flossing is done.

    _____

    _____

    _____

16. Explain the steps in brushing teeth.

    A. _____

    _____

    _____

    B. _____

    _____

    _____

    C. _____

    _____

    _____

    D. _____

    _____

    _____

17. You are giving oral care to an unconscious person. To prevent aspiration, you need to:

    A. _____

    _____

    B. _____

    _____

    C. _____

    _____

18. You are using a sponge swab to give oral hygiene to an unconscious person. Explain why you need to make sure the sponge is tight on the

    stick. _____

    _____

19. A _____ is

    an artificial tooth or a set of artificial teeth.

20. A resident removed her dentures and placed them under her pillow. While you were straightening the person's pillow, the dentures fell off the bed and broke. What should you do?

    _____

    _____

21. A patient wears an upper denture. You need to remove the denture for the person. Explain how

    you would do so. _____

    _____

    _____

    _____

    _____

22. List 8 benefits of bathing.

    A. _____

    B. _____

    C. _____

    D. _____

    E. _____

    F. _____

    G. _____

    H. _____

23. The bathing method for each person depends on:

    A. _____

    B. _____

    C. _____

24. You are giving a person a tub bath. What observations do you need to report and record?

    A. _____

    B. _____

    C. _____

    D. _____

    E. _____

    F. _____

    G. _____

    H. _____

    I. _____

    J. _____

25. Do not use powder near persons with

    respiratory disorders because _____

    _____

    _____.

26. To safely apply powder, you need to:

    A. _____

    B. _____

    C. _____

    D. _____

27. Explain why you should allow the person to use the bathroom, commode, bedpan, or urinal before bathing. _____
_____
_____
_____

28. You are giving a patient a complete bed bath. Why should you wait to remove the person's gown or pajamas until after you wash his face, ears, and neck?
_____
_____
_____

29. Bed baths are usually needed by persons who are:

    A. _____
    B. _____
    C. _____
    D. _____

30. A partial bath involves bathing the
    _____,
    _____,
    _____,
    _____,
    _____, and
    _____.

31. You protect the person's privacy during a shower by:

    A. _____
    B. _____

32. Before assisting with a shower or tub bath, what information do you need from the nurse and the care plan?

    A. _____
    B. _____
    C. _____
    D. _____
    E. _____
    F. _____
    G. _____
    H. _____

33. Before giving a back massage, you need to observe the skin for:

    A. _____
    B. _____
    C. _____
    D. _____

34. List 3 methods used to warm lotion before applying it.

    A. _____
    B. _____
    C. _____

35. Back massages are dangerous for persons with certain:

    A. _____
    B. _____
    C. _____
    D. _____
    E. _____

36. Which position is best for giving a back massage?
    _____

37. You need to give a back massage to a 90-year-old resident. The person has arthritis in her hips and knees. Which position will likely be most comfortable for the person?
    _____

38. Perineal care involves _____
    _____
    _____.

39. Explain why perineal care is given. _____
    _____
    _____

40. When is perineal care given?

    A. _____
    B. _____

41. When giving perineal care, work from
    _____ to
    _____.

42. When giving perineal care, what observations do you need to report and record?

    A. _____

    B. _____

    C. _____

    D. _____

43. You are giving perineal care to a male patient. Explain how you will clean the tip of his penis.

    _____

    _____

    _____

    _____

44. To protect the person's right to privacy, do the following:

    A. _____

    B. _____

    C. _____

    D. _____

    E. _____

45. Provide the abbreviation for each of the following words:

    A. Centigrade _____

    B. Fahrenheit _____

    C. Identification _____

Multiple Choice

Circle the **BEST** Answer

46. Before giving oral hygiene, you need the following information from the nurse and the care plan *except*
    A. The type of oral hygiene to give
    B. The type of toothbrush to use
    C. If flossing is needed
    D. How much help the person needs

47. Which action is *incorrect* when flossing the person's teeth?
    A. Hold the floss between the middle fingers of each hand.
    B. Start at the upper back tooth on the right side.
    C. Move the floss gently up and down between the teeth.
    D. Use a new piece of floss for each tooth.

48. When providing mouth care to the unconscious person, which is *correct?*
    A. Use your fingers to hold the mouth open.
    B. Position the person on his or her back.
    C. Use a hard bristle toothbrush.
    D. Explain what you are doing step-by-step.

49. How often is mouth care given to unconscious persons?
    A. At least every 2 hours
    B. At least every 4 hours
    C. Every 6 hours
    D. Twice a day

50. You are giving mouth care to an unconscious person. Which action is *incorrect?*
    A. Provide for privacy.
    B. Place a towel under the person's face.
    C. Place a kidney basin under the chin.
    D. With the tongue blade, use force to separate the upper and lower teeth.

51. When cleaning dentures, which is *correct?*
    A. Use hot water.
    B. Firmly hold them over a basin of water lined with a towel.
    C. Use a sponge swab to clean them.
    D. Store them dry in a container with a lid.

52. Which is *not* a rule for bathing?
    A. Follow the care plan for bathing method.
    B. Allow personal choice whenever possible.
    C. Cover the person for warmth and privacy.
    D. Briskly rub the person dry with a clean towel.

53. Which is *not* a rule for bathing?
    A. Protect the person from falling.
    B. Use good body mechanics at all times.
    C. Use hot water and soap.
    D. Keep bar soap in the soap dish between latherings.

54. A person with dementia becomes agitated when you try to give him a tub bath. Which measure might be helpful?
    A. Trying to hurry the person to get the bath over with as soon as possible
    B. Explaining to the person that there is nothing to be afraid of
    C. Trying the bath later
    D. Getting help to force the person into the tub

55. Persons with dementia may feel threatened by bathing procedures.
    A. True
    B. False

56. Water temperature for a complete bed bath is usually between:
    A. 95° F and 100° F
    B. 100° F and 110° F
    C. 110° F and 115° F
    D. 115° F and 120° F

57. When giving a complete bed bath, do the following *except*
    A. Place the bed in the lowest horizontal position
    B. Lower the head of the bed
    C. Cover the person for warmth
    D. Change the water if it is soapy or cool
58. To wash around the person's eyes
    A. Use warm soapy water
    B. Wipe from the outer to the inner aspect of the eye
    C. Clean around the near eye first
    D. Use a clean part of the washcloth for each stroke
59. Risks from tub baths and showers include
    A. Falls, chilling, and burns
    B. Dementia, confusion, and restlessness
    C. Skin breakdown and infection
    D. Hypertension and shortness of breath
60. You are giving a resident a tub bath. Which is *correct?*
    A. The bath should last 30 minutes.
    B. The tub bath may cause the person to feel faint and weak.
    C. Use bath oils in the water.
    D. Drain the tub after the person gets out of the tub.
61. Shower chair wheels are locked during the shower.
    A. True
    B. False
62. Which is *not* a safety measure for tub baths and showers?
    A. Clean and disinfect the tub or shower before and after use.
    B. Place needed items within the person's reach.
    C. Place the signal light within the person's reach.
    D. Have the person use the towel bars for support.
63. When giving a shower, turn hot water on first, then the cold water.
    A. True
    B. False
64. Fill the tub before the person gets into it.
    A. True
    B. False
65. A resident can bathe alone in the tub. How often do you need to check on the person?
    A. At least every 5 minutes
    B. At least every 15 minutes
    C. Whenever you have time
    D. Only when the person turns on the signal light

66. When giving a back massage, do the following *except*
    A. Warm the lotion before applying
    B. Use firm strokes
    C. Always keep your hands in contact with the person's skin
    D. Massage bony areas that are reddened
67. A back massage is safe for all persons.
    A. True
    B. False
68. When giving a back massage, use fast movements to relax the person.
    A. True
    B. False
69. After giving a back massage, what do you need to report and record?
    A. The type of lotion used
    B. How you warmed the lotion
    C. How long the massage lasted
    D. Breaks in the skin and reddened areas
70. When giving perineal care, which action is *correct?*
    A. Cover the person with a drawsheet.
    B. Use hot water.
    C. Rinse thoroughly.
    D. Rub the area dry after rinsing.
71. When giving perineal care, you need to use a clean part of the washcloth for each stroke.
    A. True
    B. False
72. You protect the person's right to privacy by
    A. Exposing the person during bathing procedures
    B. Allowing visitors to stay in the room when giving care
    C. Providing care with the room door open
    D. Covering persons who are taken to and from tubs and shower rooms

CASE STUDY

A resident of Pine View Nursing Center is alert and can make her needs known. The person is continent of bowel and bladder. You are assigned to care for the person today. Your assignment sheet tells you that the person:

- Uses a wheelchair to get around
- Eats all of her meals in the dinning room
- Has an upper and lower denture
- Needs a whirlpool tub bath today
  - She likes her bath at 10 AM.
- Gets a back massage after her bath

Answer the following questions:

1. What care do you need to give the person before breakfast?

2. What care do you need to give the person after breakfast?

3. Before assisting the person with a bath, what information do you need from the nurse and the care plan?

4. When assisting the person with a bath, what observations do you need to make?

5. How will you promote the person's right to privacy?

6. How will you promote the person's right to personal choice?

ADDITIONAL LEARNING ACTIVITIES

1. Discuss the importance of hygiene and cleanliness in your personal life.
   A. Explain how important it is for you to feel clean and free from unpleasant odors when you are around other people.

   B. List the personal care routines you practice daily to promote cleanliness.

2. Has illness ever prevented you from carrying out your daily hygiene routines? Explain.

   A. Discuss how this affected your personal comfort.

3. To help you learn and practice the following procedures, view the following CD Companion Skills:
   A. Brushing the Person's Teeth
   B. Providing Mouth Care for the Unconscious Person
   C. Providing Denture Care
   D. Giving a Complete Bed Bath
   E. Giving a Back Massage
   F. Giving Female and Male Perineal Care

4. The procedures in this chapter require you to provide personal care to another person. The procedures must be performed in a way that respects the person's privacy and dignity. It will help you to understand how the person feels if you practice the procedures with a classmate. Take your turn being the patient or resident. Under the supervision of your instructor, use the procedure checklist provided on pp. 234-254 to practice the procedures in Chapter 15. Use a simulator to practice female and male perineal care.
   A. After practicing each procedure, discuss your experience.

16 ASSISTING WITH GROOMING

STUDY QUESTIONS

Matching
Match each term with the correct definition.

1. _____ Hair loss
2. _____ Excessive amounts of dry, white flakes from the scalp
3. _____ Excessive body hair
4. _____ A skin disorder caused by a female mite
5. _____ Being in or on a host
6. _____ Infestation with wingless insects: lice
7. _____ Prevents or slows down blood clotting

A. Hirsutism
B. Alopecia
C. Anticoagulant
D. Pediculosis
E. Dandruff
F. Infestation
G. Scabies

Fill in the Blanks

8. The nursing process reflects the person's:

   A. _____

   B. _____

   C. _____

   D. _____

   E. _____

9. Hirsutism results from

   _____

   _____

   _____.

10. Lice spread to others through:

    A. _____

    B. _____

    C. _____

    D. _____

    E. _____

    F. _____

    G. _____

    H. _____

11. Common sites for scabies are

    _____

    _____

    _____.

    Other sites include

    _____

    _____

    _____.

12. Brushing and combing hair are part of

    _____,

    _____, and

    _____ care.

13. _____ chooses
    how to brush, comb, and style hair.

14. You have finished brushing a resident's hair.
    What observations do you need to report and
    record?

    A. _____

    B. _____

    C. _____

    D. _____

    E. _____

F. _____

G. _____

H. _____

15. Describe the following:

   A. Nits (lice eggs attached to hair shafts)

      _____

      _____

      _____

   B. Lice

      _____

      _____

      _____

16. A resident is dressed for the day. The person asks you to brush her hair. Explain why you should place a towel across the person's back and shoulders before you begin.

   _____

17. The nurse tells you which shampoo method to use. The shampoo method depends on:

   A. _____
   B. _____
   C. _____

18. List 4 shampoo methods.

   A. _____
   B. _____
   C. _____
   D. _____

19. You have finished shampooing a patient's hair. What observations do you need to report and record?

   A. _____
   B. _____
   C. _____
   D. _____
   E. _____
   F. _____
   G. _____
   H. _____
   I. _____

20. A patient uses medicated shampoo. When you are finished shampooing the person's hair, what should you do with the shampoo?

   _____

   _____

   _____

21. You need to shampoo a resident's hair. The person has scalp sores. You need to wear

   _____.

22. An 80-year-old resident cannot tip his head back. You are shampooing the person's hair in the tub. How would you keep shampoo out of the person's eyes while shampooing his hair?

   _____

   _____

   _____

   _____

23. What type of shaver is used for a person taking an anticoagulant drug? _____

   _____

24. When using a safety razor, shave in the direction of hair growth when shaving _____

   _____.

25. Explain why you should not use a safety razor to shave a person with dementia.

   _____

   _____

   _____

   _____

26. When shaving a person, what observations do you need to report at once?

   A. _____
   B. _____
   C. _____

27. Where are used razor blades and disposable shavers disposed of?

   _____

28. Never trim or shave a beard or mustache without _____.

29. When giving foot care, what observations do you need to report and record?

    A. _____

    B. _____

    C. _____

    D. _____

30. You do not cut or trim toenails if a person:

    A. _____

    B. _____

    C. _____

    D. _____

31. How are fingernails trimmed?

    _____

    _____

    _____

32. List the rules to follow when changing clothes and hospital gowns.

    A. _____

    B. _____

    C. _____

    D. _____

    E. _____

    F. _____

33. Before assisting with dressing, what information do you need from the nurse and the care plan?

    A. _____

    B. _____

    C. _____

    D. _____

    E. _____

    F. _____

34. Before changing a gown, what information do you need from the nurse and the care plan?

    A. _____

    B. _____

35. Write the meaning of the following abbreviations:

    A. IV _____

    B. C _____

    C. ID _____

Multiple Choice

Circle the **BEST** answer

36. Infestation of the scalp with lice is
    A. Pediculosis capitis
    B. Pediculosis pubis
    C. Pediculosis corporis
    D. Dandruff

37. Brushing and combing hair is
    A. Done whenever needed
    B. Done when you have time
    C. Not your responsibility
    D. Always done by the patient or resident

38. When giving hair care, which action is *correct?*
    A. You decide how to style the hair.
    B. Brush or comb from the scalp to the hair ends.
    C. Cut matted and tangled hair.
    D. Braid long hair to keep it neat.

39. Before shampooing a person's hair, you need the following information from the nurse and the care plan *except*
    A. When to shampoo the person's hair
    B. What method to use
    C. The person's position restrictions or limits
    D. How long the person's hair is

40. A patient has limited range of motion in her neck. The person is not shampooed
    A. In bed
    B. In the shower
    C. In the tub
    D. At the sink or on a stretcher

41. A person receives a cut during shaving. Which action is *correct?*
    A. Apply after-shave lotion to the cut.
    B. Apply direct pressure to the cut.
    C. Put a dressing on the cut.
    D. Put a piece of tissue on the cut.

42. A resident has a beard. Which action is *incorrect?*
    A. Wash and comb the beard daily.
    B. Ask the person how to groom his beard.
    C. Trim the person's beard once a week.
    D. Wash the beard whenever mouth or nose drainage is present.

43. Use nail clippers to cut fingernails. Never use scissors.
    A. True
    B. False
44. Nails are easier to trim and clean
    A. In the morning
    B. Before the bath
    C. Right after soaking or bathing
    D. At bedtime
45. When trimming fingernails, which action is *correct?*
    A. Let the fingernails soak for 30 minutes before starting.
    B. Clip the fingernails in a curved shape.
    C. Shape the nails with an emery board or a nail file.
    D. Use a scissors.
46. Feet are soaked for
    A. 5 to 10 minutes
    B. 15 to 20 minutes
    C. 25 to 30 minutes
    D. 30 minutes
47. You are assisting a person with dementia to dress. Which action is *not* helpful?
    A. Let the person choose what to wear from two or three outfits.
    B. Choose clothing that is easy to get on and off.
    C. Stack clothes in the order that they will be put on.
    D. Dress the person as quickly as possible.

48. You must allow for personal choice and independence when assisting with dressing and undressing.
    A. True
    B. False
49. If there is injury or paralysis, the gown is removed from
    A. The strong side first
    B. The weak side first
    C. The right side first
    D. The left side first
50. A patient has an IV in his right arm. The person has an IV pump and a standard gown. You are changing the person's gown. Which is *correct?*
    A. The person's right arm is put through the sleeve first.
    B. The person's left arm is put through the sleeve first.
    C. The person's gown is not changed until he no longer has the IV.
    D. The person's right arm is not put through the sleeve.
51. You need to follow the person's grooming routines whenever possible.
    A. True
    B. False
52. You promote courteous and dignified care by
    A. Combing the person's hair the way you like it
    B. Making sure clothing is properly fastened
    C. Encouraging a man to shave off his beard
    D. Exposing the person when changing garments

CASE STUDY

A patient is recovering from surgery on her right knee. Today is the person's bath day. She also wants her hair shampooed. The person has thick, long curly hair, which she usually wears up. She dresses in regular clothes during the day and wears a nightgown to bed. The person needs some assistance with dressing and undressing.

Answer the following questions:

1. Before you assist the person to shampoo her hair, what information do you need from the nurse and the care plan?

2. When assisting the person with shampooing, what safety measures will you practice?

3. How will you brush or comb the person's hair?

4. Who will choose what the person wears?

ADDITIONAL LEARNING ACTIVITIES

1. List the grooming activities you perform every day. Answer these questions:

   A. How important are your grooming routines?

   B. When you are performing your grooming activities, how important is personal choice?

   C. When you are performing your grooming activities, how important is privacy?

   D. How might you feel if you were unable to perform your grooming activities?
   (1) How would you want to be treated?
   (2) Role-play weakness on one side of the body.
   (3) Role-play that the person is not able to help.
   (4) Take your turn being the patient or resident.

   B. Did you feel safe and secure during the procedures?

   C. How might your experience affect how you help others with grooming and dressing activities?

2. View the CD Companion: Skills to help you learn and practice the following procedures:
   A. Brushing and Combing the Person's Hair
   B. Shampooing the Person's Hair
   C. Giving Nail and Foot Care
   D. Undressing the Person
   E. Dressing the Person

3. Carefully review the procedures in Chapter 16. Under the supervision of your instructor, use the procedure checklists on pp. 255-269 to practice each procedure.
   A. Practice dressing and undressing procedures with classmates or family members.
   (1) Use different types of clothing. (For example: clothes that open in front and clothes that open in back, button and pullover shirts, pants with zippers and buttons, and pants that pull on.)

17 ASSISTING WITH URINARY ELIMINATION

STUDY QUESTIONS

Matching

Match each term with the correct definition.

1. _____ Small amounts of urine leak from a bladder that is always full

2. _____ The loss of urine at predictable intervals when the bladder is full

3. _____ When urine leaks during exercise and certain movements that cause pressure on the bladder

4. _____ Urine is lost in response to a sudden, urgent need to void

5. _____ The need to void at once

6. _____ The person has bladder control but cannot use the toilet in time

7. _____ Voiding at frequent intervals

8. _____ The involuntary loss or leakage of urine

A. Overflow incontinence
B. Urinary frequency
C. Functional incontinence
D. Urinary urgency
E. Stress incontinence
F. Reflex incontinence
G. Urge incontinence
H. Urinary incontinence

Fill in the Blanks

9. The urinary system removes _____ from the blood and maintains the body's

_____.

10. List 7 factors affecting urine production.

    A. _____

    B. _____

    C. _____

    D. _____

    E. _____

    F. _____

    G. _____

11. When assisting with urination, you need to observe urine for:

    A. _____

    B. _____

    C. _____

    D. _____

    E. _____

12. A patient is recovering from hip replacement surgery. What type of bedpan will the person use?

    _____

13. Explain how you will promote safety when handling bedpans and their contents.

    A. _____

    B. _____

14. A resident cannot assist in getting on the bedpan. How will you give the person the bedpan?

    A. _____

    B. _____

    C. _____

    D. _____

    E. _____

    F. _____

15. A person you assist with the bedpan is unable to clean her genital area. Describe how you will clean the person's genital area.

_____

_____

_____

_____

_____

16. Men use _____ to void.

17. Before assisting with urinals, what information do you need from the nurse and the care plan?

A. _____

B. _____

C. _____

D. _____

E. _____

F. _____

G. _____

H. _____

18. Explain why you need to empty urinals promptly.

_____

_____

_____

_____

_____

19. A resident stands to use the urinal. How will you give him the urinal?

A. _____

B. _____

C. _____

D. _____

20. A _____ is a chair or wheelchair with an opening for a container.

21. When assisting with commodes, what information do you need from the nurse and the care plan?

A. _____

B. _____

C. _____

D. _____

E. _____

F. _____

G. _____

22. After you transfer a person to the commode, how can you provide warmth and promote privacy?

_____

_____

23. List 7 causes of functional incontinence.

A. _____

B. _____

C. _____

D. _____

E. _____

F. _____

G. _____

24. A person has stress incontinence and urge incontinence. This is called _____.

25. What should you do if incontinence is a new problem for a patient or resident?

_____

_____

26. A resident is incontinent of urine. You help prevent urinary tract infections by:

A. _____

B. _____

C. _____

27. _____ is the process of inserting a catheter.

28. This type of urinary catheter is left in the bladder. ____

29. Persons with catheters are at high risk for ____.

30. A resident has an indwelling catheter. Why do you need to keep the drainage bag below the person's bladder? ____

31. After giving catheter care, what observations do you need to report and record?
    A. ____
    B. ____
    C. ____
    D. ____
    E. ____
    F. ____

32. When using a safety pin and rubber band to secure tubing to the bottom linens, what safety measures are needed?
    A. ____
    B. ____
    C. ____
    D. ____

33. Explain why a closed drainage system is used for an indwelling catheter. ____

34. What should you do if a urinary drainage system is accidentally disconnected?
    A. ____
    B. ____
    C. ____
    D. ____

E. ____
F. ____
G. ____

35. You empty a person's urinary drainage bag at the end of your shift. What observations do you need to report and record?
    A. ____
    B. ____
    C. ____
    D. ____
    E. ____

36. A patient is embarrassed about having a catheter. What measures can help promote the person's mental comfort? ____

37. A ____ is a soft sheath that slides over the penis.

38. Never use adhesive tape to secure a condom catheter because ____.

39. You should not apply a condom catheter if ____.

40. You are applying a condom catheter. The man becomes aroused. What should you do? ____

41. What is the goal of a bladder training program? ____

42. Leaving a person on the bedpan for a long time is likely to cause ____.

43. If your state and agency allow you to insert urinary catheters:

   A. The procedure must _____

   _____.

   B. You must have the necessary _____

   _____.

   C. You must know how to use _____

   _____.

   D. A nurse must be available to _____

   _____.

Multiple Choice

Circle the **BEST** answer

44. How much urine does the healthy adult produce each day?
   A. About 500 mL
   B. About 700 mL
   C. About 1500 mL
   D. About 3000 mL

45. Which is *not* a rule for normal elimination?
   A. Follow Standard Precautions and the Bloodborne Pathogen Standard.
   B. Limit the amount of fluid intake to 1500 mL daily.
   C. Follow the person's voiding routines and habits.
   D. Help the person to the bathroom when the request is made.

46. You promote normal elimination by
   A. Setting new voiding routines
   B. Asking the person to hurry
   C. Providing only small amounts of fluid
   D. Providing privacy

47. Normal urine
   A. Is pale yellow, straw colored, or amber
   B. Does not have an odor
   C. Is cloudy
   D. Contains particles

48. To place a fracture pan correctly, the smaller end is placed under the buttocks.
   A. True
   B. False

49. Before assisting with the bedpan, you need the following information from the nurse and the care plan *except*
   A. How to position the bedpan
   B. If you can leave the room
   C. If the nurse needs to observe the results
   D. What observations to report

50. Remind men to place urinals on the overbed table after use.
   A. True
   B. False

51. Nervous system disorders and injuries are common causes of
   A. Stress incontinence
   B. Urge incontinence
   C. Functional incontinence
   D. Reflex incontinence

52. Which is *not* a nursing measure for persons with urinary incontinence?
   A. Increase fluid intake at bedtime.
   B. Provide good skin care.
   C. Answer signal lights promptly.
   D. Observe for signs of skin breakdown.

53. You feel impatient when caring for a person with incontinence. Which action is *correct*?
   A. Tell a co-worker to take care of the person for you.
   B. Wait to provide care until you feel less stressed.
   C. Talk to the nurse at once.
   D. Tell the person how you feel.

54. You observe a resident with dementia urinating in the trash can. Which action is *correct*?
   A. Remove the trash can from the person's room.
   B. Tell the person to urinate in the bathroom.
   C. Tell the person to empty the trash can into the toilet.
   D. Check with the nurse and the care plan for measures to help the person.

55. When a person has dementia, which measure can help keep the person clean and dry?
   A. Remind the person where the bathroom is.
   B. Provide all fluids before 5:00 PM.
   C. Follow the person's bathroom routine as closely as possible.
   D. Tell the person to ask to use the bathroom when the urge to void is felt.

56. Catheters are used for the following reasons *except*
   A. As a first choice to treat incontinence
   B. For persons who are too weak or disabled to use the bedpan, urinal, commode, or toilet
   C. To protect wounds and pressure ulcers from urine
   D. To allow hourly urinary output measurements

57. When caring for a person with an indwelling catheter, you need to do the following *except*
   A. Keep the catheter connected to the drainage tubing
   B. Attach the drainage bag to the bed rail
   C. Coil the drainage tubing on the bed and secure it to the bottom linen
   D. Report leaks to the nurse at once

58. To apply a condom catheter correctly, you need to do the following *except*
    A. Roll the sheath onto the penis
    B. Leave a 1-inch space between the penis and the end of the catheter
    C. Apply tape completely around the penis
    D. Make sure the condom is not twisted
59. You do not know how to apply the condom catheter used at your agency. What should you do?
    A. Ask the patient or resident how to apply it.
    B. Read the instructions before you apply it.
    C. Ask the nurse to show you the correct application.
    D. Use an incontinence product for the person instead.
60. The abbreviation for milliliter is
    A. ML
    B. Ml
    C. ml
    D. mL

CROSSWORD

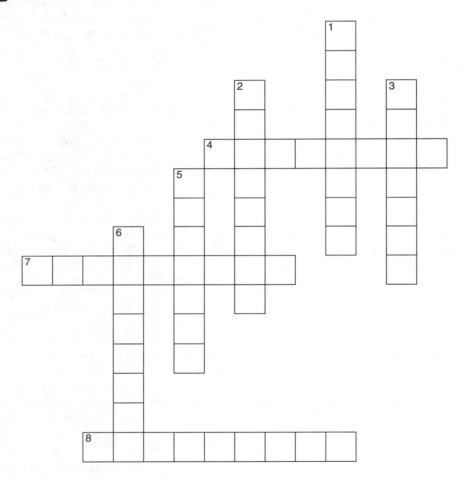

Across
4. Scant amount of urine
7. Blood in the urine
8. The process of emptying urine from the bladder

Down
1. Frequent urination at night
2. Abnormally large amounts of urine
3. Urination
5. Painful or difficult urination
6. A tube used to drain or inject fluid through a body opening

CASE STUDY

A 70-year-old hospital patient has an indwelling catheter. The person is alert and can assist with her daily care. She likes to make her own decisions. The person walks with a walker and is out of bed most of the day. Her husband visits every day at 1300.

Answer the following questions:

1. Before giving catheter care, what information do you need from the nurse and the care plan?

2. When giving catheter care, what observations do you need to report and record?

3. What safety measures do you need to practice?

4. How often do you need to give catheter care?

5. How will you protect the person's right to privacy?

6. How will you promote the person's independence?

ADDITIONAL LEARNING ACTIVITIES

1. Think of your personal voiding patterns.
   A. List the factors that affect your daily patterns.

   B. Discuss how changes in your personal patterns affect your comfort.

2. View the CD Companion: Skills to help you learn and practice the following procedures:
   A. Giving the Bedpan
   B. Giving Catheter Care

3. Carefully review and practice the procedure for giving the bedpan. Work with a classmate. Use a regular bedpan and a fracture pan.
   A. Use the procedure checklist provided on pp. 270-271 as a guide.

B. Wear clothing to practice. Take your turn being the patient or resident. Discuss your experience.

(1) Did you have concerns about dignity and privacy?

(2) Was the experience physically comfortable? Explain.

(3) Was it difficult to position the bedpan correctly? Explain.

(4) How might it feel to be left on a bedpan for 15 minutes or longer?

4. Carefully review and practice all the procedures in this chapter. Use a simulator when appropriate. Use the procedure checklists provided on pp. 270-280. If you are embarrassed by any of these procedures, discuss your feelings with your instructor or a nurse.

18 ASSISTING WITH BOWEL ELIMINATION

STUDY QUESTIONS

Matching

Match each term with the correct definition.

1. _____ The inability to control the passage of feces and gas through the anus

2. _____ The process of excreting feces from the rectum through the anus (bowel movement)

3. _____ The prolonged retention and buildup of feces in the rectum

4. _____ The semi-solid mass of waste products in the colon that is expelled through the anus

5. _____ The excessive formation of gas or air in the stomach and intestines

6. _____ Excreted feces

A. Flatulence
B. Stool
C. Fecal impaction
D. Fecal incontinence
E. Defecation
F. Feces

Fill in the Blanks

7. Stools are normally _____,

_____,

_____,

_____,

and _____.

They normally have an_____.

8. _____,
causes black or tarry stools.

9. What observations about stools do you need to report to the nurse?

A. _____

B. _____

C. _____

D. _____

E. _____

F. _____

G. _____

H. _____

10. List 9 factors that affect the frequency, consistency, color, and odor of stools.

A. _____

B. _____

C. _____

D. _____

E. _____

F. _____

G. _____

H. _____

I. _____

11. Explain why providing privacy is important when meeting the person's elimination needs.

_____

_____

_____

_____

12. Explain how aging affects bowel elimination.

    _____

    _____

    _____

    _____

13. _____
    results if constipation is not relieved.

14. You are caring for a person with diarrhea. You need to:

    A. _____

    B. _____

    C. _____

    D. _____

15. Causes of diarrhea include _____

    _____

    _____.

16. *Clostridium difficile (C. difficile)* is _____

    _____

    _____.

17. How can you spread *C. difficile?*

    _____

    _____

    _____

    _____.

18. List 7 causes of fecal incontinence.

    A. _____

    B. _____

    C. _____

    D. _____

    E. _____

    F. _____

    G. _____

19. The person with fecal incontinence may need the following:

    A. _____

    B. _____

    C. _____

    D. _____

20. List 6 causes of flatulence.

    A. _____

    B. _____

    C. _____

    D. _____

    E. _____

    F. _____

21. What are the two goals of bowel training?

    A. _____

    B. _____

22. Doctors order enemas to _____

    _____

    _____

    _____.

23. Describe the following types of enemas:

    A. Tap water enema _____

    _____

    _____

    B. Soapsuds enema _____

    _____

    _____

    C. Saline enema _____

    _____

    _____

24. You are giving a cleansing enema. You need to stop tube insertion if:

    A. _____

    B. _____

    C. _____

25. After giving a saline enema, what do you need to report and record?

    A. _____

    B. _____

    C. _____

    D. _____

    E. _____

    F. _____

    G. _____

26. Enemas are dangerous for _____

    _____

    _____ .

27. To prevent cramping when giving an enema, you need to:

    A. _____

    B. _____

28. The doctor orders *"enemas until clear."* This

    means _____

    _____

    _____ .

29. To give a small volume enema, squeeze and roll up the plastic bottle from the bottom. You should not release pressure on the bottle because

    _____

    _____

    _____ .

30. After giving an oil retention enema, you need to do the following:

    A. _____

    _____

    _____

    B. _____

    _____

    _____

    C. _____

    _____

    _____

    D. _____

    _____

    _____

31. Describe the following:

    A. A permanent colostomy _____

    _____

    _____

    B. A temporary colostomy _____

    _____

    _____

32. If a colostomy is near the start of the colon, stools

    are _____ .

33. List four measures that help prevent ostomy pouch odors.

    A. _____

    B. _____

    C. _____

    D. _____

34. A resident wears an ostomy pouch. You need to assist the person with a tub bath. Why should you delay the bath for 1 to 2 hours after applying

    a new pouch? _____

    _____ .

35. Write the meanings of the following abbreviations:

    A. BM _____

    B. oz _____

    C. SSE _____

Multiple Choice
Circle the **BEST** answer

36. Normal stools are
    A. Black in color
    B. Soft, formed, and moist
    C. Hard and marble sized
    D. Liquid and pale in color

37. Safety and comfort during bowel elimination are promoted by the following *except*
    A. Positioning the person in a normal sitting or squatting position
    B. Covering the person for warmth and privacy
    C. Allowing time for a BM
    D. Allowing visitors to stay in the room

38. Which will *not* promote safety and comfort during bowel elimination?
    A. Follow Standard Precautions and the Bloodborne Pathogen Standard.
    B. Place the signal light and toilet tissue within the person's reach.
    C. Leave the room. Check on the person in 15 minutes.
    D. Dispose of stools promptly.
39. Warm fluids decrease peristalsis.
    A. True
    B. False
40. A patient's stool is black in color and has a tarry consistency. What should you do?
    A. Ask if the person has had anything unusual to eat.
    B. Ask the nurse to observe the stool.
    C. Dispose of the stool and report the color to the nurse.
    D. Ask a co-worker if this is normal for the person.
41. You need to follow Standard Precautions and the Bloodborne Pathogen Standard when in contact with stools.
    A. True
    B. False
42. Which is a common cause of constipation?
    A. A high fiber diet
    B. Regular exercise
    C. Increased fluid intake
    D. Ignoring the urge to have a BM
43. Which is a sign of fecal impaction?
    A. Liquid feces seeping from the anus
    B. Black, tarry stools
    C. Increased flatulence
    D. Frequent passage of soft stools
44. *Clostridium difficile* is a microbe found in
    A. Water
    B. Food
    C. Feces
    D. The air
45. A resident has fecal incontinence. Which statement is *correct?*
    A. The person has dementia.
    B. A bowel training program will cure the person's incontinence.
    C. You need to provide good skin care.
    D. The person has an intestinal disease.
46. Which action will *not* help produce flatus?
    A. Lying quietly in the supine position
    B. Walking
    C. Moving in bed
    D. The left side-lying position

47. Which measure does *not* promote comfort and safety when giving an enema to an adult?
    A. Have the person void first.
    B. Lubricate the enema tip before inserting it.
    C. Insert the enema tubing 6 inches.
    D. Give the solution slowly.
48. The preferred position for giving enemas is
    A. Fowler' or semi-Fowler's
    B. The left side-lying or Sims'
    C. Prone
    D. Dorsal recumbent
49. All states and agencies allow nursing assistants to give enemas.
    A. True
    B. False
50. The doctor orders "enemas until clear." You need to ask the nurse how many enemas to give.
    A. True
    B. False
51. It usually takes 10 to 15 minutes to give 750 to 1000 mL of enema solution.
    A. True
    B. False
52. After giving an oil retention enema, do the following *except*
    A. Position the person in the supine position
    B. Urge the person to retain the enema for the time ordered
    C. Place extra waterproof pads on the bed if needed
    D. Check the person often while the person retains the enema
53. A resident has a colostomy. Which statement is *incorrect?*
    A. Good skin care is very important.
    B. Colostomies can be permanent or temporary.
    C. Feces and flatus pass through a stoma located on the abdominal wall.
    D. The entire large intestine has been removed.
54. A resident has an ileostomy. Which statement is *correct?*
    A. Part of the colon is removed.
    B. Stool consistency ranges from liquid to solid.
    C. A skin barrier is not needed around the stoma.
    D. Good skin care is required.
55. Ostomy pouches are changed
    A. When completely full
    B. Every shift and when they leak
    C. Every 3 to 7 days and when they leak
    D. After each meal

56. Used ostomy pouches are flushed down the toilet.
    A. True
    B. False

57. Leaving a person sitting in feces is neglect. It is a form of physical abuse.
    A. True
    B. False

CROSSWORD

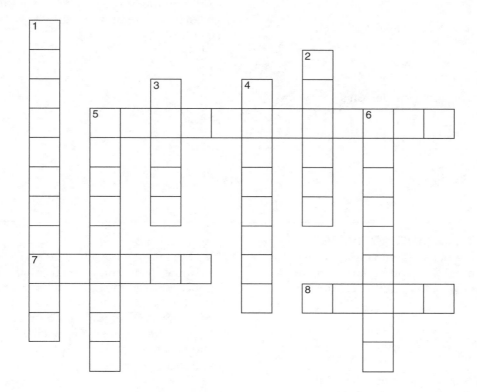

Across

5. The passage of a hard, dry stool
7. A surgically created opening
8. An opening

Down

1. A cone-shaped, solid drug that is inserted into a body opening; it melts at body temperature
2. Gas or air passed through the anus
3. The introduction of fluid into the rectum and lower colon
4. The frequent passage of liquid stools
5. A surgically created opening between the colon and abdominal wall
6. A surgically created opening between the ileum and the abdominal wall

CASE STUDY

A 50-year-old patient in Valley View Hospital is scheduled for bowel x-rays in the morning. The person's doctor ordered saline enemas until clear. The RN has delegated the task of giving the enemas to you.

Answer the following questions:

1. How is a saline enema prepared?

2. How will you promote the person's safety and comfort?

3. How will you protect the person's right to privacy?

4. After giving the enema, what measures do you need to take to promote the person's safety and comfort?

ADDITIONAL LEARNING ACTIVITIES

1. Think of your personal elimination routines.
   A. Explain how important these routines are to your physical and psychological comfort.

   B. Are you aware of how your diet, fluid intake, and level of activity affect your bowel elimination routines? Explain.

   C. Have you had personal experience with constipation or diarrhea? How did the experience affect your comfort?

2. If available at your school or place of work, examine several types of colostomy and ileostomy pouches. Read the manufacturer's instructions. Practice handling the pouches and applying them on yourself and a willing classmate.
3. Handle the various types of enema equipment and become familiar with how each is used. This will increase your comfort and confidence.

NOTE: Remember that some states and agencies do not allow nursing assistants to give enemas.

4. Carefully review the procedures in Chapter 18.
   A. Under the supervision of your instructor, practice each procedure. Use a simulator when appropriate. Use the procedure checklists provided on pp. 281-285 as a guide.
   B. If any of these procedures embarrass you, discuss your feelings with your instructor.

NOTE: Remember that some states and agencies do not allow nursing assistants to give enemas.

19 ASSISTING WITH NUTRITION AND FLUIDS

STUDY QUESTIONS

Matching

Match each term with the correct definition.

1. _____ Difficulty swallowing
2. _____ Breathing fluid, food, vomitus, or an object into the lungs
3. _____ The amount of energy produced when the body burns food
4. _____ The processes involved in the ingestion, digestion, absorption, and use of foods and fluids by the body
5. _____ The swelling of body tissues with water
6. _____ A decrease in the amount of water in body tissues
7. _____ The loss of appetite
8. _____ Giving nutrients into the gastro-intestinal tract through a feeding tube
9. _____ The process of giving a tube feeding
10. _____ The number of drops per minute
11. _____ The backward flow of stomach contents into the mouth
12. _____ Giving fluids through a needle or catheter inserted into a vein
13. _____ A substance that is ingested, digested, absorbed, and used by the body

A. Dehydration
B. Gavage
C. Anorexia
D. Calorie
E. Regurgitation
F. Intravenous (IV) therapy
G. Aspiration
H. Nutrition
I. Edema
J. Flow rate
K. Nutrient
L. Dysphagia
M. Enteral nutrition

Fill in the Blanks

14. The person's diet affects _____

_____.

15. Good nutrition is needed for _____

_____.

16. Nutrients are grouped into _____,

_____, _____,

_____,

_____, and _____.

17. When using MyPlate, calories are balanced by

A. _____

B. _____.

18. When using MyPlate, which food group or groups have these health benefits?

A. Build and maintain bone mass throughout life

_____

B. Provides B vitamins and vitamin E

_____

C. May prevent constipation

_____

D. May reduce risk of kidney stones

_____

E. May prevent certain birth defects

_____

F. Provides nutrients needed for health and body maintenance

_____

19. _____ is the most important nutrient.

20. _____ provide energy and fiber for bowel elimination.

21. List 8 factors affecting nutrition and eating habits.

    A. _____

    B. _____

    C. _____

    D. _____

    E. _____

    F. _____

    G. _____

    H. _____

22. Explain how illness can affect eating and nutrition. _____

    _____

    _____

    _____

    _____

23. Doctors order special diets for the following reasons:

    A. _____

    B. _____

    C. _____

24. Explain what happens when there is too much sodium in the body. _____

    _____

    _____

    _____

25. Sodium controlled diets involve:

    A. _____

    B. _____

    C. _____

26. _____ is produced and secreted by the pancreas. It lets the body use sugar.

27. Explain why it is important for persons with diabetes to eat at regular times each day.

    _____

    _____

28. You are feeding a person with dysphagia. What observations do you need to report at once?

    _____

    _____

29. Fluid balance is needed for health. The amount of _____ and the amount of _____ must be equal.

30. List 6 common causes of dehydration.

    A. _____

    B. _____

    C. _____

    D. _____

    E. _____

    F. _____

31. Your assignment sheet tells you that a patient has an order to restrict fluids to 1500 mL per day. What care measures are needed?

    _____

    _____

    _____

    _____

    _____

32. A patient has an order for thickened liquids. The thickness ordered depends on _____

    _____.

33. To provide for comfort, the meal setting must be free of _____

    _____.

34. You are preparing a resident for breakfast. The person will eat breakfast in bed. After you assist with eyeglasses, hearing aids, oral hygiene, elimination, and hand washing you need to:

    A. _____

    _____

    B. _____

    _____

    C. _____

    _____

35. Nursing centers have dining programs to meet resident needs. With _____

_____,

residents eat at a dinning room table with four to six others. Food is served as in a restaurant. Residents are oriented and can feed themselves.

36. Describe low-stimulation dinning. _____

_____

_____

37. Explain why it is important to prepare the person for a meal before serving the meal tray.

_____

_____

_____

_____

38. A person's food was not served within 15 minutes. What should you do? _____

_____

_____

_____

_____

39. Before serving meal trays, what information do you need from the nurse and the care plan?

A. _____

B. _____

C. _____

D. _____

40. After feeding a person, what observations do you need to report and record?

A. _____

B. _____

C. _____

D. _____

41. A resident eats slowly. The person complains that food will not go down. The person frequently coughs after swallowing. These are

signs and symptoms of _____.

42. A resident has finished eating. The nurse tells you to check for pocketing. You need to check:

A. _____

B. _____

C. _____

43. A patient has dysphagia. To prevent aspiration the person is positioned in a chair or in the semi-Fowler's position for at least

_____ after eating.

44. When are snacks served? _____

_____

45. Before passing drinking water, what information do you need from the nurse and the care plan?

A. _____

B. _____

C. _____

46. Define the following terms:

A. Naso-gastric (NG) tube _____

_____

_____

B. Gastrostomy tube _____

_____

_____

47. _____

_____

are risks from enteral nutrition.

48. Why is it important for the RN to check tube placement before a tube feeding? _____

_____

_____

_____

49. Why is the left side-lying position avoided after a tube feeding? _____

_____

50. A patient is receiving nutrients through an NG tube. How often is oral hygiene provided?

_____

51. Explain why NG tubes are secured to the person's nose and to the person's garment.

_____

_____

_____

52. A patient is receiving IV therapy. When giving the person a bath, you check the flow rate. You need to tell the RN at once if:

   A. _____

   B. _____

   C. _____

   D. _____

53. Write the meaning of the following abbreviations:

   A. GI _____

   B. IV _____

   C. mg _____

   D. NPO _____

Labeling

54. Using the numbers on a clock, describe each food item and where it is located on the plate.

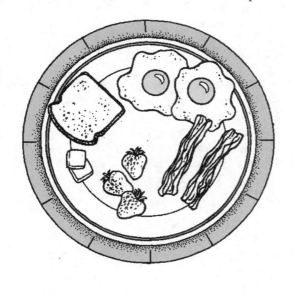

_____

_____

_____

_____

55. Label the IV equipment.

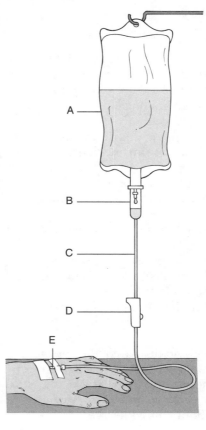

   A. _____

   B. _____

   C. _____

   D. _____

   E. _____

Multiple Choice

Circle the **BEST** Answer

56. Poor diet and poor eating habits
   A. Decrease the risk for disease
   B. Cause healing problems
   C. Do *not* affect mental function
   D. Decrease the risk for accidents

57. One gram of protein has
   A. 4 calories
   B. 6 calories
   C. 8 calories
   D. 9 calories

58. One gram of fat has
   A. 4 calories
   B. 6 calories
   C. 8 calories
   D. 9 calories

59. All of these are food groups in MyPlate *except*
    A. Grains
    B. Vegetables
    C. Fruits
    D. Oils
60. An example of moderate physical activity in MyPlate would be
    A. Bicycling at less than 10 miles per hour
    B. Freestyle swimming laps
    C. Chopping wood
    D. Running and jogging at 5 miles per hour
61. All of the following are included in MyPlate *except*:
    A. Eating high fat foods
    B. Making half of your plate fruits and vegetables
    C. Increasing the amount of meat and fish in your diet.
    D. Drinking water instead of sugary drinks
62. The amount needed from each food group in MyPlate depends on
    A. The ethnic background of the person
    B. The age, sex, and physical activity of the person
    C. The likes and dislikes of the person
    D. The budget available to the person
63. Whole wheat grains in the grain group include
    A. Bulgur, oatmeal, and brown rice
    B. White flour and white rice
    C. Black beans, lentils, and split peas
    D. Potatoes, green bananas, and water chestnuts
64. When choosing from the protein food group, foods that may reduce the risk of heart disease include
    A. Whole eggs
    B. Processed meats
    C. Salmon, trout, and herring
    D. Regular ground beef and chicken with skin
65. During illness
    A. Appetite increases
    B. Fewer nutrients are needed
    C. Nutritional needs increase to fight infection and heal tissue
    D. The person will prefer protein foods
66. Which vitamins are stored by the body?
    A. The B complex vitamins
    B. Vitamin C and the B complex vitamins
    C. Vitamins A, D, E, and K
    D. Vitamin B_{12} and the B complex vitamins
67. This nutrient is needed for all body processes.
    A. Water
    B. Protein
    C. Carbohydrate
    D. Fat

68. Which is *not* an OBRA requirement for food served in nursing centers?
    A. Food is nourishing and tastes good.
    B. Hot food is served hot and cold food is served cold.
    C. Each person receives at least three meals and three snacks a day.
    D. The center provides needed assistive devices and utensils.
69. Which food is allowed on a clear liquid diet?
    A. Creamed cereal
    B. Plain puddings
    C. Eggnog
    D. Gelatin
70. Diabetes is a chronic disease from a lack of insulin. Insulin lets the body use
    A. Sugar
    B. Fat
    C. Protein
    D. Minerals
71. To promote safety and comfort when feeding a person with dysphagia, you must
    A. Feed the person only liquids
    B. Position the person in the semi-Fowler's position in bed
    C. Give thickened liquids using a straw
    D. Feed the person according to the care plan
72. Food spills out of a person's mouth while eating. This is a sign of
    A. Dementia
    B. Toothache
    C. Infection
    D. Dysphagia
73. Which is *not* a sign or symptom of dysphagia?
    A. Food pockets in the person's cheeks.
    B. The person eats very fast.
    C. The person regurgitates food after eating.
    D. The person is hoarse after eating.
74. For normal fluid balance, how many mL of water are needed per day?
    A. 1000 to 1500
    B. 1500 to 2000
    C. 2000 to 2500
    D. 2500 to 3000
75. Body water increases with age.
    A. True
    B. False
76. You notice an NPO sign above a patient's bed. This means
    A. All of the person's fluids are given with a straw
    B. The person cannot eat or drink anything
    C. Water is offered in small amounts
    D. The person cannot have solid food

77. A resident has an order for thickened liquids. This means that all liquids are thickened, including water.
    A. True
    B. False
78. To prepare a person for meals, you need the following information from the nurse and the care plan *except*
    A. How much help the person needs
    B. Where the person will eat
    C. A list of the person's favorite foods
    D. How to position the person
79. A resident needs help eating. The person eats at a horseshoe table in the dinning room. Two other residents also sit at the table. Which type of dinning program is this?
    A. Social dinning
    B. Family dinning
    C. Assistive dinning
    D. Low-stimulation dinning
80. Always check food temperature after re-heating.
    A. True
    B. False
81. When feeding a person, do the following *except*
    A. Serve food and fluids in the order the person prefers
    B. Use a fork to feed the person
    C. Offer fluids during the meal
    D. Sit facing the person
82. When feeding a visually impaired person, you need to
    A. Tell the person what is on the tray
    B. Describe the aroma of each food item
    C. Describe the color and consistency of each food item
    D. Offer fluids only at the end of the meal
83. Aspiration precautions include
    A. Feeding the person liquids through a straw
    B. Positioning the person in Fowler's position or upright in a chair for meals and snacks
    C. Checking the person's mouth before each meal for pocketing
    D. Positioning the person supine after each meal and snack
84. A calorie count is being kept for a patient. Which is *correct*?
    A. On a flow sheet, note what the person ate and how much.
    B. Weigh the food on the person's tray before and after eating.

C. Measure the number of calories in each food item.
D. Ask the dietitian to check the person's tray after each meal.
85. When providing drinking water, which action is *incorrect*?
    A. Make sure the water pitcher is labeled with the person's name and room and bed number.
    B. Do not touch the rim or inside of the water cup or pitcher.
    C. Do not let the ice scoop touch the rim or inside of the water cup or pitcher.
    D. Keep the ice scoop in the ice container or dispenser.
86. A resident is receiving nutrition through an NG tube. The person complains of nausea and discomfort during the tube feeding. What should you do?
    A. Measure the person's vital signs.
    B. Report the person's complaints to the nurse at once.
    C. Stop the tube feeding until the person feels better.
    D. Give the person cool water orally.
87. You have an alarm on an IV infusion pump. What should you do?
    A. Turn the pump off.
    B. Adjust the controls on the pump.
    C. Close the regulator clamp.
    D. Tell the nurse at once.
88. You are *never* responsible for starting or maintaining IV therapy.
    A. True
    B. False
89. A patient complains of pain at the IV site. The area around the IV site is swollen. What should you do?
    A. Turn off the IV infusion pump.
    B. Place a dressing over the IV insertion site.
    C. Apply heat to the area.
    D. Tell the nurse at once.
90. The OBRA survey team makes sure that
    A. Residents eat all meals in the dining room
    B. Needed help is provided during meals
    C. Tablecloths are used at all meals
    D. At least three menu choices are offered at each meal

CASE STUDY

An 80-year-old resident of Pine View Nursing Center with diabetes and high blood pressure needs assistance to get ready for meals. The person wears eyeglasses and a hearing aid in her right ear. She has upper and lower dentures, which she cares for herself. She is continent of bowel and bladder. She needs help with transfers to and from the toilet. She uses a wheelchair to get to the dining room and can push the wheelchair herself. She needs help preparing her food, but can eat by herself. The person sits at a dining room table with three other residents. She always prays before meals.

The person requires diabetes meal planning.

You help her get ready for the noon meal and help prepare her food when she is in the dining room. She complains that her food is not appetizing. She tells you that her portions are too small. She also tells you that she had bread and dessert for every meal when she was doing her own cooking.

Answer the following questions:

1. What factors might affect the person's eating and nutrition?

2. What is involved in diabetes meal planning?

3. What information will you report to the nurse when the person is finished eating? Why is this information important?

4. To whom will you report the person's complaints? When will you report her complaints?
   A. How might this information be used in the care planning process?

ADDITIONAL LEARNING ACTIVITIES

1. Discuss with a classmate the importance of food in your daily life. Besides meeting physical needs, what role does food play in your life?
   A. Discuss how your culture and religion affect the food you eat.

   B. Discuss the role food plays in your social life.

   C. Discuss why you enjoy some foods and dislike others.

2. Has illness ever affected your appetite or your ability to eat certain foods? Explain.

   A. Discuss your experience. How might your experience help you provide better care?

3. Review the MyPlate food guidance system (pp. 323-327 in the textbook).

   A. Based on the MyPlate food guidance system, are you making wise food choices?

4. Discuss the special needs of persons with dementia. List ways that you can help meet their nutritional needs.

5. View the CD Companion: Skills to help you learn and practice the Feeding the Person procedure.

6. Carefully review the procedures in this chapter.
   A. Use the procedure checklists on pp. 286-292 as a guide.
   B. Practice feeding a classmate using various food thicknesses.

C. Take your turn being fed by a classmate. Discuss your experience. Answer these questions:
   (1) How does it feel to be fed by another person?

   (2) Did you enjoy your meal? Explain.

   (3) Were you fed too fast or too slow?

   (4) Was the amount given with each bite right for you?

   (5) Were liquids offered during the meal?

   (6) Did your food remain at the right temperature throughout the meal?

   (7) How might your experience affect the care you give?

20 ASSISTING WITH ASSESSMENT

STUDY QUESTIONS

Matching

Match each term with the correct definition.

1. _____ The amount of heat in the body that is a balance between the amount of heat produced and the amount lost by the body

2. _____ Elevated body temperature

3. _____ A slow pulse rate; the rate is less than 60 beats per minute

4. _____ The pressure in the arteries when the heart is at rest

5. _____ Blood pressure measurements that remain above a systolic pressure of 140 mm Hg or a diastolic pressure above 90 mm Hg

6. _____ When the systolic blood pressure is below 90 mm Hg and the diastolic pressure is below 60 mm Hg

7. _____ The beat of the heart felt at an artery as a wave of blood passes through the artery

8. _____ The amount of force exerted against the walls of an artery by the blood

9. _____ The number of heartbeats or pulses felt in 1 minute

10. _____ Breathing air into (inhalation) and out of (exhalation) the lungs

11. _____ An instrument used to listen to the sounds produced by the heart, lungs, and other body organs

12. _____ Pressure in the arteries when the heart contracts

13. _____ A rapid heart rate; the heart rate is over 100 beats per minute

14. _____ Temperature, pulse, respirations, and blood pressure

15. _____ A cuff and measuring device used to measure blood pressure

16. _____ Means to ache, hurt, or be sore

A. Hypertension
B. Blood pressure
C. Respiration
D. Pulse
E. Stethoscope
F. Tachycardia
G. Hypotension
H. Diastolic pressure
I. Bradycardia
J. Pulse rate
K. Sphygmomanometer
L. Vital signs
M. Pain
N. Body temperature
O. Systolic pressure
P. Fever

Fill in the Blanks

17. Vital signs reflect these three body processes:

    A. _____

    B. _____

    C. _____

18. Accuracy is essential when you _____,

    _____, and

    _____

    vital signs.

19. Vital signs show even minor changes in a person's condition. They also tell about response to treatment and often signal life-threatening events. Therefore you must report the following at once:

    A. _____

    B. _____

20. List the sites for measuring body temperature.

    A. _____

    B. _____

    C. _____

    D. _____

    E. _____

21. List the normal range for body temperature for the:

    A. Rectal site _____

    B. Oral site _____

    C. Tympanic membrane site _____

    D. Axillary site _____

22. Oral temperatures are *not* taken if the person:

    A. _____

    B. _____

    C. _____

    D. _____

    E. _____

    F. _____

    G. _____

    H. _____

    I. _____

    J. _____

23. A patient has heart disease. Which temperature sites can you use? _____

    _____

    _____

24. Which temperature site is *not* used for children under 4 or 5 years of age? _____

    _____

25. How should you shake down a glass thermometer? _____

    _____

    _____

    _____

26. What do the short lines on a Fahrenheit thermometer mean? _____

27. What does each long line on a centigrade thermometer mean? _____

28. List four special measures needed when taking a rectal temperature with a glass thermometer.

    A. _____

    B. _____

    C. _____

    D. _____

29. The covered probe of a tympanic membrane thermometer is gently inserted into the

    _____.

30. How is temperature measured using a temporal artery thermometer? _____

    _____

    _____

31. _____ and

    _____

    thermometers are used to measure temperatures for persons who are confused and resist care.

32. After measuring temperature, what observations do you need to report and record?

    A. _____

    B. _____

33. When measuring a rectal temperature, how is the person positioned?_____

_____

34. Which site is used most often for taking a pulse?

_____

35. Which pulse is taken with a stethoscope?

_____

36. To use a stethoscope, do the following:

A. _____

_____

_____

B. _____

_____

_____

C. _____

_____

_____

D. _____

_____

_____

E. _____

_____

_____

37. Stethoscope diaphragms tend to be _____.

You need to _____
the diaphragm in your hand before applying it
to the person.

38. The normal adult pulse rate is between

_____ beats per minute.

39. The rhythm of the pulse should be regular. This means _____

_____

_____

40. Where is the radial artery located? _____

_____

41. You should not use your thumb to take a pulse because _____

_____

_____

_____.

42. Apical pulses are taken for persons who:

A. _____

B. _____

C. _____

43. Describe normal respirations. _____

_____

44. The healthy adult has _____
respirations per minute.

45. When are respirations counted?

_____

46. After counting respirations, what observations do you need to report and record?

A. _____

B. _____

C. _____

D. _____

E. _____

F. _____

47. Respirations are usually counted for 30 seconds. The number is multiplied by 2. You need to count respirations for 1 minute if:

A. _____

B. _____

C. _____

D. _____

48. _____ and

_____

are used to measure blood pressure.

49. Blood pressure is measured in _____

_____

50. What should you do if a mercury manometer breaks? _____

_____

_____

51. Before measuring blood pressure, what information do you need from the nurse and the care plan?

    A. _____

    B. _____

    C. _____

    D. _____

    E. _____

    F. _____

    G. _____

    H. _____

    I. _____

52. When measuring a blood pressure, how should you position the person's arm? _____

    _____

    _____

53. Describe the following types of pain:

    A. Acute pain _____

    _____

    _____

    _____

    B. Chronic pain _____

    _____

    _____

    _____

54. A resident complains of pain in her lower abdomen. What other information about the person's pain does the nurse need?

    A. _____

    B. _____

    C. _____

    D. _____

    E. _____

    F. _____

    G. _____

55. Intake and output (I&O) records are used to

    _____

    _____.

They also are kept when _____

_____.

56. Output includes _____

    _____

57. A measuring container for fluids is called a

    _____.

58. Measure intake as follows:

    A. _____

    _____

    B. _____

    _____

    C. _____

    _____

    D. _____

    _____

    E. _____

    _____

    F. _____

    _____

    G. _____

    _____

    H. _____

59. Before measuring weight and height, what information do you need from the nurse and the care plan?

    A. _____

    _____

    B. _____

    _____

    C. _____

    _____

    D. _____

    _____

60. Write the meanings of the following abbreviations:

    A. C _____

    B. Hg _____

C. I&O _____

D. mL _____

E. mm _____

F. mm Hg _____

Labeling

61. Record the readings on the thermometers shown.

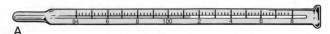

A

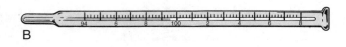

B

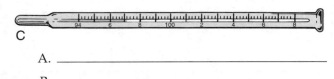

C

A. _____

B. _____

C. _____

62. Label the pulse sites.

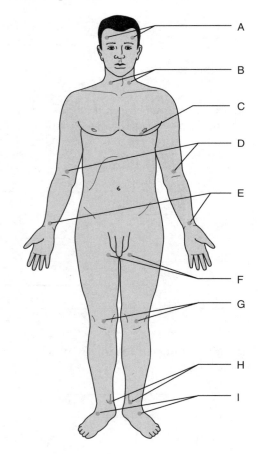

A. _____

B. _____

C. _____

D. _____

E. _____

F. _____

G. _____

H. _____

I. _____

63. Label the parts of a stethoscope.

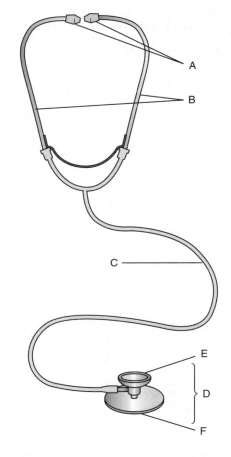

A. _____

B. _____

C. _____

D. _____

E. _____

F. _____

64. Place an X at the apical pulse site.

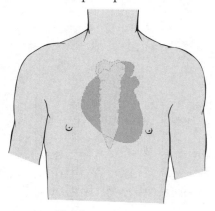

65. Fill in the drawing so that the dials show the
correct blood pressure.
A. 152/86 mm Hg
B. 104/68 mm Hg

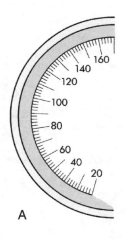

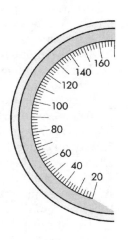

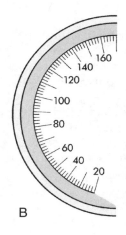

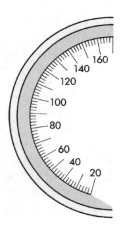

66. Fill in the drawing so the mercury column shows the correct blood pressure.
    A. 152/86 mm Hg
    B. 198/100 mm Hg

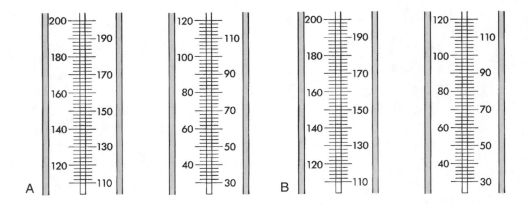

Multiple Choice
Circle the **BEST** Answer

67. Unless otherwise ordered, vital signs are taken
    A. After the person's bath
    B. With the person at rest lying or sitting
    C. After breakfast
    D. After performing range-of-motion exercises

68. You are unsure of a person's pulse rate. What should you do?
    A. Ask the person what the usual rate is.
    B. Wait 15 minutes and take it again.
    C. Record a previous measurement.
    D. Ask the nurse to take the person's pulse again.

69. Do *not* take a rectal temperature if
    A. The person is unconscious
    B. The person has just had a bath
    C. The person is receiving oxygen
    D. The person has diarrhea

70. The least reliable temperature site is the
    A. Oral site
    B. Axillary site
    C. Tympanic membrane site
    D. Rectal site

71. When using a glass thermometer, which measure will help prevent infection?
    A. Use only the person's thermometer.
    B. Rinse the thermometer under warm running water.
    C. Dry the thermometer from the bulb to the stem with tissue.
    D. After cleaning, store the thermometer in the person's bedside stand.

72. You are taking a rectal temperature with a glass thermometer. Which is *incorrect?*
    A. Privacy is important.
    B. The thermometer is lubricated before insertion.
    C. The thermometer is held in place.
    D. The thermometer remains in the rectum for one minute.

73. Axillary temperatures
    A. Are more reliable than oral temperatures
    B. Are taken right after bathing the person
    C. Are taken for 3 minutes
    D. Are used when other routes cannot be used

74. The force of a pulse relates to
    A. How regular the pulse is
    B. The strength of the pulse
    C. The number of beats per minute
    D. The number of skipped beats

75. Which pulse rate would you report to the nurse at once?
    A. 60 beats per minute
    B. 72 beats per minute
    C. 90 beats per minute
    D. 104 beats per minute

76. The apical pulse is located
    A. In the middle of the sternum
    B. On the right side of the chest slightly above the nipple
    C. On the left side of the chest slightly below the nipple
    D. One inch below and to the left of the sternum

77. An apical pulse is counted for
    A. 30 seconds
    B. 1 minute
    C. 2 minutes
    D. 5 minutes
78. When counting respirations, count each rise of the chest as one respiration and each fall of the chest as one respiration.
    A. True
    B. False
79. The period of heart muscle contraction is called
    A. Systole
    B. Diastole
    C. Blood pressure
    D. Aneroid
80. The normal range for diastolic pressure is
    A. Greater than 80 mm Hg
    B. Less than 80 mm Hg
    C. Greater than 120 mm Hg
    D. Less than 120 mm Hg
81. The normal range for systolic pressure is
    A. Greater than 80 mm Hg
    B. Less than 80 mm Hg
    C. Greater than 120 mm Hg
    D. Less than 120 mm Hg
82. Which is *not* a guideline for measuring blood pressure?
    A. Avoid taking blood pressure on an injured arm.
    B. Let the person rest for 10 to 20 minutes before measuring blood pressure.
    C. Measure blood pressure with the person sitting or lying.
    D. Apply the cuff over clothing.
83. Blood pressure is normally measured
    A. In the radial artery
    B. At the apical site
    C. In the brachial artery
    D. In the popliteal artery

84. You are having problems hearing a person's blood pressure measurement. What should you do?
    A. Report what you think you heard.
    B. Ask a co-worker what the person's usual blood pressure is.
    C. Tell the nurse.
    D. Ask the person what his usual blood pressure is.
85. Pain is personal. It differs for each person.
    A. True
    B. False
86. Pain felt in a body part that is no longer there is
    A. Chronic pain
    B. Radiating pain
    C. False pain
    D. Phantom pain
87. Appetite changes and difficulty sleeping can suggest that a person is having pain.
    A. True
    B. False
88. One ounce equals
    A. 30 mL
    B. 50 mL
    C. 90 mL
    D. 100 mL
89. Which is *not* measured as intake?
    A. Gravy
    B. Milk
    C. Gelatin
    D. Orange juice
90. Which is *correct* when measuring weight and height?
    A. The person wears pajamas, a robe, and shoes for warmth and comfort.
    B. After breakfast is the best time to weigh the person.
    C. Balance the scale at zero before weighing the person.
    D. The person voids after being weighed.

CASE STUDY

An 80-year-old resident of Valley View Nursing Center shares a room. The person is receiving continuous oxygen by mask. She has a dressing on her lower left arm. The person is able to communicate her needs. The nurse has delegated measuring and recording the person's vital signs to you. When you enter the person's room, you notice that she is drinking a cup of coffee.

Answer the following questions:

1. What sites can you use to measure the person's temperature?

2. Which arm will you use to measure the person's pulse and blood pressure?

3. What observations about the person's pulse do you need to report and record?

4. What pulse rates do you need to report at once?

5. How can you promote the person's right to personal choice?

6. How can you protect the person's right to privacy?

ADDITIONAL LEARNING ACTIVITIES

1. View the CD Companion: Skills to help you learn and practice the following procedures:
   A. Taking a Temperature With a Glass Thermometer
   B. Taking a Temperature With an Electronic Thermometer
   C. Taking a Radial Pulse
   D. Counting Respirations
   E. Measuring Blood Pressure
   F. Measuring Intake and Output
   G. Measuring Weight and Height

   (2) Take radial pulses on various persons. Do you notice differences in rate, rhythm, and force?

   (3) Take a person's pulse before and after exercise. Notice and record the differences in rate, rhythm, and force.

2. Under the supervision of your instructor, practice the procedures in Chapter 20 with a classmate. Use the procedure checklists on pp. 293-304 as a guide. Practice with various partners. Take your turn being the patient or resident.
   Use a simulator for practicing rectal temperature.
   A. Temperature
      (1) Practice reading a glass thermometer.
      (2) If available, practice taking temperatures with different types of thermometers. Discuss the advantages and disadvantages of each.

   B. Pulse
      (1) Practice with various classmates. Locate the following pulse sites: carotid, apical, brachial, radial, femoral, popliteal, and dorsalis pedis.

   C. Respirations
      (1) Practice with various people. Note differences in respiratory rates. Do the respiratory rate and depth of respirations change with exercise?

   D. Blood pressure
      (1) Practice with various people.
      (2) Take and record blood pressures before and after exercise.
      (3) Take and record blood pressures with the person lying, sitting, and standing.
      (4) If available, practice using different types of blood pressure equipment.

STUDY QUESTIONS

Matching

Match each term with the correct definition.

1. _____ Sugar in the urine

2. _____ Blood in the urine

3. _____ Bloody sputum

4. _____ Samples collected and tested to prevent, detect, and treat disease

5. _____ A substance that appears in urine from rapid breakdown of fat for energy

6. _____ Mucus from the respiratory system that is expectorated through the mouth

A. Hematuria
B. Sputum
C. Glucosuria (glycosuria)
D. Hemoptysis
E. Acetone (ketone body or ketone)
F. Specimens

Fill in the Blanks

7. All specimens sent to the laboratory require

_____.

8. Before collecting a urine specimen, what information do you need from the nurse and the care plan?

A. _____

B. _____

C. _____

D. _____

E. _____

F. _____

G. _____

H. _____

I. _____

9. To identify the person when collecting a specimen, you need to _____

_____

_____

_____.

10. A _____ is collected for a routine urinalysis.

11. To help ensure accuracy, where should you label the specimen container? _____

_____

12. The midstream specimen is also called

_____

_____.

13. The nurse asks you to collect a midstream specimen. Before going to the person's room, what equipment and supplies do you need to collect?

A. _____

B. _____

C. _____

D. _____

E. _____

F. _____

14. You are collecting a midstream urine specimen from a female. How is the person's perineal area cleansed? _____

_____

_____

_____

_____

_____

15. _____ is another term for a double-voided specimen.

16. Double-voided specimens are used to test urine for _____ .

17. _____ measures if urine is acidic or alkaline.

18. A _____ specimen is needed to test urine pH.

19. _____ specimens are best for testing urine for glucose and ketones.

20. When is testing urine for glucose and ketones usually done? _____

_____

21. Unseen blood is called _____

_____ .

22. When testing urine specimens, what observations do you need to report and record?

    A. _____

    B. _____

    C. _____

    D. _____

    E. _____

    F. _____

23. How can you make sure that you use reagent strips correctly? _____

_____

_____

24. When internal bleeding is suspected, stool specimens are checked for _____ . Stools also are studied for _____ ,

_____ , _____ ,

and _____ .

25. What information do you need from the nurse before collecting a stool specimen?

    A. _____

    B. _____

    C. _____

    D. _____

    E. _____

26. When collecting specimens, you must follow:

    A. _____

    B. _____

    C. _____

27. Sputum specimens are studied for

    _____ , _____ ,

    and _____ .

28. Mouthwash is not used to rinse the mouth before collecting a sputum specimen because

_____

_____ .

29. The nurse asks you to collect a sputum specimen. What observations do you need to report and record?

    A. _____

    B. _____

    C. _____

    D. _____

    E. _____

    F. _____

    G. _____

    H. _____

    I. _____

30. When collecting a sputum specimen from a person who has or may have TB, you need to follow Standard Precautions and the Bloodborne Pathogen Standard. The doctor may order

_____ .

31. When collecting specimens, you promote comfort and privacy by:

    A. _____

    _____

    B. _____

    _____

    C. _____

    _____

    D. _____

    _____

    E. _____

    _____

32. You made an error in procedure when collecting a stool specimen. What should you do?

    _____

    _____

    _____

33. Write the meaning of each of the following abbreviations:

    A. mL _____

    B. I & O _____

    C. oz _____

    D. TB _____

Multiple Choice
Circle the **BEST** Answer

34. Which is *not* a rule for collecting specimens?
    A. Follow the rules of medical asepsis.
    B. Use the correct container.
    C. Label the container accurately.
    D. Collect the specimen when you have time.

35. What type of specimen is collected for a routine urinalysis?
    A. A random specimen
    B. A midstream specimen
    C. A fresh-fractional specimen
    D. A double-voided specimen

36. A random urine specimen is collected in the morning before breakfast.
    A. True
    B. False

37. A sterile container is used for a midstream specimen.
    A. True
    B. False

38. A double-voided specimen is needed to test urine for occult blood.
    A. True
    B. False

39. The body needs insulin to
    A. Maintain fluid balance
    B. Use protein for tissue repair
    C. Produce urine
    D. Use sugar for energy

40. What kind of urine specimen is needed to test for blood?
    A. A clean-catch specimen
    B. A double-voided specimen
    C. A routine specimen
    D. An early morning specimen

41. The normal pH of urine is
    A. 2.0 to 3.5
    B. 4.6 to 8.0
    C. 10.2 to 10.8
    D. 10.5 to 12.2

42. When testing urine with reagent strips, you need to wear gloves.
    A. True
    B. False

43. Stool specimens must *not* be contaminated with urine.
    A. True
    B. False

44. Which statement about collecting sputum specimens is *incorrect?*
    A. The person coughs up sputum from the bronchi and trachea.
    B. The person rinses the mouth with water before coughing up sputum.
    C. Privacy is important.
    D. It is easier to collect a specimen in the evening.

CASE STUDY

You have been assigned to assist with the care of a 60-year-old patient. Your assignment includes collecting:
- A urine specimen to check for blood
- A stool specimen to check for occult blood

The person is able to assist in obtaining the specimens. The RN will test the urine and stool specimens.

Answer the following questions:

1. What information do you need from the nurse before collecting each specimen?

2. What safety measures do you need to practice when collecting each specimen?

3. What instructions do you need to give the person about the urine specimen?

4. What type of urine specimen do you need to collect?

ADDITIONAL LEARNING ACTIVITIES

1. The nurse asks you to collect a double-voided specimen.
   A. What additional information do you need from the nurse before you collect the specimen?

   B. What equipment and supplies do you need to collect?

   C. How will you explain the procedure to the person?

   D. What are the steps involved in collecting the specimen?

   E. What observations do you need to report and record?

2. Under the supervision of your instructor, practice the procedures in Chapter 21. Use the procedure checklists on pp. 305-315 as a guide.

22 ASSISTING WITH EXERCISE AND ACTIVITY

STUDY QUESTIONS

Matching
Match the following terms with the correct definitions.

1. _____ Moving a body part away from the midline of the body
2. _____ Moving a body part toward the midline of the body
3. _____ The lack of joint mobility caused by abnormal shortening of a muscle
4. _____ Turning the joint
5. _____ The foot is bent; bending the foot down at the ankle
6. _____ Turning the joint outward
7. _____ The act of walking
8. _____ Turning the joint upward
9. _____ The decrease in size or the wasting away of tissue
10. _____ Bending a body part
11. _____ Excessive straightening of a body part
12. _____ The foot falls down at the ankle; permanent plantar flexion
13. _____ Abnormally low blood pressure when the person suddenly stands up
14. _____ Straightening a body part
15. _____ Turning the joint downward
16. _____ The movement of a joint to the extent possible without causing pain
17. _____ Turning the joint inward
18. _____ Bending the toes and foot up at the ankle

A. Adduction
B. Dorsiflexion
C. Hyperextension
D. Orthostatic hypotension
E. Pronation
F. Internal rotation
G. Abduction
H. External rotation
I. Contracture
J. Flexion
K. Plantar flexion
L. Supination
M. Atrophy
N. Extension
O. Range of motion (ROM)
P. Rotation
Q. Footdrop
R. Ambulation

Fill in the Blanks

19. Inactivity, whether mild or severe, affects

_____

_____.

It also affects mental well-being.

20. A resident with dementia resists your efforts to assist with exercises. What should you do?

_____

_____

_____

_____

21. List 5 reasons bedrest is ordered.

A. _____

B. _____

C. _____

D. _____

E. _____

22. Define these types of bedrest:

A. Strict bedrest _____

_____

_____

B. Bedrest _____

_____

_____

C. Bedrest with commode privileges

_____

_____

_____

D. Bedrest with bathroom privileges

_____

_____

_____

23. List 10 complications of bedrest.

A. _____

B. _____

C. _____

D. _____

E. _____

F. _____

G. _____

H. _____

I. _____

J. _____

24. Postural relates to _____.

25. _____ is key to preventing orthostatic hypotension.

26. To check for postural hypotension, ask the person these questions:

A. _____

B. _____

C. _____

D. _____

27. What is the purpose of footboards?

_____

_____

_____

28. Trochanter rolls prevent the hips and legs from

_____

_____.

29. Handrolls or handgrips prevent _____

_____.

30. Splints keep the _____,

_____,

_____,

_____,

_____, and _____

in normal position.

31. _____ keep the weight of top linens off the feet and toes.

32. _____ range-of-motion exercises are done by the person.

33. You have been delegated range-of-motion exercises. What information do you need from the nurse and the care plan?

   A. _____

   B. _____

   C. _____

   D. _____

   E. _____

   F. _____

   G. _____

34. When can you perform range-of-motion exercises to a person's neck? _____

   _____

   _____

35. List and describe the range-of-motion exercises performed to the forearms.

   A. _____

   B. _____

36. List and describe the range-of-motion exercises performed to the hips.

   A. _____

   B. _____

   C. _____

   D. _____

   E. _____

   F. _____

37. The nurse asks you to assist a patient with ambulation. The person is weak and unsteady. What safety measures are needed?

   _____

   _____

   _____

   _____

   _____

38. After assisting with ambulation, what observations do you need to report and record?

   A. _____

   B. _____

   C. _____

   D. _____

   E. _____

39. Before assisting with ambulation, you need to talk to the person about the activity. Why is this important? _____

   _____

   _____

40. You will assist a patient with ambulation. How should you encourage the person to stand?

   _____

   _____

41. You are helping a resident to walk. Where should you walk? _____

   _____

   _____

42. Explain why loose clothes are unsafe for a person using crutches. _____

   _____

   _____

   _____

   _____

43. Canes help provide _____

   and _____.

44. A resident uses a cane for ambulation. The person's left leg is weak. In which hand is the cane held? _____

45. Braces are used to:

   A. _____

   B. _____

   C. _____

46. You are applying a knee brace to a patient's left knee. What observations do you need to report to the nurse at once?

    A. _____

    B. _____

47. The _____ tells you when to apply and remove a brace.

48. To promote the person's activity, exercise, and well-being, you can:

    A. _____
    _____
    _____

    B. _____
    _____
    _____

    C. _____
    _____
    _____

    D. _____
    _____
    _____

    E. _____
    _____
    _____

49. OBRA requires activity programs for nursing center residents. Activities must
    _____
    _____
    _____.

50. Write the meaning of each of the following abbreviations:

    A. ID _____

    B. ADL _____

    C. ROM _____

Multiple Choice
Circle the **BEST** Answer

51. Exercise and activity are promoted in all persons to the extent possible.
    A. True
    B. False

52. Complications of bedrest include the following *except*
    A. Pneumonia
    B. Muscle atrophy
    C. Pressure ulcers
    D. Dorsiflexion

53. Bedboards are used to
    A. Prevent the mattress from sagging
    B. Prevent plantar flexion
    C. Prevent orthostatic hypotension
    D. Strengthen the feet

54. Where are hip abduction wedges placed?
    A. At the foot of the bed
    B. Between the person's legs
    C. Alongside the person's body
    D. Under the mattress

55. Trochanter rolls prevent
    A. Plantar flexion
    B. Footdrop
    C. External rotation of the hips
    D. Contractures of the knees

56. Who performs active-assistive range-of-motion exercises?
    A. The person
    B. The person with some help from another person
    C. A health team member
    D. The physical therapist

57. You are assisting a patient with range-of-motion exercises. Which is *incorrect?*
    A. Exercise only the joints the nurse tells you to exercise.
    B. Expose only the body part being exercised.
    C. Move the joint slowly, smoothly, and gently.
    D. Move the joint slightly beyond the point of pain.

58. You are assisting a resident with ambulation. Which is *incorrect?*
    A. The person wears non-skid shoes.
    B. Make sure the person's feet are flat on the floor.
    C. Stand on the person's weak side while he gains balance.
    D. Encourage the person to walk slowly and to slide his feet.

59. Which is *not* a safety measure for using crutches?
    A. Replace worn or torn crutch tips.
    B. Check wooden crutches for cracks.
    C. Have the person wear comfortable bedroom slippers.
    D. Keep crutches within the person's reach.
60. When using a cane to walk
    A. The cane tip is about 16 inches to the side of the foot
    B. The grip is level with the waist
    C. The cane is held on the strong side
    D. The strong leg is moved forward first
61. A walker gives more support than a cane.
    A. True
    B. False

62. To promote the person's dignity and mental comfort during exercise, you need to
    A. Provide for privacy
    B. Do as much as possible for the person
    C. Discuss the person's exercise program with the person's family
    D. Tell the person everything will be OK
63. OBRA requires activity programs for nursing center residents. Which is *incorrect?*
    A. Activities are important for physical and mental well-being.
    B. The right to personal choice is protected.
    C. The person must participate in at least one activity each day.
    D. Listen and suggest options the person may like.

CASE STUDY

You have received the following information about a resident from end-of-shift report and your assignment sheet:

- The person is in bed most of the day. He needs help to get out of bed. He is often unsteady when getting out of bed.
- The person needs help to walk three times a day. He uses a wheeled walker and wears a brace over his right ankle.
- The person receives active-assistive range-of-motion exercises to both knees and ankles. He is able to move up in bed and turn using a trapeze.

Answer the following questions:

1. For what complications is the person at risk?

A. What measures can help decrease these risks?

2. What additional information do you need from the nurse and the care plan before you:
   A. Help the person with ambulation?

   B. Assist with range-of-motion exercises?

3. What safety measures are practiced when assisting the person out of bed?

4. What safety measures are practiced when helping the person with ambulation?

5. What information do you need to report and record about range-of-motion exercises?

6. When putting on and removing the person's brace, what do you need to report to the nurse at once?

7. How will you promote personal choice when providing care?

8. How will you promote the person's right to privacy when assisting with range-of-motion exercises?

ADDITIONAL LEARNING ACTIVITIES

1. Make a list of activities in your daily life that provide range-of-motion exercises.
   A. How do these activities promote your physical, social, and mental well being?

   B. How can you use daily activities to promote ROM for patients and residents?

2. View the CD Companion: Skills to help you learn and practice the following procedures:
   A. Performing Range-of-Motion Exercises
   B. Helping the Person to Walk

3. Practice active range-of-motion exercises. Use the procedure checklists on pp. 316-319 as a guide. This will help you better understand the ROM of each joint.

4. Under the supervision of your instructor, practice the procedures in Chapter 22. Use the procedure checklists on pp. 316-321 as a guide.
   A. Take your turn being the patient or resident.
   B. Discuss your experience.

23 ASSISTING WITH WOUND CARE

STUDY QUESTIONS

Matching

Match each term with the correct definition.

1. _____ A soft pad applied over a body area

2. _____ To narrow

3. _____ An open sore on the lower leg and foot caused by decreased blood flow through arteries or veins

4. _____ Scraping the skin, causing an open area

5. _____ When the skin sticks to a surface while deeper tissues move downward

6. _____ To expand or open wider

7. _____ A localized injury to the skin and/or underlying tissue usually over a bony prominence

8. _____ A break or rip in the skin; the epidermis separates from the underlying tissues

9. _____ A blood clot

10. _____ A break in the skin or mucous membrane

11. _____ A blood clot that travels through the vascular system until it lodges in a vessel

A. Constrict
B. Shearing
C. Pressure ulcer
D. Dilate
E. Thrombus
F. Friction
G. Circulatory ulcer
H. Wound
I. Skin tear
J. Embolus
K. Compress

Fill in the Blanks

12. _____ is an accident or violent act that injures the skin, mucous membranes, bones, and organs.

13. A wound is a portal of entry for _____ _____. _____ is a major threat.

14. Wound care involves _____ _____ _____.

15. Skin tears are caused by _____ _____ _____.

16. Pressure ulcers are a result of _____ _____ _____.

17. A bony prominence is _____ _____ _____.

18. _____, _____, or _____ are other terms for pressure ulcers.

19. List 8 risk factors for skin breakdown and pressure ulcers.

   A. _____

   B. _____

   C. _____

   D. _____

   E. _____

   F. _____

   G. _____

   H. _____

20. Persons at risk for pressure ulcers are those who:

   A. _____

   B. _____

   C. _____

   D. _____

   E. _____

   F. _____

   G. _____

   H. _____

   I. _____

   J. _____

21. In persons with light skin, the first sign of a

   pressure ulcer is _____

   _____. In persons with

   dark skin, skin color may _____

   _____.

22. List 5 common sites for pressure ulcers in obese persons.

   A. _____

   B. _____

   C. _____

   D. _____

   E. _____

23. Explain how these devices help prevent or treat pressure ulcers:

   A. Bed cradle _____

   _____

   _____

   _____

   B. Heel and foot elevators _____

   _____

   _____

   _____

24. _____ is
   a condition in which there is death of tissue.

25. An ulcer is _____

   _____

   _____.

26. Common sites for venous ulcers (stasis ulcers)

   are _____

   _____

   _____.

27. Arterial ulcers are found _____

   _____

   _____.

28. A diabetic foot ulcer is _____

   _____

   _____.

29. How do elastic stockings help prevent blood

   clots? _____

   _____

   _____

30. An embolus from a vein lodges in a lung. This

   is a _____.

31. A pulmonary embolus can cause severe respiratory problems and death. You need to

   report _____
   to the nurse at once.

32. Persons at risk for thrombi include those who:

   A. _____

   B. _____

   C. _____

   D. _____

   E. _____

33. Before you apply elastic stockings, what information do you need from the nurse and the care plan?

   A. _____

   B. _____

   C. _____

   D. _____

   E. _____

   F. _____

34. Explain why elastic stockings are applied before the person gets out of bed. _____

   _____

   _____

   _____

35. When applying elastic stockings, why is it important to remove twists, creases, and wrinkles? _____

   _____

   _____

36. When applying elastic bandages, you need to start at _____

   _____

37. You are applying an elastic bandage to a patient's right leg. You should expose the person's toes because _____.

38. A resident has an elastic bandage on her left arm. The person complains of pain and tingling in her fingers. What should you do? _____

   _____

   _____

39. List 7 functions of wound dressings.

   A. _____

   B. _____

   C. _____

   D. _____

   E. _____

   F. _____

   G. _____

40. Tape is not applied to circle the entire body part because _____

   _____

41. A patient has a lot of pain during dressing changes. What measure will help promote the person's comfort? _____

   _____

   _____

   _____

42. Remove tape by pulling it _____

   _____

43. Binders are applied to the _____,

   _____, or

   _____.

44. How do binders promote healing? _____

   _____

   _____

   _____

   _____

45. What type of binders secure dressings in place after rectal and perineal surgeries? _____

   _____

46. An incorrectly applied binder can cause:

   A. _____

   B. _____

   C. _____

   D. _____

47. You need to reapply a binder if:

   A. _____

   B. _____

48. You need to change binders that are _____

   _____

49. What are the functions of heat applications?

   _____

   _____

   _____

   _____

50. When heat is applied to the skin, blood vessels in the area _____.

51. When heat is applied to the skin, burns are a risk. What signs and symptoms do you need to report at once? _____
_____
_____

52. When applying heat to an area, you need to observe for pale skin because _____
_____
_____
_____

53. Which persons are at risk for burns from heat applications?

    A. _____

    B. _____

    C. _____

54. A hot soak involves _____
_____

55. Provide the temperature ranges in Fahrenheit and centigrade for each of the following:

    A. Hot _____

    B. Tepid _____

    C. Cold _____

56. Cold applications are used to:

    A. _____

    B. _____

    C. _____

57. Explain what happens when cold is applied for a long time. _____
_____
_____
_____

58. List 8 observations you need to report and record when applying heat or cold applications.

    A. _____

    B. _____

    C. _____

    D. _____

    E. _____

    F. _____

    G. _____

    H. _____

59. You are assisting a patient with a sitz bath. How will you promote the person's safety?
_____
_____
_____
_____

60. An aquathermia pad is placed in a flannel cover because _____
_____
_____

61. Before applying an elastic bandage, changing a dressing, or applying heat and cold, you need to make sure that:

    A. _____

    B. _____

    C. _____

    D. _____

    E. _____

    F. _____

62. A patient has an abdominal wound. The wound is draining and requires frequent dressing changes. List 4 measures that promote the person's comfort and interaction with family and friends.

    A. _____

    B. _____

    C. _____

    D. _____

Multiple Choice
Circle the **BEST** Answer

63. Any injury that results from pressure or pressure in combination with shear and/or friction is
    A. A skin tear
    B. A pressure ulcer
    C. An intentional wound
    D. A chronic wound
64. Which measure helps prevent skin tears?
    A. Wearing rings with large stones
    B. Restricting fluids
    C. Dressing the person as quickly as possible
    D. Keeping your fingernails short and smoothly filed
65. Which measure helps prevent pressure ulcers?
    A. Repositioning the person every 4 hours
    B. Raising the head of the bed 45 to 60 degrees when the person is in bed
    C. Positioning the person in the 30-degree lateral position
    D. Vigorously rubbing the skin dry after bathing
66. Remind persons sitting in chairs to shift their positions
    A. Whenever they think about it
    B. Before and after meals
    C. Every hour
    D. Every 15 minutes
67. A frame placed on the bed and over the person to keep top linens off the feet is a
    A. Bed cradle
    B. Heel elevator
    C. Flotation pad
    D. Trochanter roll
68. Open sores on the lower legs and feet caused by poor blood flow through the veins are
    A. Arterial ulcers
    B. Pressure ulcers
    C. Epidermal ulcers
    D. Stasis ulcers
69. Which action will *not* help prevent circulatory ulcers?
    A. Having the person use elastic garters to hold socks in place
    B. Keeping linens clean, dry, and wrinkle free
    C. Keeping pressure off the heels
    D. Reporting changes in skin color
70. Which measure helps prevent circulatory ulcers?
    A. Having the person sit with the legs crossed
    B. Dressing the person in tight clothes
    C. Making sure shoes fit well
    D. Massaging pressure points
71. When applying elastic stockings, the opening in the toe area is over the top of the toes.
    A. True
    B. False

72. After applying an elastic bandage to a patient's right leg, you need to check the color and temperature of the leg
    A. Every 15 minutes
    B. Every hour
    C. Every 2 hours
    D. Every shift
73. When applying a non-sterile dressing, which action is *correct*?
    A. Telling the person how you feel about the wound
    B. Removing the dressing so the person can see the soiled side
    C. Telling the person to look at the wound
    D. Touching only the outer edges of the old and new dressings
74. When applying tape to secure a dressing, which is *correct*?
    A. Tape is applied to secure the top and bottom of the dressing.
    B. Tape is applied to secure the top, middle, and bottom of the dressing.
    C. Tape should encircle the entire body part whenever possible.
    D. The tape extends 1 inch on each side of the dressing.
75. Montgomery ties are used to secure a dressing. Which is *incorrect*?
    A. The adhesive strips are removed with each dressing change.
    B. Cloth ties are secured over the dressing.
    C. The cloth ties are undone for dressing changes.
    D. The adhesive strips are removed when soiled.
76. Heat is *not* applied to a joint replacement site.
    A. True
    B. False
77. Moist heat has greater and faster effects than dry heat.
    A. True
    B. False
78. Which is a moist cold application?
    A. Ice bag
    B. Ice collar
    C. Ice glove
    D. Cold compress
79. The prolonged application of cold has the same effects as heat applications.
    A. True
    B. False
80. You have applied an ice pack to a resident's left knee. How often do you need to check the skin at the application site?
    A. Frequently
    B. Every 5 minutes
    C. Every 10 minutes
    D. Every 15 minutes

81. Heat and cold are applied for no longer than
    A. One hour
    B. 30 minutes
    C. 15 to 20 minutes
    D. 5 to 10 minutes
82. To correctly and safely apply an aquathermia pad
    A. Keep the heating unit below the pad and connecting hoses
    B. Make sure hoses are free of kinks and bubbles
    C. Place the pad under the person
    D. Secured the pad with pins

83. Cold applications are used for the following *except* to
    A. Reduce pain
    B. Reduce bleeding
    C. Increase circulation to an area
    D. Prevent swelling
84. What is the correct abbreviation for centigrade?
    A. Cent
    B. CE
    C. Ct
    D. C

Labeling
85. Place an x on the pressure points for each position.

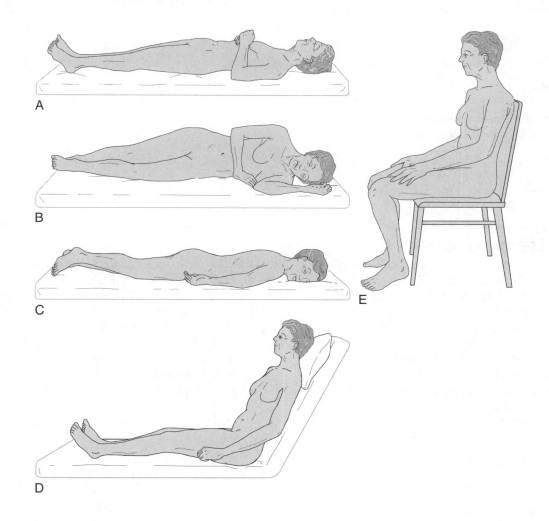

CASE STUDY

A 50-year-old patient at Valley View Hospital has red hair and fair skin. Her doctor has ordered sitz baths following rectal surgery. The doctor has also ordered elastic bandages to both legs. The RN has assigned you to apply the elastic bandage and to assist with the person's sitz bath.

Answer the following questions:

1. What additional information do you need before you apply the elastic bandages?

2. What safety measures are needed when applying elastic bandages?

3. After applying the elastic bandages, what observations do you need to report and record?

4. For what complications from the sitz bath is the person at risk?

A. What measures can help prevent these complications?

B. To promote the person's comfort and safety, what questions might you ask?

ADDITIONAL LEARNING ACTIVITIES

1. If available, handle the various types of dressings commonly used for wound care. Practice opening packages and applying various types of dressings. Practice applying and removing various types of tape. The greater your skill, the better care you can provide.
2. If available, handle the various types of heat and cold applications commonly used in health care agencies. Practice opening packages and applying various types of applications. The greater your skill, the better care you can provide.
3. View the CD Companion: Skills to help you learn and practice the Applying Elastic Stockings procedure.
4. Under the supervision of your instructor, practice the procedures in this chapter. Use the procedure checklists on pp. 322-330 as a guide. Take your turn being the patient or resident.
   A. Discuss ways to promote the person's safety, comfort, and dignity when performing each procedure.

24 ASSISTING WITH OXYGEN NEEDS

STUDY QUESTIONS

Matching
Match each term with the correct definition.

1. _____ A tasteless, odorless, and colorless gas required for life
2. _____ The amount (percent) of hemoglobin containing oxygen
3. _____ A machine that removes oxygen from the air
4. _____ Bluish color to the skin, mucous membranes, and nail beds
5. _____ Slow breathing; respirations are fewer than 12 per minute

A. Bradypnea
B. Oxygen
C. Oxygen concentration
D. Oxygen concentrator
E. Cyanosis

Fill in the Blanks

6. Early signs of low levels of oxygen (O_2) are

   _____,

   _____, and

   _____.

7. Describe normal respirations. _____

   _____

   _____

   _____

8. Describe Cheyne-Stokes respirations.

   _____

   _____

   _____

9. Kussmaul respirations are _____

   _____

   _____.

10. Breathing is usually easier in these positions.

    A. _____

    B. _____

11. A patient has difficulty breathing. The person prefers sitting up and leaning over a table to breathe. This position is called _____

    _____.

    What can you do to increase the person's

    comfort? _____

    _____

12. How do deep-breathing and coughing exercises help persons with respiratory problems?

    A. _____

    B. _____

13. How often are deep-breathing and coughing

    exercises usually done? _____

    _____

    _____

14. The nurse delegates deep-breathing and coughing exercises to you. What information do you need from the nurse and the care plan?

    A. _____

    B. _____

    C. _____

    D. _____

    E. _____

15. If the person has a productive cough,

_____ and

_____

are needed.

16. Oxygen is treated as a _____.

17. Pulse oximetry measures _____

_____

_____.

18. _____ is
the amount (percent) of hemoglobin containing
oxygen.

19. List and briefly describe 4 ways that oxygen is
supplied.

A. _____

_____

_____

B. _____

_____

_____

C. _____

_____

_____

D. _____

_____

_____

20. Describe the following devices used to give
oxygen.

A. Nasal cannula _____

_____

_____

_____

B. Simple face mask _____

_____

_____

_____

21. List two complications that can occur when
using a nasal cannula.

A. _____

B. _____

22. The oxygen flow rate is measured in

_____.

23. Which health team members are responsible for

setting the oxygen flow rate? _____

_____

_____

24. Write the meaning of each of the following
abbreviations:

A. L/min _____

B. O$_2$ _____

Multiple Choice

Circle the **BEST** Answer

25. Oxygen is a gas. It has no taste, odor, or color.
    A. True
    B. False

26. In healthy adults, how often do normal
respirations occur?
    A. 12 to 20 times per minute
    B. 20 to 30 times per minute
    C. 5 to 10 times per minute
    D. 35 times per minute

27. A bluish color to the skin, lips, mucous
membranes, and nail beds is
    A. Dyspnea
    B. Cannula
    C. Cyanosis
    D. Oxygen concentration

28. To promote oxygenation, position changes are
needed
    A. When the person complains of difficulty
       breathing
    B. When the person requests a position change
    C. At least every 2 hours
    D. As often as you have time

29. Respiratory hygiene and cough etiquette include
the following *except*
    A. Covering the nose and mouth when coughing
       and sneezing
    B. Using tissues to contain respiratory secretions
    C. Disposing of tissues in the nearest waste
       container after use
    D. Washing the person's hands every 2 hours
       while awake

30. You are assisting a resident with deep-breathing and coughing exercises. Which is *incorrect?*
    A. Have the person place the hands over the rib cage.
    B. Have the person take a deep breath in through the nose.
    C. Ask the person to hold the breath for 2 to 3 seconds.
    D. Ask the person to exhale slowly through the nose.
31. Which is *not* a rule for oxygen safety?
    A. Remove the oxygen device when assisting the person with ambulation.
    B. Make sure the oxygen device is secure but not tight.
    C. Check for signs of irritation from the device.
    D. Make sure there are no kinks in the tubing.
32. The nurse tells you that a patient's oxygen flow rate needs to be at 2 liters per minute. When getting the person up to sit in the chair, you note that the flow rate is at 4 liters per minute. What should you do?
    A. Remind the person not to change the flow rate.
    B. Tell the nurse at once.
    C. Change the oxygen flow rate to 2 liters per minute.
    D. Check the care plan as soon as you have time.

33. The normal range for oxygen concentration is
    A. 80% to 100%
    B. 85% to 100%
    C. 90% to 100%
    D. 95% to 100%
34. Which is *not* a sensor site for pulse oximetry?
    A. The earlobes
    B. The fingers
    C. The abdomen
    D. The toes
35. Liquid oxygen is very cold. It can freeze the skin.
    A. True
    B. False
36. Smoking is allowed when a person uses oxygen, as long as the person smokes in the designated smoking area.
    A. True
    B. False
37. Always check the oxygen level when you are with or near persons using oxygen tanks or liquid oxygen systems.
    A. True
    B. False

CROSSWORD

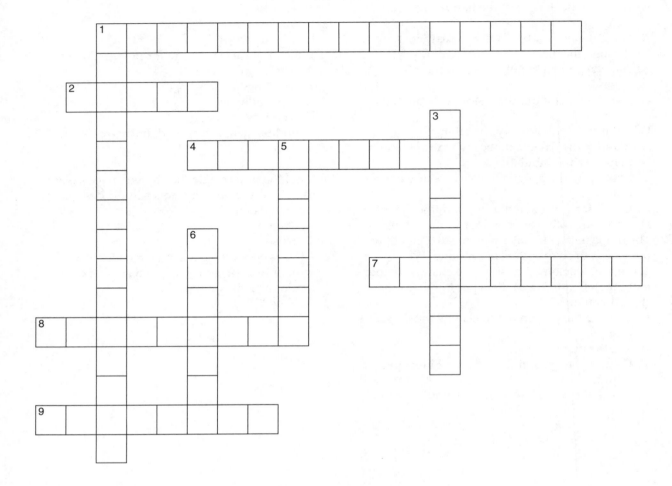

Across

1. Respirations are rapid and deeper than normal
2. Lack or absence of breathing
4. Breathing deeply and comfortably only when sitting
7. The amount of oxygen in the blood is less than normal
8. Slow breathing; respirations are fewer than 12 per minute
9. The amount of oxygen given

Down

1. Respirations are slow, shallow, and sometimes irregular
3. Rapid breathing; respirations are more than 20 per minute
5. Cells do not have enough oxygen
6. Difficult, labored, or painful breathing

CASE STUDY

A patient with pneumonia is in a private room. The person has difficult and painful breathing (dyspnea). The person's doctor has ordered:

- Humidified oxygen by nasal cannula at 3 liters per minute
- Position changes every 2 hours while awake
- Deep-breathing and coughing exercises every 2 hours while awake

You have been assigned to care for the person today.

Answer the following questions:

1. After assisting with deep-breathing and coughing exercises, what observations do you need to report and record?

2. How will you promote the person's comfort?

3. The person has a productive cough. What precautions are needed? How can you explain the needed precautions to the person?

4. What observations do you need to report to the nurse about the person's oxygen therapy?

5. How will you protect the person's right to privacy?

ADDITIONAL LEARNING ACTIVITIES

1. If available, handle the various types of oxygen administration devices. Place each device on yourself and observe how each feels and your comfort level.

2. Position yourself in the orthopneic position and note how it feels.

3. Review the following:
   A. The safety measures for fire and the use of oxygen in Chapter 8 in the textbook.
   B. The rules for oxygen safety listed in this chapter
      - Knowing and following these rules is needed to provide safe and effective care.

4. Under the supervision of your instructor, practice the procedure in this chapter. Use the procedure checklist on p. 331 as a guide. Take your turn being the patient or resident.
   A. Discuss ways to promote the person's safety, comfort, and dignity when performing the procedure.

25 ASSISTING WITH REHABILITATION AND RESTORATIVE NURSING CARE

STUDY QUESTIONS

Matching

Match each term with the correct definition.

1. _____ The inability to have normal speech

2. _____ The activities usually done during a normal day in a person's life

3. _____ The process of restoring the person to his or her highest possible level of physical, psychological, social, and economic function

4. _____ An artificial replacement for a missing body part

5. _____ Difficulty swallowing

6. _____ Any lost, absent, or impaired physical or mental function

7. _____ Care that helps persons regain health, strength, and independence

8. _____ A nursing assistant with special training in restorative nursing and rehabilitation skills

A. Prosthesis
B. Restorative nursing care
C. Activities of daily living (ADL)
D. Aphasia
E. Rehabilitation
F. Disability
G. Restorative aide
H. Dysphagia

Fill in the Blanks

9. The focus of rehabilitation is on _____ _____.

   When improved function is not possible, the goal is to _____ _____.

10. Restorative nursing programs do the following:

    A. _____

    B. _____

11. Restorative nursing programs may involve measures that promote:

    A. _____

    B. _____

    C. _____

    D. _____

    E. _____

    F. _____

12. The person with a disability needs to adjust

    _____,

    _____,

    _____ and

    _____.

13. Explain why rehabilitation usually takes longer in older persons than in other age-groups.

    _____

    _____

    _____

    _____

14. List three complications that must be prevented for rehabilitation to be successful.

    A. _____

    B. _____

    C. _____

15. If not used, muscles will _____.

16. The health team evaluates the person's ability to perform activities of daily living (ADL). Sometimes _____ _____ are needed for self-care.

17. Some persons need bladder training. The method depends on _____ _____.

18. A patient is learning how to use an artificial left arm. The goal is for the prosthesis to _____ _____ _____.

19. Rehabilitation is a team effort. _____ is the key team member.

20. All members of the rehabilitation team help the person regain _____ and _____.

21. Explain why family members are important. _____ _____ _____ _____ _____

22. Every part of your job focuses on. _____ _____ _____.

23. Successful rehabilitation and restorative care improve the person's quality of life. To promote the person's quality of life, you need to:

    A. _____
    B. _____
    C. _____
    D. _____
    E. _____
    F. _____
    G. _____

24. Protecting the person's privacy protects _____ and promotes _____.

25. You want to become a restorative aide. What qualities are required?

    _____
    _____
    _____
    _____
    _____
    _____

26. Independence to the extent possible is a goal of rehabilitation and restorative care. List 5 measures that promote independence.

    A. _____
    B. _____
    C. _____
    D. _____
    E. _____

27. You need to assist a resident to apply a leg brace. Why should you practice applying the brace on yourself first?

    _____

28. The abbreviation ADL means _____ _____.

Multiple Choice
Circle the **BEST** Answer

29. Restorative nursing and rehabilitation both focus on
    A. The person's strengths
    B. Promoting independence
    C. Regaining physical abilities
    D. The whole person

30. When does rehabilitation start?
    A. When the person enters a rehabilitation hospital
    B. When the person goes home with home care
    C. When the person seeks health care
    D. When it is ordered by the doctor

31. Which measure will *not* help prevent complications?
    A. Good alignment
    B. Maintaining the same position for 4 hours
    C. Range-of-motion exercises
    D. Good skin care
32. Successful rehabilitation depends on the person's attitude.
    A. True
    B. False
33. You promote a person's rehabilitation by
    A. Doing as much as possible for the person
    B. Helping the person focus on remaining abilities
    C. Telling the person to work harder
    D. Focusing on what the person cannot do
34. A patient is feeling discouraged with his slow progress. Which action is *incorrect*?
    A. Remind the person of even small progress.
    B. Give support and encouragement.
    C. Give the person sympathy.
    D. Stress the person's strengths and abilities.
35. A resident is receiving physical therapy. You hear a caregiver shouting at the person in an angry voice. What should you do?
    A. Report what you heard to the nurse at once.
    B. Tell the caregiver to stop shouting.
    C. Tell the person's family what you heard.
    D. Do nothing. It is none of your business.
36. A patient wants to skip her exercises scheduled for 2:00 PM because she is tired. What should you do?
    A. Let the person take a nap.
    B. Allow the person to do only half the amount required.
    C. Check the person's care plan.
    D. Report the problem to the nurse.
37. A patient is making slow progress learning how to use a transfer board. The person tells you that he is tired and is not going to work today. You feel yourself getting impatient. What should you do?
    A. Tell the person that he will never get better if he does not keep trying.
    B. Ask a co-worker to work with the person today.
    C. Leave the room and come back when you are less impatient.
    D. Discuss your feelings with the nurse.
38. Nursing teamwork involves providing emotional support to each other.
    A. True
    B. False

CASE STUDY

A 60-year-old widow works as a secretary for a lawyer. As the result of a stroke, the person's right side is paralyzed. She has facial drooping and her speech is affected. She has trouble expressing herself. The person needs assistance with all ADL. She is currently receiving rehabilitation in a skilled nursing center. Her goal is to learn to walk and to care for herself so she can go home. She worries that she will not be able to work as a secretary again.

The person works hard with the rehabilitation team. She tells you that she is embarrassed by her appearance. She wants to eat in her room because she is "messy." She told the nurse that she does not want visitors until she is doing better.

Answer the following questions:

1. How does the person's stroke affect her physically, psychologically, socially, and financially?

2. What effect does the stroke have on the person's self-image?

3. How can the health team protect the person's right to:
   A. Privacy?

   B. Personal choice?

C. Be free from abuse and mistreatment?

4. How can the health team help the person deal with her emotions?

ADDITIONAL LEARNING ACTIVITIES

1. If available handle various self-help devices used in the rehabilitation process. Becoming familiar with these devices will help you provide effective and safe care.

2. Visit a medical supply business and look at the self-help devices and other rehabilitation equipment available.

26 CARING FOR PERSONS WITH COMMON HEALTH PROBLEMS

STUDY QUESTIONS

Matching

Match each term with the correct definition.

1. _____ The surgical replacement of a joint
2. _____ Difficulty expressing or sending out thoughts
3. _____ Paralysis on one side of the body
4. _____ High sugar in the blood
5. _____ Low sugar in the blood
6. _____ Malignant tumor
7. _____ Paralysis in the legs and trunk
8. _____ Paralysis in the arms, legs, and trunk
9. _____ Difficulty understanding language
10. _____ Inflammation of the mouth

A. Receptive aphasia
B. Quadriplegia
C. Paraplegia
D. Hemiplegia
E. Hypoglycemia
F. Hyperglycemia
G. Stomatitis
H. Expressive aphasia
I. Arthroplasty
J. Cancer

Fill in the Blanks

11. _____ tumors do not spread to other body parts.

12. List the 10 cancer risk factors described by the National Cancer Institute.

A. _____
B. _____
C. _____
D. _____
E. _____
F. _____
G. _____
H. _____
I. _____
J. _____

13. List and briefly describe 3 common cancer treatments.

A. _____
_____
_____

B. _____
_____
_____

C. _____
_____
_____

14. List and briefly describe the 2 types of arthritis.

A. _____
_____
_____
_____

B. _____
_____
_____
_____

15. Treatment for osteoarthritis involves:

  A. _____

  B. _____

  C. _____

  D. _____

  E. _____

  F. _____

16. Treatment goals for rheumatoid arthritis are to:

  A. _____

  B. _____

  C. _____

17. A person has rheumatoid arthritis. Why is weight control important? _____

  _____

  _____

18. With_____,
the bone becomes porous and brittle. Bones are fragile and break easily.

19. List 7 risk factors for osteoporosis.

  A. _____

  B. _____

  C. _____

  D. _____

  E. _____

  F. _____

  G. _____

20. Describe these types of fractures:

  A. Closed fracture _____

  _____

  _____

  B. Open fracture _____

  _____

  _____

21. The signs and symptoms of a fracture include:

  A. _____

  B. _____

  C. _____

  D. _____

  E. _____

  F. _____

22. Reduction or fixation means _____

  _____

  _____.

23. A new cast is applied to a person's right leg. You must not cover the cast with blankets or other material because _____

  _____.

24. A patient with a cast on his left arm complains of numbness in his fingers. This signals _____

  _____.

25. A patient requires a total hip replacement to repair a fractured hip. After surgery, these hip movements are avoided:

  A. _____

  B. _____

  C. _____

  D. _____

26. A patient requires surgery to repair a fractured right hip. List 4 life-threatening problems that can occur after surgery.

  A. _____

  B. _____

  C. _____

  D. _____

27. _____ is the removal of all or part of an extremity.

28. Stroke is _____

  _____.

  It also is called _____

  _____.

29. What are the two major types of strokes?

     A. _____

     B. _____

30. List 5 warning signs of stroke.

     A. _____

     _____

     _____

     B. _____

     _____

     _____

     C. _____

     _____

     _____

     D. _____

     _____

     _____

     E. _____

     _____

     _____

31. Briefly describe Parkinson's disease. _____

     _____

     _____

     _____

32. Signs and symptoms of Parkinson's disease include:

     A. _____

     B. _____

     C. _____

     D. _____

     E. _____

33. _____ is a chronic disease in which the myelin in the brain and spinal cord is destroyed.

34. _____ attacks the nerve cells that control voluntary muscles. It is commonly called Lou Gehrig's disease.

35. _____ occurs when a sudden trauma damages the brain.

36. Disabilities from traumatic brain injury depend on _____

     _____.

37. Common causes of spinal cords injuries are:

     A. _____

     B. _____

     C. _____

     D. _____

38. Hearing loss is _____

     _____

     _____.

     Deafness is _____

     _____

     _____.

39. List 5 signs of hearing loss.

     A. _____

     B. _____

     C. _____

     D. _____

     E. _____

40. List 4 simple measures to try when a hearing aid does not seem to be working properly.

     A. _____

     B. _____

     C. _____

     D. _____

41. Briefly describe what occurs with glaucoma.

     _____

     _____

     _____

     _____.

42. Treatment for glaucoma involves _____

     _____.

43. With _____ the lens of the eye becomes cloudy.

44. _____ is the only treatment for cataract.

45. _____ is a touch reading and writing system that uses raised dots.

46. What two aids are used worldwide to assist blind persons to move about safely?

   A. _____

   B. _____

47. How can you protect a person's eyeglasses from breakage or other damage? _____

_____

_____

_____

48. Contact lenses are cleaned, removed, and stored according to _____

_____.

49. With hypertension, the _____ _____ is too high.

50. Pre-hypertension is _____

_____

_____.

51. List 4 risk factors for hypertension you *cannot* change.

   A. _____

   B. _____

   C. _____

   D. _____

52. The _____ supply the heart with blood.

53. The most common cause of coronary artery disease is _____.

54. The major complications of coronary artery disease (CAD) are _____,

_____,

_____,

and _____.

55. Coronary artery disease (CAD) can be treated. The goals of treatment are to:

   A. _____

   B. _____

   C. _____

   D. _____

   E. _____

56. Angina is chest pain from _____

_____.

It is described as _____

_____

_____.

57. With _____, blood flow to the heart muscle is suddenly blocked. Part of the heart muscle dies.

58. _____ occurs when the heart is weakened and cannot pump blood normally. Blood backs up and tissue congestion occurs.

59. When the left side of the heart cannot pump blood normally, blood backs up into the

_____.

The person has _____

_____.

60. A very severe form of heart failure is _____

_____.

This is an emergency.

61. List the two disorders grouped under chronic obstructive pulmonary disease (COPD).

   A. _____

   B. _____

62. _____ is the most important risk factor for COPD.

63. Bronchitis means _____

_____.

64. In emphysema, the _____ enlarge and become less elastic.

65. The most common cause of emphysema is

_____.

66. With _____,
the airways become inflamed and narrow. Extra
mucus is produced.

67. Pneumonia is _____

_____.

It is caused by _____

_____.

68. Tuberculosis (TB) is spread by _____

_____
with coughing, sneezing, speaking, singing, or
laughing.

69. List 7 signs and symptoms of TB.

A. _____

B. _____

C. _____

D. _____

E. _____

F. _____

G. _____

70. TB is detected by _____

and _____.

71. Vomiting means _____

_____.

72. A resident is vomiting. You turn the person's

head well to one side to prevent _____.

73. Vomitus that looks like coffee grounds contains

_____.

74. Many people have small pouches in the colon.

Each pouch is called a _____.

75. The condition of having pouches in the colon is

called _____.

The pouches can become infected or inflamed.

This is called _____.

76. _____
is an inflammation of the liver.

77. Hepatitis A is spread by _____.

78. The hepatitis B virus is present in _____

_____.

79. The hepatitis B virus is spread by:

A. _____

B. _____

C. _____

D. _____

E. _____

80. List 4 common causes of urinary tract infections.

A. _____

B. _____

C. _____

D. _____

81. Cystitis is _____.

82. _____

_____

_____ are
signs and symptoms of cystitis.

83. _____ is
inflammation of the kidney pelvis.

84. Cystitis and pyelonephritis are treated with

_____ and

_____.

85. The prostate enlarges as men get older. This is

called _____.

86. The enlarged prostate presses against the

_____.

This causes _____.

87. A sexually transmitted disease (STD) is spread

by _____

_____.

88. Using _____
helps prevent the spread of STDs, especially HIV
and AIDS.

89. _____ is
the most common endocrine disorder.

90. List and briefly describe the three types of diabetes.

A. _____

_____

_____

_____

B. _____

_____

_____

_____

C. _____

_____

_____

_____

91. Type 1 diabetes is treated with _____,

_____,

and _____.

92. Causes of hypoglycemia include:

A. _____

B. _____

C. _____

D. _____

E. _____

F. _____

G. _____

93. AIDS is caused by a virus. The virus is called the

_____.

94. The AIDS virus is transmitted mainly by:

A. _____

_____

B. _____

_____

C. _____

_____

D. _____

_____

95. Write the meaning of each of the following abbreviations:

A. AIDS _____

B. ALS _____

C. BPH _____

D. CAD _____

E. COPD _____

F. MI _____

G. MS _____

H. TIA _____

I. UTI _____

Multiple Choice
Circle the **BEST** Answer

96. Which measure will *not* help prevent osteoporosis?
    A. Bedrest
    B. Calcium and vitamin supplements
    C. Exercising weight-bearing joints
    D. Not smoking

97. When caring for a person in traction, do the following *except*
    A. Keep the person in good alignment
    B. Remove the traction when making the person's bed
    C. Keep the weights off the floor
    D. Give skin care as directed

98. Care of a person following surgery to repair a fractured right hip includes the following *except*
    A. Keeping the operated leg adducted at all times
    B. Giving good skin care
    C. Preventing external rotation of the right hip
    D. Applying elastic stockings as directed

99. With this condition, there is death of tissue.
    A. Amputation
    B. Gangrene
    C. Aphasia
    D. Emesis

100. A patient's right foot is amputated. The person complains of pain in his right foot. This is
    A. A delusion
    B. Sclerosis
    C. Phantom limb pain
    D. Radiating pain

101. All stroke-like symptoms signal the need for emergency care.
    A. True
    B. False
102. When caring for a person with a stroke, do the following *except*
    A. Perform range-of-motion exercises to prevent contractures
    B. Approach the person from the strong side.
    C. Keep the bed in the flat position to promote breathing
    D. Encourage deep breathing and coughing
103. In the United States, the leading cause of disability in adults is
    A. Cancer
    B. Heart attack
    C. Stroke
    D. Parkinson's disease
104. When caring for a person with a stroke, which is *correct?*
    A. Keep the bed in the flat position.
    B. Turn and reposition the person every 4 hours.
    C. Do all ADL for the person.
    D. Assist with range-of-motion exercises as directed.
105. A person has Parkinson's disease. It is important to do everything for the person.
    A. True
    B. False
106. A person has multiple sclerosis. Which is *incorrect?*
    A. There is no cure.
    B. Muscle weakness and difficulty with balance occur.
    C. Symptoms usually start after age 50.
    D. The person's condition worsens over time.
107. Which statement about ALS is *correct?*
    A. It is rapidly progressive and fatal.
    B. Symptoms usually start after age 65.
    C. The mind and memory are usually affected.
    D. The disease usually causes bowel and bladder incontinence.
108. Which statement about ALS is *incorrect?*
    A. ALS has no cure.
    B. Some drugs slow the progression of the disease.
    C. Damage cannot be reversed.
    D. Bedrest is recommended.
109. With spinal cord injuries, the higher the level of injury, the fewer functions lost.
    A. True
    B. False
110. A person who wears a hearing aid hears better because
    A. The hearing problem is cured
    B. Background noise is decreased
    C. The person's ability to hear improves
    D. The hearing aid makes sounds louder
111. To care for a hearing aid properly, do the following *except*
    A. Follow the manufacturer's instructions
    B. Wash the mold in soapy water every day
    C. Remove the battery at night
    D. When not in use, turn the hearing aid off
112. To communicate with a hearing-impaired person, do the following
    A. Shout loudly
    B. Approach the person from behind
    C. Speak clearly, distinctly, and slowly
    D. Stand or sit in dim light
113. Which is *not* a symptom of cataract?
    A. Severe eye pain
    B. Cloudy vision
    C. Sensitivity to light
    D. Poor vision at night
114. Age-related macular degeneration (AMD)
    A. Is a complication of diabetes
    B. Affects peripheral vision
    C. Blurs central vision
    D. Causes halos around lights and double vision
115. When caring for a blind person, you must avoid using the words *see, look,* or *read.*
    A. True
    B. False
116. When caring for a blind person, which action will *not* promote safety?
    A. Provide lighting as the person prefers.
    B. Orient the person to the room.
    C. Keep doors partly open.
    D. Tell the person when you are leaving the room.
117. When assisting a blind person to walk, which action is *correct?*
    A. Tell the person which arm is offered.
    B. Walk slightly behind the person.
    C. Guide the person in front of you.
    D. Walk very slowly.
118. A touch reading and writing system that uses raised dots is
    A. Retinopathy
    B. Glaucoma
    C. Aphasia
    D. Braille

119. The leading causes of death in the United States are
    A. Infections
    B. Pulmonary diseases
    C. Cardiovascular disorders
    D. Cancers
120. Which is *not* a risk factor for hypertension?
    A. Tobacco use
    B. A high-salt diet
    C. Regular exercise
    D. Being over-weight
121. Angina is relieved by
    A. Exercise and fresh air
    B. Food and fluids
    C. Continuous oxygen
    D. Rest and nitroglycerin
122. Which is *not* a sign or symptom of myocardial infarction?
    A. Sudden, severe chest pain
    B. Indigestion and nausea
    C. Warm, dry, flushed skin
    D. Fear, apprehension, and a feeling of doom
123. This occurs when the right side of the heart cannot pump blood normally.
    A. Blood backs up into the lungs.
    B. The feet and ankles swell.
    C. A high sodium diet is ordered.
    D. The dorsal recumbent position is preferred.
124. Heart failure cannot be treated.
    A. True
    B. False
125. Not smoking is the best way to prevent COPD.
    A. True
    B. False
126. This condition is usually triggered by allergies.
    A. Emphysema
    B. Chronic bronchitis
    C. Asthma
    D. Pneumonia
127. Vomitus is measured as output.
    A. True
    B. False
128. With hepatitis C, the person always has symptoms.
    A. True
    B. False
129. Which occurs only in people infected with hepatitis B?
    A. Hepatitis A
    B. Hepatitis C
    C. Hepatitis D
    D. Hepatitis E

130. Hepatitis C is spread by
    A. Blood contaminated with the hepatitis C virus
    B. Food contaminated with feces
    C. Poor hygiene
    D. Water contaminated with feces
131. Renal calculi are
    A. Particles in the urine
    B. Kidney stones
    C. Waste products
    D. Pus in the urine
132. Which statement about renal failure is *incorrect?*
    A. The person has urinary frequency and urgency.
    B. The person's kidneys do not function or are severely impaired.
    C. Waste products are not removed from the blood.
    D. The body retains fluid.
133. A patient has diabetes. Which statement is *correct?*
    A. The person's body cannot produce or use insulin properly.
    B. The person is obese.
    C. The person cannot eat a balanced diet.
    D. The person needs a diet low in protein.
134. Which is a cause of hyperglycemia?
    A. Vomiting
    B. Too much insulin
    C. Eating too much food
    D. Increased exercise
135. The immune system can cause diseases by attacking the body's own normal cells, tissues, and organs.
    A. True
    B. False
136. The AIDS virus is spread through
    A. Sneezing and coughing
    B. Holding hands and hugging
    C. Insect bites
    D. Blood, semen, vaginal secretions, and breast milk
137. All persons infected with HIV have symptoms.
    A. True
    B. False
138. A resident infected with the AIDS virus does not have symptoms. The person cannot spread the disease.
    A. True
    B. False
139. Persons over age 50 do not spread HIV.
    A. True
    B. False

CROSSWORD

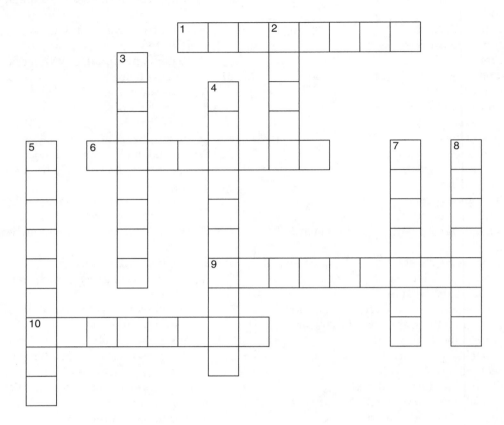

Across

1. A bladder infection
6. A broken bone
9. Joint inflammation
10. Hair loss

Down

2. A new growth of abnormal cells
3. Loss of appetite
4. The spread of cancer to other body parts
5. A tumor that grows fast and invades and destroys other tissues
7. The food and fluids expelled from the stomach through the mouth; emesis
8. The total or partial loss of the ability to use or understand language

CASE STUDY

A 55-year-old male patient is being treated for colon cancer. He had surgery to remove a tumor and is now receiving radiation therapy. He is married and has two teenage children. He is a teacher at the high school. His wife works part time as a check-out clerk at the local grocery store.

Answer the following questions:

1. How might the person feel about having cancer?

2. What measures by the health team are helpful?

3. What are the side effects of radiation therapy?

Following hip replacement surgery, a 75-year-old woman is receiving rehabilitation at a skilled nursing center. The person fell in her driveway and fractured her right hip. She is a retired nurse. She lives alone in her home. She does volunteer work at the hospital 2 days a week.

1. What complications is the person at risk for?

2. What care measures are needed after hip replacement surgery?

ADDITIONAL LEARNING ACTIVITIES

1. Review each of the common health problems discussed in this chapter.
   A. Identify how each problem affects the person's physical, psychological, social, and spiritual needs.

   B. List the risk factors for each of the health problems discussed in this chapter.
      (1) Identify the risk factors that can be controlled and the risk factors that cannot be controlled.

   (2) List any life-style changes you can make to decrease your risks for any of the common health problems discussed in this chapter.

27 CARING FOR PERSONS WITH MENTAL HEALTH PROBLEMS

STUDY QUESTIONS

Matching

Match each term with the correct definition.

1. _____ A recurrent, unwanted thought, idea, or image

2. _____ False beliefs and suspicions about a person or situation

3. _____ An intense fear

4. _____ To kill oneself

5. _____ A false belief

6. _____ A state of severe mental impairment

7. _____ The response or change in the body caused by any emotional, physical, social, or economic factor

8. _____ Seeing, hearing, smelling, or feeling something that is not real

9. _____ A vague, uneasy feeling in response to stress

10. _____ An intense or sudden feeling of fear, anxiety, terror, or dread

A. Delusion
B. Paranoia
C. Stress
D. Anxiety
E. Psychosis
F. Hallucination
G. Panic
H. Obsession
I. Phobia
J. Suicide

Fill in the Blanks

11. Mental health and mental illness involve

_____ .

12. Define the following terms:

A. Mental _____

_____

_____

B. Mental health _____

_____

_____

C. Mental illness _____

_____

_____

13. List 5 causes of mental health disorders.

A. _____

B. _____

C. _____

D. _____

E. _____

14. _____ and

_____

are used to relieve anxiety.

15. Defense mechanisms are _____

_____

_____ .

16. Name these common phobias:

A. _____
means fear of being in an open, crowded, or public space.

B. _____
means fear of water.

17. A compulsion is _____
_____.

18. _____ occurs
after a terrifying ordeal. It involved physical
harm or the threat of physical harm.

19. A flashback is _____
_____
_____.

20. Define the following terms:

    A. Delusion of grandeur _____
    _____
    _____

    B. Delusion of persecution _____
    _____
    _____

21. Persons with schizophrenia may have disorders
of movement. These include:

    A. _____

    B. _____

    C. _____

    D. _____

    E. _____

22. To regress means _____
_____

23. A person hallucinates. For good communication:

    A. Remember to _____
    _____

    B. Do not _____
    _____

    C. Do not _____
    _____

24. Mood relates to _____.

25. The person with bipolar disorder has
_____
_____
_____

26. _____
involves the body, mood, and thoughts. The
person is very sad.

27. Why might depression in an older person *not* be
treated? _____
_____
_____
_____

28. Personality disorders involve _____
_____.

29. Maladaptive means _____
_____.

30. Describe antisocial personality disorder.
_____
_____
_____
_____
_____
_____

31. The person with _____
has problems with moods, interpersonal
relationships, self-image, and behavior. The
person has intense bouts of anger, depression,
and anxiety.

32. _____ or
_____
occurs when a person overuses or depends on
alcohol or drugs.

33. Alcoholism includes these symptoms:

    A. _____

    B. _____

    C. _____

    D. _____

34. Older persons are at risk for falls, vehicle
crashes, and other injuries from drinking alcohol
because they have:

    A. _____

    B. _____

    C. _____

35. Drug abuse is _____
_____
_____.

36. Drug addiction is _____
_____
_____.

37. A person has tolerance to a substance. This means:

A. _____
_____
_____

B. _____
_____
_____

38. _____ is the physical and mental response after stopping or severely reducing the use of a substance that was used regularly.

39. Suicide is most often linked to:

A. _____
B. _____
C. _____

40. If a person mentions or talks about suicide, you need to:

A. _____
B. _____
C. _____

41. Define suicide contagion. _____
_____
_____

42. Treatment of mental health problems involves
_____
_____
_____.

This is done through _____
_____
_____.

43. When interacting with persons with mental health problems, do the following:

A. _____
B. _____
C. _____
D. _____
E. _____
F. _____

44. The abbreviation PTSD means
_____
_____.

Multiple Choice
Circle the **BEST** Answer

45. Which statement about anxiety is *incorrect?*
    A. Anxiety is an abnormal response to stress.
    B. Often anxiety occurs when a person's needs are not met.
    C. Signs and symptoms depend on the degree of anxiety.
    D. Defense mechanisms are used to relieve anxiety.

46. A man has a disagreement with his boss. When he gets home, he shouts at his son. Which defense mechanism is he using?
    A. Projection
    B. Displacement
    C. Regression
    D. Denial

47. A woman does not want to visit her mother. She complains of a stomachache. Which defense mechanism is she using?
    A. Compensation
    B. Conversion
    C. Projection
    D. Regression

48. A man always checks every door in his house exactly five times before leaving. He becomes very anxious if he is unable to do so. This is
    A. Compulsion
    B. Phobia
    C. Paranoia
    D. Flashback

49. A woman believes that she is the mother of Christ. This is
    A. A hallucination
    B. Paranoia
    C. A phobia
    D. A delusion

50. People with schizophrenia tend to be violent.
    A. True
    B. False
51. Which statement about bipolar disorder is *incorrect?*
    A. The disorder also is called manic-depressive illness.
    B. The disorder tends to run in families.
    C. The disorder usually develops in early childhood.
    D. The disorder requires life-long management.
52. Depression is common in older people.
    A. True
    B. False
53. Alcoholism can be treated but not cured.
    A. True
    B. False
54. Which statement about alcohol is *incorrect?*
    A. It affects alertness and reaction time.
    B. Over time, heavy drinking damages the heart and blood vessels.
    C. It speeds up brain activity.
    D. It can cause forgetfulness and confusion.
55. Which statement about drug abuse and addiction is *incorrect?*
    A. Social and mental functions are affected.
    B. They are linked to crimes and violence.
    C. They are linked to motor vehicle crashes.
    D. Only illegal drugs are abused.

CASE STUDY

A person you are caring for suddenly becomes angry. The person shows signs of increased anxiety. She is pacing back and forth in front of you. She begins to raise her voice and speak rapidly.

Answer the following question:
1. What should you do to protect yourself?

ADDITIONAL LEARNING ACTIVITIES

1. Many communities offer support groups for families and friends of persons with mental health problems. Find out what programs and services are available in your community. The phone book yellow pages and the Internet are resources.

    B. Whom should you contact?

    C. What support resources are available in your community?

2. A friend or family member thinking of suicide may confide in you. The person may ask you not to tell anyone about his or her thoughts.
    A. What should you do?

28 CARING FOR PERSONS WITH CONFUSION AND DEMENTIA

STUDY QUESTIONS

Matching

Match each term with the correct definition.

1. _____ A false belief

2. _____ The loss of cognitive function that interferes with routine personal, social, and occupational activities

3. _____ Signs, symptoms, and behaviors of Alzheimer's disease (AD) increase during hours of darkness

4. _____ Seeing, hearing, smelling, or feeling something that is not real

5. _____ False dementia

6. _____ A state of temporary but acute mental confusion

A. Pseudodementia
B. Dementia
C. Delirium
D. Sundowning
E. Hallucination
F. Delusion

Fill in the Blanks

7. Cognitive function involves:

   A. _____

   B. _____

   C. _____

   D. _____

   E. _____

   F. _____

8. The treatment of acute confusion (delirium) is aimed at _____.

9. List 8 early warning signs of dementia.

   A. _____

   B. _____

   C. _____

   D. _____

   E. _____

   F. _____

   G. _____

   H. _____

10. Treatable causes of dementia include:

    A. _____

    B. _____

    C. _____

    D. _____

    E. _____

    F. _____

    G. _____

11. Multi-infarct dementia is caused by _____.

12. _____ is the most common type of permanent dementia.

13. _____ is the most common mental health problem in older persons.

14. Depression is often overlooked in older persons because

    _____

    _____

    _____.

15. The classic sign of Alzheimer's disease (AD) is

    _____

    _____.

16. The Alzheimer's Association describes these 7 stages of AD:

    A. _____

    B. _____

    C. _____

    D. _____

    E. _____

    F. _____

    G. _____

17. What is the purpose of *MedicAlert + Safe Return*? _____

    _____

    _____

18. List 10 common behaviors in persons with AD.

    A. _____

    B. _____

    C. _____

    D. _____

    E. _____

    F. _____

    G. _____

    H. _____

    I. _____

    J. _____

19. Briefly describe catastrophic reactions.

    _____

    _____

    _____

20. Explain how caregivers can cause agitation and restlessness when caring for a person with AD.

    _____

    _____

    _____

21. Aggressive and combative behaviors include

    _____

    _____

    _____.

22. Persons with AD scream to communicate. Possible causes include:

    A. _____

    B. _____

    C. _____

    D. _____

    E. _____

    F. _____

23. Sexual behaviors are labeled abnormal because of _____.

24. Persons with AD are not oriented to person, place, and time. Therefore, sexual behaviors may involve _____

    _____

    _____.

25. What are some nonsexual reasons a person with dementia may touch or rub the genitals?

    A. _____

    B. _____

    C. _____

26. A resident at Valley View Nursing Center has AD. Why is it important to report any changes in the person's usual behavior to the nurse?

    _____

    _____

    _____.

27. Impaired communication is a common problem among persons with AD and other dementias. To promote communication, you need to avoid the following:

    A. _____

    B. _____

    C. _____

28. Some nursing centers have special secured units for persons with AD and other dementias. What is the purpose of these units? _____

    _____

    _____

    _____

29. Persons in the early stages of AD may live at home with family. Long-term care is needed when:

    A. _____

    B. _____

    C. _____

    D. _____

    E. _____

30. Many adult children are in the *sandwich generation*.

    This means _____

    _____

    _____

    _____.

31. Many caregivers join AD support groups. What is the purpose of these groups? _____

    _____

    _____

    _____

    _____

32. Maintaining the day-night cycle is important when caring for confused persons. List measures that might help maintain the day-night cycle.

    A. _____

    B. _____

    C. _____

33. Write the definition of each abbreviation:

    A. AD _____

    B. ADL _____

    C. OBRA _____

Multiple Choice
Circle the **BEST** Answer

34. Cognitive relates to
    A. Beliefs
    B. Changes in the brain
    C. Social function
    D. Knowledge

35. Which is *not* a change in the nervous system from aging?
    A. Reaction times are slower.
    B. Delirium occurs.
    C. Taste and smell decrease.
    D. Sleep patterns change.

36. Which statement about acute confusion is *incorrect?*
    A. Treatment is aimed at the cause.
    B. It occurs suddenly.
    C. It usually is permanent.
    D. It can occur from infection.

37. Dementia is a normal part of aging.
    A. True
    B. False

38. Delirium is an emergency.
    A. True
    B. False

39. Which statement about delirium is *incorrect?*
    A. It is common in older persons with acute or chronic illnesses.
    B. Hypoglycemia is a cause.
    C. It signals physical illness in persons with dementia.
    D. It usually lasts longer than 6 months.

40. Which statement about Alzheimer's disease (AD) is *correct?*
    A. It is usually diagnosed before age 60.
    B. The disease is sudden in onset.
    C. The cause is unknown.
    D. It is a normal part of aging.

41. AD is often described in terms of 3 stages. A person in stage 1 (mild AD)
    A. Is disoriented to time and place
    B. Has fecal and urinary incontinence
    C. Has problems with movement and gait
    D. Cannot swallow

42. A person is confused. Which of the following measures is *not* helpful?
    A. Provide care in a calm, relaxed manner.
    B. Explain everything in great detail.
    C. Use touch to communicate.
    D. Tell the person the date and time each morning.

43. A person is confused. Which of the following measures is *not* helpful?
    A. Change the person's routine for staff convenience.
    B. Encourage the person to take part in self-care.
    C. Discuss current events with the person.
    D. Explain what you are going to do and why.

44. A resident has AD. You promote the person's safety by
    A. Restraining the person
    B. Explaining safety rules to the person
    C. Changing the person's room frequently
    D. Placing safety plugs in electric outlets

45. You are caring for a person with AD. Which action causes increased agitation?
    A. Rushing the person
    B. Keeping noise levels low
    C. Speaking in a calm, gentle voice
    D. Using touch to calm the person

46. A resident with AD is screaming in the dining room. You can help by
    A. Firmly asking the person to stop
    B. Taking the person to her room and closing the door
    C. Turning on loud music
    D. Having a favorite caregiver comfort and calm the person

47. When caring for a person with hallucinations, which measure is *not* helpful?
    A. Make sure the person is wearing eyeglasses and hearing aids as needed.
    B. Distract the person with some item or activity.
    C. Use touch to calm and reassure the person.
    D. Calmly explain that the hallucinations are not real.

48. A patient resists your efforts to help him into the bathtub. The person starts to scream. Which action might be helpful?
    A. Explain to the person why a bath is needed.
    B. Get help from two co-workers to force the person into the tub.
    C. Try bathing the person later, when he is calm.
    D. To show the person that there is nothing to be afraid of, step into the tub yourself.

49. Repetitive behaviors are usually harmless.
    A. True
    B. False

50. The person with AD
    A. Chooses to be incontinent
    B. Needs your support and understanding
    C. Has control over his or her actions
    D. Can understand and follow instructions

51. Catastrophic reactions are common from
    A. Wanting to go home
    B. Too many stimuli
    C. Being hungry
    D. Elimination needs

52. Validation therapy may be part of the person's care plan. Which is *not* a principle of validation therapy?
    A. All behaviors have meaning.
    B. A person may return to the past to resolve issues and emotions.
    C. Caregivers need to listen and provide empathy.
    D. Attempts are made to bring the person back to reality.

53. Proper use of validation therapy requires special training.
    A. True
    B. False

54. The right to privacy and confidentiality is *not* important for persons with dementia.
    A. True
    B. False

55. Restraints can make confusion and demented behaviors worse.
    A. True
    B. False

56. According to OBRA, secured nursing units are physical restraints.
    A. True
    B. False

CASE STUDY

A resident on the secured nursing unit was diagnosed with AD 3 years ago. Before coming to the nursing center, she lived with her daughter. The person was admitted to the nursing center after her daughter found her wandering three blocks from home at 9 o'clock at night. The person's daughter lives a few blocks from the nursing center. She visits at least three times a week. She often brings her 3-year-old son along. She has left a picture album with family pictures for her mother.

The person frequently gets up at night and wanders about the unit. She tells you that she is looking for her baby. She repeats the question, "Where is my baby?" over and over. Sometimes she wanders into other resident rooms looking for her baby.

Answer the following questions:

1. What measures might be part of the person's care plan to:
   A. Promote safety?

   B. Promote dignity?

2. What measures might be used to deal with the wandering?

3. What can you do to protect the person's right to confidentiality and privacy?

4. What feelings might the person's daughter have about her mother's illness?

5. How might the person's daughter be involved in her mother's care?

ADDITIONAL LEARNING ACTIVITIES

1. Compare the signs and symptoms of delirium, depression, and early Alzheimer's disease.
   A. How are the signs and symptoms similar?

   B. Why is a correct diagnosis needed?

29 ASSISTING WITH EMERGENCY CARE

STUDY QUESTIONS

Matching

Match each term with the correct definition.

1. _____ The heart stops suddenly and without warning
2. _____ The excessive loss of blood in a short time
3. _____ The sudden loss of consciousness from an inadequate blood supply to the brain
4. _____ A life-threatening sensitivity to an antigen
5. _____ Breathing stops but heart action continues for several minutes
6. _____ Violent and sudden contractions or tremors of muscle groups
7. _____ Results when organs and tissues do not get enough blood

A. Hemorrhage
B. Respiratory arrest
C. Sudden cardiac arrest
D. Fainting
E. Shock
F. Seizure (convulsion)
G. Anaphylaxis

Fill in the Blanks

8. First aid is _____

_____

_____.

9. The goals of first aid are to:

A. _____

B. _____

10. For emergencies in out-of-hospital settings, the

_____

_____

is activated. To activate the Emergency Medical Services (EMS) system, do one of the following:

A. _____

B. _____

C. _____

11. You have activated the EMS system. What information do you need to give the operator?

A. _____

B. _____

C. _____

D. _____

E. _____

F. _____

12. In the hospital, a Rapid Response Team (RRT) is called to the bedside when the person shows warning signs of a life-threatening condition.

The RRT's goal is _____

_____.

13. When the heart and breathing stop, the person

is _____.

14. The American Heart Association's (AHA's) Basic Life Support courses teach the adult *Chain of Survival*. Chain of Survival actions for the adult are:

    A. _____

    B. _____

    C. _____

    D. _____

    E. _____

15. What are the 3 major signs of sudden cardiac arrest (SCA)?

    A. _____

    B. _____

    C. _____

16. A person is in respiratory arrest. If breathing is

    not restored, _____ occurs.

17. _____ must be started at once when a person has sudden cardiac arrest.

18. What are the 4 parts involved in cardiopulmonary resuscitation (CPR)?

    A. _____

    B. _____

    C. _____

    D. _____

19. CPR procedures require

    _____,

    _____, and

    _____.

20. The head tilt-chin lift method opens the airway. Describe how to perform the head tilt-chin lift method.

    A. _____

    _____

    _____

    B. _____

    _____

    _____

C. _____

    _____

    _____

    _____

D. _____

    _____

    _____

E. _____

    _____

    _____

21. Rescue breaths are given when there is a pulse but no breathing or only gasping. To give rescue breaths:

    A. _____

    B. _____

    C. _____

    D. _____

22. With CPR each breath should take 1 second. You

    should see the chest _____

    _____.

23. When giving mouth-to-mouth breathing, you need to pinch the person's nostrils shut. Why is

    this done? _____

    _____

    _____

24. What is the purpose of the barrier device used in mouth-to-barrier device rescue breathing?

    _____

    _____

    _____

25. During CPR, _____ force blood through the circulatory system.

26. Before starting chest compressions, check for

    _____.

27. To give chest compressions, how should your hands and arms be positioned? _____

_____

_____

_____

_____

28. How far is the sternum depressed when doing chest compressions on an adult?

_____

29. When giving chest compressions, the American Heart Association recommends that you:

A. _____

B. _____

C. _____

D. _____

30. The abbreviations for ventricular fibrillation are

_____ or

_____ .

31. What occurs with ventricular fibrillation?

_____

_____

_____

_____

32. When a person is in V-fib, _____ is used to deliver a shock to the heart.

33. Where will you learn about using an automated external defibrillator? _____

_____

_____

34. CPR is done if the person _____

_____

_____ .

35. Before staring CPR in an adult, check to see if the person is responding by: _____

_____

_____

_____ .

36. The recovery position is used when _____

_____

_____ .

37. Do not use the recovery position if the person

_____

_____ .

38. List 5 signs and symptoms of internal hemorrhage.

A. _____

B. _____

C. _____

D. _____

E. _____

39. Bleeding from an _____ occurs in spurts. There is a steady flow of blood from a _____ .

40. If direct pressure over the bleeding site does not control external bleeding, what should you do?

_____

41. Signs and symptoms of shock include:

A. _____

B. _____

C. _____

D. _____

E. _____

F. _____

G. _____

42. When a person has signs and symptoms of shock, the following measures are needed:

A. Keep the person _____ .

B. Maintain an open _____ .

C. Control _____ .

D. Begin _____ if cardiac arrest occurs.

43. Signs and symptoms of anaphylaxis include:

    A. _____

    B. _____

    C. _____

    D. _____

    E. _____

    F. _____

    G. _____

    H. _____

44. List and briefly describe the 3 major types of seizures.

    A. _____

       _____

       _____

    B. _____

       _____

       _____

    C. _____

       _____

       _____

45. Describe the two phases of a generalized tonic-clonic seizure (grand mal seizure).

    A. _____

       _____

       _____

    B. _____

       _____

       _____

46. _____,

    _____, and

    _____

    are warning signals for fainting.

47. Stroke occurs when _____

    _____

    _____.

48. A stroke may be caused by:

    A. _____

    B. _____

    C. _____

49. Signs of stroke depend on _____

    _____.

50. Emergency care for a stroke includes:

    A. Positioning the person _____

       _____

       _____.

    B. Raising the _____

       without flexing the _____.

51. During an emergency, your main concern is

    _____

    _____.

52. Write the meaning of each abbreviation:

    A. BLS _____

    B. CPR _____

    C. EMS _____

    D. RRT _____

    E. AED _____

    F. SCA _____

Multiple Choice
Circle the **BEST** Answer

53. When providing emergency care, it is important to do the following *except*
    A. Check for signs of life-threatening problems
    B. Move the person to a comfortable position
    C. Call for help
    D. Keep the person warm

54. For CPR, the airway is opened by
    A. Turning the head to the side
    B. Lifting the head up and tilting it forward
    C. Sitting the person up
    D. The head tilt-chin lift method

55. Which artery is used to check for a pulse before starting chest compressions?
    A. The radial artery
    B. The brachial artery
    C. The carotid artery
    D. The femoral artery

56. For chest compressions to be effective, the person
    A. Must be in a sitting position
    B. Must be supine and on a hard, flat surface
    C. Must be flat and on a soft surface
    D. Is positioned with pillows

57. A patient is in ventricular fibrillation. Defibrillation as soon as possible increases the person's chance of survival.
    A. True
    B. False
58. Hands-Only CPR is used to educate
    A. Persons not trained in basic life support
    B. Doctors
    C. RNs
    D. All health care professionals
59. During two-person CPR, Rescuer 2 gives
    A. 1 breath after every 5 chest compressions
    B. 1 breath after every 10 chest compressions
    C. 2 breaths after every 30 chest compressions
    D. 1 breath at the same rate as chest compressions
60. For internal hemorrhage, do the following *except*
    A. Keep the person warm until help arrives
    B. Keep the person flat
    C. Keep the person quiet until help arrives
    D. Give the person fluids
61. To control external hemorrhage, do the following *except*
    A. Elevate the affected part
    B. Remove any objects that have pierced or stabbed the person
    C. Place a sterile dressing directly over the wound
    D. Apply pressure with your hand directly over the bleeding site

62. To prevent or treat shock, do the following *except*
    A. Maintain an open airway
    B. Control bleeding
    C. Keep the person warm
    D. Keep the person in Fowler's position
63. Which action will protect the person from injury during a generalized tonic-clonic seizure?
    A. Lower the person to the floor.
    B. Turn the person onto his or her back.
    C. Restrain body movements during the seizure.
    D. Put your fingers or an object between the person's teeth.
64. Emergency care for fainting includes the following *except*
    A. Have the person sit or lie down
    B. Loosen tight clothing
    C. If the person is lying down, raise the legs
    D. Give the person sips of cool water
65. There is no need to protect the person's right to privacy during an emergency.
    A. True
    B. False

CASE STUDY

While a resident is eating lunch in the dinning room, you notice that the left side of the person's face is drooping and he is leaning to the left. The person is having difficulty swallowing and has slurred speech.

Answer the following questions:

1. The person is having signs of

   _____.

2. What are some possible causes?

3. What does emergency care involve?

4. How would you protect the person's right to privacy?

ADDITIONAL LEARNING ACTIVITIES

1. Identify the EMS system in your community.
   A. Check the phone book yellow pages and the Internet.

   B. Do you know how to activate the EMS system in an emergency?

2. Are you and your family prepared to respond to emergency situations in your home?
   A. Are emergency phone numbers easily found?

   B. Do members of your family know what information to give the operator in an emergency?

   C. Do you and your family know basic life support procedures?

3. Do you know which agencies in your community offer classes in basic life support procedures and first aid? Check the following agencies in your community.
   A. Hospitals
   B. Nursing centers
   C. Community colleges
   D. The American Heart Association
   E. The American Red Cross
   F. The National Safety Council

4. If possible, enroll in a Basic Life Support class. Your instructor can help you with this process.

30 CARING FOR THE DYING PERSON

STUDY QUESTIONS

Matching

Match each term with the correct definition.

1. _____ Care that focuses on the physical, emotional, social, and spiritual needs of dying persons and their families

2. _____ Care of the body after death

3. _____ The belief that the spirit or soul is reborn in another human body or in another form of life

4. _____ The examination of the body after death

5. _____ A document about measures that support or maintain life when death is likely

6. _____ The stiffness or rigidity of skeletal muscles that occurs after death

7. _____ An illness or injury from which the person will not likely recover

8. _____ A document stating a person's wishes about health care when that person cannot make his or her own decisions

9. _____ Gives the power to make health care decisions to another person

A. Post-mortem care
B. Rigor mortis
C. Hospice care
D. Durable power of attorney for health care
E. Living will
F. Advance directive
G. Terminal illness
H. Reincarnation
I. Autopsy

Fill in the Blanks

10. Explain why it is important for you to understand the dying process. _____

_____

_____

_____

11. A patient you are caring for is dying. Your religious beliefs about death differ from those of your patient. Effective communication with the person involves _____

_____

_____

_____

_____.

12. List 4 fears adults may have when facing death.

A. _____

B. _____

C. _____

D. _____

13. Adults often resent death because it affects

_____,

_____,

_____,

and _____.

14. Why might some older persons welcome death?

_____

_____

_____

15. List the 5 stages of dying described by Dr. Elisabeth Kübler-Ross.

    A. _____

    B. _____

    C. _____

    D. _____

    E. _____

16. How can you use listening and touch to help meet the dying person's psychological, social, and spiritual needs?

    A. Listening: _____

    _____

    _____

    _____

    B. Touch: _____

    _____

    _____

    _____

17. When a patient or resident asks to visit with a

    spiritual leader, you need to _____

    _____

    _____ .

18. _____ is

    one of the last functions lost. Always assume

    that the person can _____ .

19. Which position is usually best for breathing

    problems? _____

20. List 8 measures that promote the dying person's physical comfort.

    A. _____

    B. _____

    C. _____

    D. _____

    E. _____

    F. _____

    G. _____

    H. _____

21. The goal of hospice care is to _____

    _____

    _____ .

22. _____ and

    _____ give

    persons the right to accept or refuse medical treatment and to make advance directives.

23. A living will may instruct doctors:

    A. _____

    B. _____

24. The doctor wrote a "do not resuscitate" (DNR) order for a resident. What does this mean?

    _____

    _____

    _____

25. List 6 signs that signal death is near.

    A. _____

    _____

    _____

    B. _____

    _____

    _____

    C. _____

    _____

    _____

    D. _____

    _____

    E. _____

    _____

    _____

    F. _____

    _____

26. The signs of death include:

    A. _____

    B. _____

27. Which health team member determines that

    death has occurred? _____

28. When does post-mortem care begin?

    _____

    _____

29. Post-mortem care is done to _____

    _____.

30. What is the purpose of an autopsy? _____

    _____

31. When assisting with post-mortem care, what information do you need from the nurse?

    A. _____

    B. _____

    C. _____

    D. _____

    E. _____

32. A patient you are caring for has an advance directive that is against your religious values.

    What should you do? _____

    _____

    _____

    _____

33. List the dying person's rights under OBRA.

    A. _____

    B. _____

    C. _____

    D. _____

    E. _____

    F. _____

34. Write the meaning of each of the following abbreviations:

    A. CPR _____

    B. DNR _____

Multiple Choice

Circle the **BEST** Answer

35. Attitudes and beliefs about death usually stay the same throughout a person's life.
    A. True
    B. False

36. Infants and toddlers do not understand the nature or meaning of death.
    A. True
    B. False

37. Children between the ages of 2 and 6 years
    A. Know that death is final
    B. Often think they will die
    C. Often blame themselves when someone dies
    D. Are not curious about death

38. The person in the bargaining stage of dying
    A. Is very sad
    B. Makes promises in exchange for more time
    C. Is calm and at peace
    D. Feels anger and rage

39. The person in the stage of acceptance
    A. Refuses to believe that he or she is dying
    B. Bargains for more time
    C. Is very sad
    D. Is calm and at peace

40. A resident is dying. The person asks you to stay and talk in the middle of the night. Which is *correct?*
    A. Tell the person to go back to sleep.
    B. Call the person's family.
    C. Call a pastor to talk with the person.
    D. Let the person express feelings and emotions.

41. A person's pastor is visiting at 11:00 PM. You need to
    A. Stay in the room while the pastor visits
    B. Provide for privacy
    C. Tell the nurse at once
    D. Ask the person why the pastor is visiting so late

42. A patient is unconscious. When providing care, do the following *except*
    A. Assume that the person can hear you
    B. Speak in a whisper
    C. Offer words of comfort
    D. Avoid topics that could upset the person

43. When caring for a dying person, you promote comfort by
    A. Playing cheerful music
    B. Asking a lot of questions to keep the person talking
    C. Providing care quickly, so the person can be alone
    D. Providing good skin care and personal hygiene

44. A darkened room is comforting to the dying person.
   A. True
   B. False
45. The family goes through stages like the dying person.
   A. True
   B. False
46. When an autopsy is to be done, post-mortem care is *not* done.
   A. True
   B. False
47. Post-mortem care involves the following *except*
   A. Pronouncing the person dead
   B. Positioning the body in normal alignment before rigor mortis sets in
   C. Preparing the body for viewing by the family
   D. Bathing soiled areas

48. When providing post-mortem care, you must practice Standard Precautions and follow the Bloodborne Pathogen Standard.
   A. True
   B. False
49. The right to confidentiality does *not* apply after death.
   A. True
   B. False
50. The dying person has the right to receive kind and respectful care before and after death.
   A. True
   B. False

CASE STUDY

You are caring for a 59-year-old male patient receiving hospice care. The person currently sleeps most of the time. His verbal communication is minimal. He occasionally opens his eyes. His wife stays with him most of the day. She has spent the past two nights at his bedside. She says prayers and talks to her husband about important events in their lives. His son from another state arrived 3 days ago. The person's daughter lives in the same town and visits several times a day. She often washes his face and applies lotion to his feet. She tells him that she loves him and that she will miss him.

After his son arrived, the person told his wife that he was ready to die and that he was at peace with his family and with God. He discussed his will and his funeral arrangements with his wife and his children.

Answer the following questions:

1. According to Elisabeth Kübler-Ross' stages of dying, what stage is the person in? Explain.

2. What physical care needs does the person have?

3. What measures will help meet the person's psychological, social, and spiritual needs?

4. What measures will help meet the family's needs?

ADDITIONAL LEARNING ACTIVITIES

1. List your thoughts and feelings about death and dying.

   A. How do your religion, culture, and age affect your feelings about death?

   B. Have you had experience with the death of a family member or friend that affects your feelings about death and dying? Explain.

   C. How do you feel about advance directives?

2. If you have fears about caring for dying persons, discuss them with your instructor.

Relieving Choking—Adult or Child (Over 1 Year of Age)

Name: _____ Date: _____

Procedure	S	U	Comments
1. Asked the person if he or she was choking. Helped the person if nodded yes and he or she could not talk.	___	___	_____
2. Had someone call for help:			
a. In a public area, had someone activate the Emergency Medical Services (EMS) system by dialing 911; sent someone to get an automated external defibrillator (AED).	___	___	_____
b. In an agency, called the Rapid Response Team (RRT); sent someone to get the AED.	___	___	_____
3. Gave abdominal thrusts:			
a. Stood or knelt behind the person.	___	___	_____
b. Wrapped your arms around the person's waist.	___	___	_____
c. Made a fist with one hand.	___	___	_____
d. Placed the thumb side of the fist against the abdomen. The fist was slightly above the navel in the middle of the abdomen and well below the end of the sternum (breastbone).	___	___	_____
e. Grasped the fist with your other hand.	___	___	_____
f. Pressed your fist into the person's abdomen with a quick, upward thrust.	___	___	_____
g. Repeated thrusts until the object was expelled or the person became unresponsive.	___	___	_____
4. If the person was obese or pregnant, gave chest thrusts:			
a. Stood behind the person.	___	___	_____
b. Placed your arms under the person's underarms. Wrapped your arms around the person's chest.	___	___	_____
c. Made a fist. Placed the thumb side of the fist on the middle of the sternum (breastbone).	___	___	_____
d. Grasped the fist with your other hand.	___	___	_____
e. Gave thrusts to the chest until the object was expelled or the person became unresponsive.	___	___	_____
5. If the object was dislodged, encouraged the person to go to the hospital.	___	___	_____
6. If the person became unresponsive, lowered the person to the floor or ground. Positioned the person supine. Made sure the EMS or RRT was called.	___	___	_____
7. Started CPR.			
a. Did not check for a pulse. Began with compressions. Gave 30 compressions.	___	___	_____
b. Used the head tilt-chin lift method to open the airway. Opened the person's mouth wide. Looked for an object. Removed the object if found and was easily removable. Used fingers.	___	___	_____

Date of Satisfactory Completion _____ Instructor's Initials _____

Procedure—cont'd	S	U	Comments
c. Gave 2 breaths.	___	___	_____
d. Continued cycles of 30 compressions and 2 breaths. Looked for an object every time the airway was opened for rescue breaths.	___	___	_____
8. *If choking was relieved in an unresponsive person:*			
a. Checked for a response, breathing, and a pulse.	___	___	_____
(1) *If no response, normal breathing, or pulse—* continued CPR. Attached an AED.	___	___	_____
(2) *If no response and no normal breathing but there was a pulse—* gave rescue breaths. For an adult, gave 1 breath every 5 to 6 seconds. For a child, gave 1 breath every 3 to 5 seconds. Checked for a pulse every 2 minutes. If no pulse, began CPR.	___	___	_____
(3) *If the person had normal breathing and a pulse—*placed the person in the recovery position if there is no response. Continued to check the person until help arrived. Encouraged the person to go to the hospital if the person responded.	___	___	_____

Date of Satisfactory Completion _____ Instructor's Initials _____

Using a Fire Extinguisher

Name: _____   Date: _____

Procedure	**S**	**U**	**Comments**
1. Pulled the fire alarm.	___	___	_____
2. Got the nearest fire extinguisher.	___	___	_____
3. Carried it upright.	___	___	_____
4. Took it to the fire.	___	___	_____
5. Followed the word PASS:			
a. P—pulled the safety pin.	___	___	_____
b. A—aimed low. Directed the hose or nozzle at the base of the fire. Did not try to spray the tops of the flames.	___	___	_____
c. S—squeezed or pushed down on the lever, handle, or button to start the stream. Released the lever, handle, or button to stop the stream.	___	___	_____
d. S—swept the stream back and forth (side to side) at the base of the fire.	___	___	_____

Date of Satisfactory Completion _____   Instructor's Initials _____

Applying a Transfer/Gait Belt

Name: _____   Date: _____

	S	U	Comments

Quality of Life
- Knocked before entering the person's room.
- Addressed the person by name.
- Introduced yourself by name and title.
- Explained the procedure to the person before beginning and during the procedure.
- Protected the person's rights during the procedure.
- Handled the person gently during the procedure.

Procedure
1. Reviewed *Promoting Safety and Comfort: Transfer/Gait Belts*.
2. Practiced hand hygiene.
3. Identified the person. Checked the identification (ID) bracelet against the assignment sheet. Called the person by name.
4. Provided for privacy.
5. Assisted the person to a sitting position.
6. Applied the belt around the person's waist over clothing. Did not apply it over bare skin.
7. Secured the buckle. The buckle was in front.
8. Tightened the belt so it was snug. It did not cause discomfort or impair breathing. You were able to slide your open, flat hand under the belt.
9. Made sure that a woman's breasts were not caught under the belt.
10. Turned the belt so the quick-release buckle was at the person's back. The buckle was not over the spine.
11. Tucked any excess strap under the belt.

Date of Satisfactory Completion _____   Instructor's Initials _____

Helping the Falling Person

Name: _____   Date: _____

Procedure	S	U	Comments
1. Stood behind the person with your feet apart. Kept your back straight.	_____	_____	_____
2. Brought the person close to your body as fast as possible. Used the transfer/gait belt.	_____	_____	_____
Or wrapped your arms around the person's waist. If necessary, held the person under the arms.	_____	_____	_____
3. Moved your leg so the person's buttocks rested on it. Moved the leg near the person.	_____	_____	_____
4. Lowered the person to the floor. The person slid down your leg to the floor. Bent at your hips and knees as you lowered the person.	_____	_____	_____
5. Called a nurse to check the person. Stayed with the person.	_____	_____	_____
6. Helped the nurse return the person to bed. Asked other staff to help if needed.	_____	_____	_____

Post-Procedure

	S	U	Comments
7. Provided for comfort as noted on the inside of the front textbook cover.	_____	_____	_____
8. Placed the signal light within reach.	_____	_____	_____
9. Raised or lowered bed rails. Followed the care plan.	_____	_____	_____
10. Completed a safety check of the room as noted on the inside of the front textbook cover.	_____	_____	_____
11. Reported and recorded the following:			
• How the fall occurred	_____	_____	_____
• How far the person walked	_____	_____	_____
• How activity was tolerated before the fall	_____	_____	_____
• Complaints before the fall	_____	_____	_____
• How much help the person needed while walking	_____	_____	_____
12. Completed an incident report.	_____	_____	_____

Date of Satisfactory Completion _____   Instructor's Initials _____

Applying Restraints

Name: ———————————————   Date: ———————————————

Quality of Life	S	U	Comments
• Knocked before entering the person's room.	___	___	_____
• Addressed the person by name.	___	___	_____
• Introduced yourself by name and title.	___	___	_____
• Explained the procedure to the person before beginning and during the procedure.	___	___	_____
• Protected the person's rights during the procedure.	___	___	_____
• Handled the person gently during the procedure.	___	___	_____

Pre-Procedure

1. Followed *Delegation Guidelines: Applying Restraints.* Reviewed *Promoting Safety and Comfort: Applying Restraints.*
2. Collected the following as instructed:
   • Correct type and size of restraints
   • Padding for skin and bony areas
   • Bed rail pads or gap protectors (if needed)
3. Practiced hand hygiene.
4. Identified the person. Checked the ID bracelet against the assignment sheet. Called the person by name.
5. Provided for privacy.

Procedure

6. Made sure the person was comfortable and in good alignment.
7. Put the bed rail pads or gap protectors (if needed) on the bed if the person was in bed. Followed the manufacturer's instructions.
8. Padded bony areas according to the nurse's instructions and the care plan.
9. Read the manufacturer's instructions. Noted the front and back of the restraint.
10. For wrist restraints:
    a. Applied the restraint following the manufacturer's instructions. Placed the soft or foam part toward the skin.
    b. Secured the restraint so it was snug but not tight. Made sure you could slide 1 finger under the restraint. Followed the manufacturer's instructions. Adjusted the straps if the restraint was too loose or too tight. Checked for snugness again.
    c. Buckled or tied the straps to the movable part of the bed frame out of the person's reach. Used an agency-approved tie.
    d. Repeated steps 10a, b, and c for the other wrist.

Date of Satisfactory Completion ————————————   Instructor's Initials ————————————

Procedure—cont'd	S	U	Comments

11. For mitt restraints:
    a. Made sure the person's hands were clean and dry. ___ ___ _____
    b. Applied the mitt restraint. Followed the manufacturer's instructions. ___ ___ _____
    c. Secured the restraint to the bed if directed to do so by the nurse. Buckled or tied the straps to the movable part of the bed frame. Used an agency-approved tie. ___ ___ _____
    d. Made sure the restraint was snug. Slid 1 finger between the restraint and the wrist. Followed the manufacturer's instructions. Adjusted the straps if the restraint was too loose or too tight. Checked for snugness again. ___ ___ _____
    e. Repeated steps 11b, c (if directed to do so), and d for the other hand. ___ ___ _____
12. For a belt restraint:
    a. Assisted the person to a sitting position. ___ ___ _____
    b. Applied the restraint with your free hand. Followed the manufacturer's instructions. ___ ___ _____
    c. Removed wrinkles or creases from the front and back of the restraint. ___ ___ _____
    d. Brought the ties through the slots in the belt. ___ ___ _____
    e. Helped the person lie down if he or she was in bed. ___ ___ _____
    f. Made sure the person was comfortable and in good alignment. ___ ___ _____
    g. Buckled or tied the straps to the movable part of the bed frame out of the person's reach or to the chair or wheelchair. Used an agency-approved tie. ___ ___ _____
    h. Made sure the belt was snug. Slid an open hand between the restraint and the person. Adjusted the restraint if it was too loose or too tight. Checked for snugness again. ___ ___ _____
13. For a vest restraint:
    a. Assisted the person to a sitting position. ___ ___ _____
    b. Applied the restraint with your free hand. Followed the manufacturer's instructions. The "V" part of the vest crossed in front. ___ ___ _____
    c. Brought the straps through the slots. ___ ___ _____
    d. Made sure the vest was free of wrinkles in the front and back. ___ ___ _____
    e. Helped the person lie down if he or she was in bed. ___ ___ _____
    f. Made sure the person was comfortable and in good alignment. ___ ___ _____
    g. Buckled or tied the straps underneath the chair seat or to the movable part of the bed frame. Used an agency-approved tie. If secured to the bed frame, the straps were secured at waist level out of the person's reach. ___ ___ _____
    h. Made sure the vest was snug. Slid an open hand between the restraint and the person. Adjusted the restraint if it was too loose or too tight. Checked for snugness again. ___ ___ _____

Date of Satisfactory Completion _____ Instructor's Initials _____

Procedure—cont'd   S   U   **Comments**

14. For a jacket restraint:
    a. Assisted the person to a sitting position.   _____   _____   _____
    b. Applied the restraint with your free hand. Followed the   _____   _____   _____
       manufacturer's instructions. The jacket opening was
       in back.
    c. Closed the back with the zipper, ties, or hook and loop   _____   _____   _____
       closures.
    d. Made sure the side seams were under the arms.   _____   _____   _____
       Removed any wrinkles in the front and back.
    e. Helped the person lie down if he or she was in bed.   _____   _____   _____
    f. Made sure the person was comfortable and in good   _____   _____   _____
       alignment.
    g. Buckled or tied the straps underneath the chair seat   _____   _____   _____
       or to the movable part of the bed frame. Used an
       agency-approved knot. If secured to the bed frame,
       the straps were secured at waist level out of the
       person's reach.
    h. Made sure the jacket was snug. Slid an open hand   _____   _____   _____
       between the restraint and the person. Adjusted the
       restraint if it was too loose or too tight. Checked for
       snugness again.

Post-Procedure

15. Positioned the person as the nurse directed.   _____   _____   _____
16. Provided for comfort as noted on the inside of the   _____   _____   _____
    front textbook cover.
17. Placed the signal light within the person's reach.   _____   _____   _____
18. Raised or lowered bed rails. Followed the care plan and   _____   _____   _____
    the manufacturer's instructions for the restraint.
19. Unscreened the person.   _____   _____   _____
20. Completed a safety check of the room as indicated on the   _____   _____   _____
    inside of the front textbook cover.
21. Decontaminated your hands.   _____   _____   _____
22. Checked the person and the restraints at least every
    15 minutes. Reported and recorded your observations:
    a. For wrist and mitt restraints: checked the pulse, color,   _____   _____   _____
       and temperature of the restrained parts.
    b. For a vest, jacket, and belt restraint: checked the   _____   _____   _____
       person's breathing. Called the nurse at once if the
       person was not breathing or was having problems
       breathing. Made sure the restraint was
       properly positioned in the front and back.

Date of Satisfactory Completion _____   Instructor's Initials _____

Post-Procedure—cont'd   S   U   Comments

23. Did the following at least every 2 hours for at least
    10 minutes:
    a. Removed or released the restraint.   _____ _____ _____
    b. Measured vital signs.   _____ _____ _____
    c. Repositioned the person.   _____ _____ _____
    d. Met food, fluid, hygiene, and elimination needs. _____ _____ _____
    e. Gave skin care.   _____ _____ _____
    f. Performed range-of-motion exercises or helped the
       person walk. Followed the care plan.   _____ _____ _____
    g. Provided for physical and emotional comfort as noted
       on the inside of the front textbook cover. _____ _____ _____
    h. Reapplied the restraints.   _____ _____ _____
24. Completed a safety check of the room as noted on the
    inside of the front textbook cover.   _____ _____ _____
25. Reported and recorded your observations and the
    care given.   _____ _____ _____

Date of Satisfactory Completion _____ Instructor's Initials _____

View Video! **Video CLIP** **Hand Washing (NNAAP™)**

Name: _____   Date: _____

Procedure	S	U	Comments
1. Reviewed *Promoting Safety and Comfort: Hand Hygiene*.	____	____	_____
2. Made sure you had soap, paper towels, an orange stick or nail file, and a wastebasket. Collected missing items.	____	____	_____
3. Pushed watch up your arm 4 to 5 inches. If uniform sleeves were long, pushed them up.	____	____	_____
4. Stood away from the sink so that clothes did not touch the sink. Stood so the soap and faucet were easy to reach. Did not touch inside of sink at any time.	____	____	_____
5. Turned on and adjusted the water until it felt warm.	____	____	_____
6. Wet wrists and hands. Kept your hands lower than your elbows. Wet the area 3 to 4 inches above your wrists.	____	____	_____
7. Applied about 1 teaspoon of soap to hands.	____	____	_____
8. Rubbed your palms together and interlaced fingers to work up a good lather for at least 15 seconds. (Washed your hands as long as required by state competency test.)	____	____	_____
9. Washed each hand and wrist thoroughly. Cleaned well between the fingers.	____	____	_____
10. Cleaned under the fingernails. Rubbed your fingertips against your palms.	____	____	_____
11. Cleaned under the fingernails with a nail file or orange stick.	____	____	_____
12. Rinsed wrists and hands well. Water flowed from the arms to the hands.	____	____	_____
13. Repeated steps 7 through 12, if needed.	____	____	_____
14. Dried your wrists and hands with a clean, dry paper towel. Patted dry starting at your fingertips.	____	____	_____
15. Discarded the paper towels into the wastebasket.	____	____	_____
16. Turned off faucets with clean, dry paper towels. Used a clean paper towel for each faucet.	____	____	_____
17. Discarded paper towels into the wastebasket.	____	____	_____

Date of Satisfactory Completion _____   Instructor's Initials _____

Removing Gloves (NNAAP™)

Name: _____   Date: _____

Procedure	S	U	Comments
1. Reviewed *Promoting Safety and Comfort: Gloves*.	____	____	_____
2. Made sure that glove touched only glove.	____	____	_____
3. Grasped a glove just below the cuff. Grasped it on the outside.	____	____	_____
4. Pulled the glove down over your hand so it was inside out.	____	____	_____
5. Held the removed glove with the other gloved hand.	____	____	_____
6. Reached inside the other glove. Used the first two fingers of the ungloved hand.	____	____	_____
7. Pulled the glove down (inside out) over your hand and the other glove.	____	____	_____
8. Discarded the gloves into the wastebasket.	____	____	_____
9. Decontaminated your hands.	____	____	_____

Date of Satisfactory Completion _____   Instructor's Initials _____

Donning and Removing a Gown (NNAAP™)

View Video!

Name: _____   Date: _____

Procedure	S	U	Comments
1. Removed your watch and all jewelry.	____	____	_____
2. Rolled up uniform sleeves.	____	____	_____
3. Practiced hand hygiene.	____	____	_____
4. Held a clean gown out in front of you. Let it unfold. Did not shake the gown.	____	____	_____
5. Put your hands and arms through the sleeves.	____	____	_____
6. Made sure the gown covered you from your neck to your knees. It covered your arms to the end of the wrists.	____	____	_____
7. Tied the strings at the back of the neck.	____	____	_____
8. Overlapped the back of the gown. Made sure it covered your uniform. The gown was snug, not loose.	____	____	_____
9. Tied the waist strings at the back or the side.	____	____	_____
10. Put on other personal protective equipment (PPE):			
a. Mask or respirator if needed	____	____	_____
b. Goggles or face shield if needed	____	____	_____
c. Gloves (Made sure gloves covered the gown cuffs.)	____	____	_____
11. Provided care.			
12. Removed and discarded the gloves.			
13. Removed and discarded the goggles or face shield if worn.			
14. Removed the gown. Did not touch the outside of the gown.			
a. Untied the neck and waist strings.	____	____	_____
b. Pulled the gown down from each shoulder toward same hand.	____	____	_____
c. Turned the gown inside out as it was removed. Held it at the inside shoulder seams and brought your hands together.	____	____	_____
15. Held and rolled up the gown away from you. Kept it inside out.	____	____	_____
16. Discarded the gown.	____	____	_____
17. Removed and discarded mask if worn.	____	____	_____
18. Decontaminated your hands.	____	____	_____

Date of Satisfactory Completion _____   Instructor's Initials _____

Donning and Removing a Mask

Name: _____   Date: _____

Procedure	S	U	Comments
1. Practiced hand hygiene.	___	___	_____
2. Put on a gown if required.	___	___	_____
3. Picked up the mask by its upper ties. Did not touch the part that would cover your face.	___	___	_____
4. Placed the mask over your nose and mouth.	___	___	_____
5. Placed the upper strings above your ears. Tied them at the back in the middle of your head.	___	___	_____
6. Tied the lower strings at the back of your neck. The lower part of the mask was under your chin.	___	___	_____
7. Pinched the metal band around your nose. The top of the mask was snug over your nose. If eyeglasses were worn, the mask was snug under the bottom of the eyeglasses.	___	___	_____
8. Made sure the mask was snug over your face and under your chin.	___	___	_____
9. Put on goggles or a face shield if needed and if not part of the mask.	___	___	_____
10. Put on gloves.	___	___	_____
11. Provided care. Avoided coughing, sneezing, and unnecessary talking.	___	___	_____
12. Changed the mask if it became wet or contaminated.	___	___	_____
13. Removed the mask:			
a. Removed the gloves.	___	___	_____
b. Removed the goggles or face shield and gown if worn.	___	___	_____
c. Untied the lower strings of the mask.	___	___	_____
d. Untied the top strings.	___	___	_____
e. Held the top strings. Removed the mask.	___	___	_____
14. Discarded the mask.	___	___	_____
15. Decontaminated your hands.	___	___	_____

Date of Satisfactory Completion _____   Instructor's Initials _____

Moving the Person Up in Bed

Name: ————————————————   Date: ————————————————

Quality of Life	S	U	Comments
• Knocked before entering the person's room.	———	———	———————
• Addressed the person by name.	———	———	———————
• Introduced yourself by name and title.	———	———	———————
• Explained the procedure to the person before beginning and during the procedure.	———	———	———————
• Protected the person's rights during the procedure.	———	———	———————
• Handled the person gently during the procedure.	———	———	———————

Pre-Procedure

1. Followed *Delegation Guidelines:*
   a. *Preventing Work-Related Injuries*
   b. *Moving Persons in Bed*
   Reviewed *Promoting Safety and Comfort:*
   a. *Safely Handling, Moving, and Transferring the Person*
   b. *Preventing Work-Related Injuries*
   c. *Moving the Person Up in Bed*
2. Asked a co-worker to help.
3. Practiced hand hygiene.
4. Identified the person. Checked the ID bracelet against the assignment sheet. Called the person by name.
5. Provided for privacy.
6. Locked the bed wheels.
7. Raised the bed for body mechanics. Bed rails were up if used.

Procedure

8. Lowered the head of the bed to a level appropriate for the person. It was as flat as possible.
9. Stood on one side of the bed. Your co-worker stood on the other side.
10. Lowered the bed rails if up.
11. Removed the pillow as directed by the nurse. Placed a pillow upright against the headboard if the person could be without it.
12. Stood with a wide base of support. Pointed the foot near the head of the bed toward the head of the bed. Faced the head of the bed.
13. Bent your hips and knees. Kept your back straight.
14. Placed one arm under the person's shoulder and one arm under the thighs. Your co-worker did the same. Grasped each other's forearms.
15. Asked the person to grasp the trapeze.
16. Had the person flex both knees.
17. Explained the following:
    a. You will count "1, 2, 3."
    b. The move will be on "3."
    c. On "3," the person pushes against the bed with the feet if able and pulls up with the trapeze.

Date of Satisfactory Completion ———————————   Instructor's Initials ———————————

Procedure—cont'd	S	U	Comments
18. Moved the person to the head of the bed on the count of "3." Shifted your weight from your rear leg to your front leg. Your co-worker did the same.	_____	_____	_____
19. Repeated steps 12 through 18 if necessary.	_____	_____	_____

Post-Procedure

	S	U	Comments
20. Put the pillow under the person's head and shoulders. Straightened linens.	_____	_____	_____
21. Positioned the person in good alignment.	_____	_____	_____
22. Provided for comfort as noted on the inside of the front textbook cover.	_____	_____	_____
23. Placed the signal light within reach.	_____	_____	_____
24. Raised the head of the bed to a level appropriate for the person.	_____	_____	_____
25. Lowered the bed to its lowest position.	_____	_____	_____
26. Raised or lowered bed rails. Followed the care plan.	_____	_____	_____
27. Unscreened the person.	_____	_____	_____
28. Completed a safety check of the room as noted on the inside of the front textbook cover.	_____	_____	_____
29. Decontaminated your hands.	_____	_____	_____
30. Reported and recorded your observations.	_____	_____	_____

Date of Satisfactory Completion _____ Instructor's Initials _____

Moving the Person Up in Bed With an Assist Device

Name: _____   Date: _____

	S	U	Comments

Quality of Life
- Knocked before entering the person's room.
- Addressed the person by name.
- Introduced yourself by name and title.
- Explained the procedure to the person before beginning and during the procedure.
- Protected the person's rights during the procedure.
- Handled the person gently during the procedure.

Pre-Procedure
1. Followed *Delegation Guidelines:*
   a. *Preventing Work-Related Injuries*
   b. *Moving Persons in Bed*
   Reviewed *Promoting Safety and Comfort:*
   a. *Safely Handling, Moving, and Transferring the Person*
   b. *Preventing Work-Related Injuries*
   c. *Moving the Person Up in Bed*
   d. *Moving the Person Up in Bed With an Assist Device*
2. Asked a co-worker to help.
3. Practiced hand hygiene.
4. Identified the person. Checked the ID bracelet against the assignment sheet. Called the person by name.
5. Provided for privacy.
6. Locked the bed wheels.
7. Raised the bed for body mechanics. Bed rails were up if used.

Procedure
8. Lowered the head of the bed to a level appropriate for the person. It was as flat as possible.
9. Stood on one side of the bed. Your co-worker stood on the other side.
10. Lowered the bed rails if up.
11. Removed pillows as directed by the nurse. Placed a pillow upright against the headboard if the person could be without it.
12. Stood with a broad base of support. Pointed the foot near the head of the bed toward the head of the bed. Faced that direction.
13. Rolled the sides of the assist device up close to the person. (Omitted this step if device had handles.)
14. Grasped the rolled-up assist device firmly near the person's shoulders and hips. Grasped it by handles if present. Supported the head.
15. Bent your hips and knees.
16. Moved the person up in bed on the count of "3." Shifted your weight from your rear leg to your front leg.
17. Repeated steps 12 through 16 if necessary.
18. Unrolled the assist device. (Omitted this step if device had handles.)

Date of Satisfactory Completion _____   Instructor's Initials _____

Post-Procedure   S   U   Comments

19. Put the pillow under the person's head and shoulders.
20. Positioned the person in good alignment.
21. Provided for comfort as noted on the inside of the front textbook cover.
22. Placed the signal light within reach.
23. Raised the head of the bed to a level appropriate for the person.
24. Lowered the bed to its lowest position.
25. Raised or lowered bed rails. Followed the care plan.
26. Unscreened the person.
27. Completed a safety check of the room as noted on the inside of the front textbook cover.
28. Decontaminated your hands.
29. Reported and recorded your observations.

Date of Satisfactory Completion _____ Instructor's Initials _____

Moving the Person to the Side of the Bed

Name: _____   Date: _____

Quality of Life	S	U	Comments
• Knocked before entering the person's room.	___	___	___
• Addressed the person by name.	___	___	___
• Introduced yourself by name and title.	___	___	___
• Explained the procedure to the person before beginning and during the procedure.	___	___	___
• Protected the person's rights during the procedure.	___	___	___
• Handled the person gently during the procedure.	___	___	___

Pre-Procedure

1. Followed *Delegation Guidelines:*
   a. *Preventing Work-Related Injuries*
   b. *Moving Persons in Bed*
   Reviewed *Promoting Safety and Comfort:*
   a. *Safely Handling, Moving, and Transferring the Person*
   b. *Preventing Work-Related Injuries*
   c. *Moving the Person to the Side of the Bed*
2. Asked a co-worker to help if using an assist device.
3. Practiced hand hygiene.
4. Identified the person. Checked the ID bracelet against the assignment sheet. Called the person by name.
5. Provided for privacy.
6. Locked the bed wheels.
7. Raised the bed for body mechanics. Bed rails were up if used.

Procedure

8. Lowered the head of the bed to a level appropriate for the person. It was as flat as possible.
9. Stood on the side of the bed to which you would move the person.
10. Lowered the bed rail near you if bed rails were used. (Both bed rails were lowered for step 15.)
11. Removed pillows as directed by the nurse.
12. Stood with your feet about 12 inches apart. One foot was in front of the other. Flexed your knees.
13. Crossed the person's arms over the person's chest.
14. Method 1—Moving the person in segments:
    a. Placed your arm under the person's neck and shoulders. Grasped the far shoulder.
    b. Placed your other arm under the mid-back.
    c. Moved the upper part of the person's body toward you. Rocked backward and shifted your weight to your rear leg.
    d. Placed one arm under the person's waist and one under the thighs.
    e. Rocked backward to move the lower part of the person toward you.
    f. Repeated the procedure for the legs and feet. Your arms were under the person's thighs and calves.

Date of Satisfactory Completion _____   Instructor's Initials _____

Procedure—cont'd	S	U	Comments
15. Method 2—Moving the person with a drawsheet:			
a. Rolled up the drawsheet close to the person.	___	___	_____
b. Grasped the rolled-up drawsheet near the person's shoulders and hips. Your co-worker did the same. Supported the person's head.	___	___	_____
c. Rocked backward on the count of "3," moving the person toward you. Your co-worker rocked backward slightly and then forward toward you while keeping the arms straight.	___	___	_____
d. Unrolled the drawsheet. Removed any wrinkles.	___	___	_____

Post-Procedure

	S	U	Comments
16. Positioned the person in good alignment.	___	___	_____
17. Provided for comfort as noted on the inside of the front textbook cover.	___	___	_____
18. Placed the signal light within reach.	___	___	_____
19. Lowered the bed to its lowest position.	___	___	_____
20. Raised or lowered bed rails. Followed the care plan.	___	___	_____
21. Unscreened the person.	___	___	_____
22. Completed a safety check of the room as noted on the inside of the front textbook cover.	___	___	_____
23. Decontaminated your hands.	___	___	_____
24. Reported and recorded your observations.	___	___	_____

Date of Satisfactory Completion _____ Instructor's Initials _____

Turning and Repositioning the Person (NNAAP™)

Name: ———————————————   Date: ———————————————

	S	U	Comments

Quality of Life
- Knocked before entering the person's room.
- Addressed the person by name.
- Introduced yourself by name and title.
- Explained the procedure to the person before beginning and during the procedure.
- Protected the person's rights during the procedure.
- Handled the person gently during the procedure.

Pre-Procedure
1. Followed *Delegation Guidelines:*
   a. *Preventing Work-Related Injuries*
   b. *Moving Persons in Bed*
   c. *Turning Persons*
   Reviewed *Promoting Safety and Comfort:*
   a. *Safely Handling, Moving, and Transferring the Person*
   b. *Preventing Work-Related Injuries*
   c. *Moving the Person to the Side of the Bed*
   d. *Turning Persons*
2. Practiced hand hygiene.
3. Identified the person. Checked the ID bracelet against the assignment sheet. Called the person by name.
4. Provided for privacy.
5. Locked the bed wheels.
6. Raised the bed for body mechanics. Bed rails were up.

Procedure
7. Lowered the head of the bed to a level appropriate for the person. It was as flat as possible.
8. Stood on the side of the bed opposite to where you would turn the person.
9. Lowered the bed rail near you.
10. Moved the person to the side near you. (Followed the procedure for *Moving the Person to the Side of the Bed*.)
11. Crossed the person's arms over the person's chest. Crossed the leg near you over the far leg.
12. Turning the person away from you:
    a. Stood with a wide base of support. Flexed the knees.
    b. Placed one hand on the person's shoulder. Placed the other on the hip near you.
    c. Rolled the person gently away from you toward the raised bed rail. Shifted your weight from your rear leg to your front leg.
13. Turning the person toward you:
    a. Raised the bed rail.
    b. Went to the other side. Lowered the bed rail.
    c. Stood with a wide base of support. Flexed your knees.
    d. Placed one hand on the person's far shoulder. Placed the other on the far hip.
    e. Rolled the person toward you gently.

Date of Satisfactory Completion ————————————   Instructor's Initials ————————————

Procedure—cont'd	S	U	Comments
14. Positioned the person. Followed the nurse's directions and the care plan. The following is common:			
a. Placed a pillow under the head and neck.	_____	_____	_____
b. Adjusted the shoulder. The person did not lie on an arm.	_____	_____	_____
c. Placed a small pillow under the upper hand and arm.	_____	_____	_____
d. Positioned a pillow against the back.	_____	_____	_____
e. Flexed the upper knee. Positioned the upper leg in front of the lower leg.	_____	_____	_____
f. Supported the upper leg and thigh on pillows. Made sure the ankle was supported.	_____	_____	_____

Post-Procedure

	S	U	Comments
15. Provided for comfort as noted on the inside of the front textbook cover.	_____	_____	_____
16. Placed the signal light within reach.	_____	_____	_____
17. Lowered the bed to its lowest position.	_____	_____	_____
18. Raised or lowered bed rails. Followed the care plan.	_____	_____	_____
19. Unscreened the person.	_____	_____	_____
20. Completed a safety check of the room as noted on the inside of the front textbook cover.	_____	_____	_____
21. Decontaminated your hands.	_____	_____	_____
22. Reported and recorded your observations.	_____	_____	_____

Date of Satisfactory Completion _____ Instructor's Initials _____

Logrolling the Person

Name: _____   Date: _____

	S	U	Comments
Quality of Life			
• Knocked before entering the person's room.	___	___	_____
• Addressed the person by name.	___	___	_____
• Introduced yourself by name and title.	___	___	_____
• Explained the procedure to the person before beginning and during the procedure.	___	___	_____
• Protected the person's rights during the procedure.	___	___	_____
• Handled the person gently during the procedure.	___	___	_____

Pre-Procedure

1. Followed *Delegation Guidelines:*   ___ ___ _____
   a. *Preventing Work-Related Injuries*
   b. *Moving Persons in Bed*
   c. *Turning Persons*
   Reviewed *Promoting Safety and Comfort:*   ___ ___ _____
   a. *Safely Handling, Moving, and Transferring the Person*
   b. *Preventing Work-Related Injuries*
   c. *Turning Persons*
   d. *Logrolling*
2. Asked a co-worker to help.   ___ ___ _____
3. Practiced hand hygiene.   ___ ___ _____
4. Identified the person. Checked the ID bracelet against the   ___ ___ _____
   assignment sheet. Called the person by name.
5. Provided for privacy.   ___ ___ _____
6. Locked the bed wheels.   ___ ___ _____
7. Raised the bed for body mechanics. Bed rails were up   ___ ___ _____
   if used.

Procedure

8. Made sure the bed was flat.   ___ ___ _____
9. Stood on the side opposite to which you would turn   ___ ___ _____
   the person. Your co-worker stood on the other side.
10. Lowered the bed rails if used.   ___ ___ _____
11. Moved the person as a unit to the side of the bed near you.   ___ ___ _____
    Used the assist device. (If the person had a spinal cord
    injury, assisted the nurse as directed.)
12. Placed the person's arms across the chest. Placed a pillow   ___ ___ _____
    between the knees.
13. Raised the bed rail if used.   ___ ___ _____
14. Went to the other side.   ___ ___ _____
15. Stood near the shoulders and chest. Your co-worker stood   ___ ___ _____
    near the hips and thighs.
16. Stood with a broad base of support. One foot was in   ___ ___ _____
    front of the other.
17. Asked the person to hold his or her body rigid.   ___ ___ _____
18. Rolled the person toward you or used the assist device.   ___ ___ _____
    Turned the person as a unit.

Date of Satisfactory Completion _____   Instructor's Initials _____

Procedure—cont'd	S	U	Comments
19. Positioned the person in good alignment. Used pillows as directed by the nurse and care plan. The following is common unless the spinal cord is involved:			
a. One pillow against the back for support	_____	_____	_____
b. One pillow under the head and neck if allowed	_____	_____	_____
c. One pillow or a folded bath blanket between the legs	_____	_____	_____
d. A small pillow under the upper arm and hand	_____	_____	_____

Post-Procedure

	S	U	Comments
20. Provided for comfort as noted on the inside of the front textbook cover.	_____	_____	_____
21. Placed the signal light within reach.	_____	_____	_____
22. Lowered the bed to its lowest position.	_____	_____	_____
23. Raised or lowered bed rails. Followed the care plan.	_____	_____	_____
24. Unscreened the person.	_____	_____	_____
25. Completed a safety check of the room as noted on the inside of the front textbook cover.	_____	_____	_____
26. Decontaminated your hands.	_____	_____	_____
27. Reported and recorded your observations.	_____	_____	_____

Date of Satisfactory Completion _____   Instructor's Initials _____

Sitting on the Side of the Bed (Dangling)

Name: _____   Date: _____

	S	U	Comments

Quality of Life
- Knocked before entering the person's room.   _____ _____ _____
- Addressed the person by name.   _____ _____ _____
- Introduced yourself by name and title.   _____ _____ _____
- Explained the procedure to the person before beginning _____ _____ _____
  and during the procedure.
- Protected the person's rights during the procedure.   _____ _____ _____
- Handled the person gently during the procedure.   _____ _____ _____

Pre-Procedure
1. Followed *Delegation Guidelines:*   _____ _____ _____
   a. *Preventing Work-Related Injuries*
   b. *Dangling*
   Reviewed *Promoting Safety and Comfort:*   _____ _____ _____
   a. *Safely Handling, Moving, and Transferring the Person*
   b. *Preventing Work-Related Injuries*
   c. *Dangling*
2. Asked a co-worker to help if the person would dangle. _____ _____ _____
3. Practiced hand hygiene.   _____ _____ _____
4. Identified the person. Checked the ID bracelet against the _____ _____ _____
   assignment sheet. Called the person by name.
5. Provided for privacy.   _____ _____ _____
6. Decided what side of the bed to use.   _____ _____ _____
7. Moved furniture to provide moving space.   _____ _____ _____
8. Locked the bed wheels.   _____ _____ _____
9. Raised the bed for body mechanics. Bed rails were up _____ _____ _____
   if used.

Procedure
10. Lowered the bed rail if up.   _____ _____ _____
11. Positioned the person in a side-lying position   _____ _____ _____
    facing you. The person laid on the strong side.
12. Raised the head of the bed to a sitting position.   _____ _____ _____
13. Stood by the person's hips. Faced the foot of the bed. _____ _____ _____
14. Stood with your feet apart. The foot near the head of the _____ _____ _____
    bed was in front of the other foot.
15. Slid one arm under the person's neck and shoulders. _____ _____ _____
    Grasped the far shoulder. Placed your other hand over
    the thighs near the knees.
16. Pivoted toward the foot of the bed while moving the   _____ _____ _____
    person's legs and feet over the side of the bed. As the legs
    went over the edge of the mattress, the trunk was upright.
17. Asked the person to hold on to the edge of the mattress. _____ _____ _____
    This supported the person in the sitting position.
    If possible, raised a half-length bed rail for the person
    to grasp. Raised the bed rail on the person's strong side.
    Your co-worker supported the person at all times.
18. Did not leave the person alone. Provided support   _____ _____ _____
    at all times.

Date of Satisfactory Completion _____   Instructor's Initials _____

Procedure—cont'd	S	U	Comments
19. Checked the person's condition:			
a. Asked how the person felt. Asked if the person felt dizzy or light-headed.	_____	_____	_____
b. Checked the pulse and respirations.	_____	_____	_____
c. Checked for difficulty breathing.	_____	_____	_____
d. Noted if the skin was pale or bluish in color.	_____	_____	_____
20. Reversed the procedure to return the person to bed. (Or prepared to transfer the person to a chair or wheelchair. Lowered the bed to its lowest position so the person's feet were flat on the floor. Supported the person at all times.)	_____	_____	_____
21. Lowered the head of the bed after the person returned to bed. Helped him or her move to the center of the bed.	_____	_____	_____
22. Positioned the person in good alignment.	_____	_____	_____

Post-Procedure

	S	U	Comments
23. Provided for comfort as noted on the inside of the front textbook cover.	_____	_____	_____
24. Placed the signal light within reach.	_____	_____	_____
25. Lowered the bed to its lowest position.	_____	_____	_____
26. Raised or lowered bed rails. Followed the care plan.	_____	_____	_____
27. Returned furniture to its proper place.	_____	_____	_____
28. Unscreened the person.	_____	_____	_____
29. Completed a safety check of the room as noted on the inside of the front textbook cover.	_____	_____	_____
30. Decontaminated your hands.	_____	_____	_____
31. Reported and recorded your observations.	_____	_____	_____

Date of Satisfactory Completion _____   Instructor's Initials _____

Transferring the Person to a Chair or Wheelchair (NNAAP™)

Name: ———————————————   Date: ————————————————

Quality of Life	S	U	Comments
• Knocked before entering the person's room.			
• Addressed the person by name.			
• Introduced yourself by name and title.			
• Explained the procedure to the person before beginning and during the procedure.			
• Protected the person's rights during the procedure.			
• Handled the person gently during the procedure.			

Pre-Procedure

1. Followed *Delegation Guidelines:*
   a. *Preventing Work-Related Injuries*
   b. *Transferring Persons*
   Reviewed *Promoting Safety and Comfort:*
   a. *Transfer/Gait Belts*
   b. *Safely Handling, Moving, and Transferring the Person*
   c. *Preventing Work-Related Injuries*
   d. *Transferring Persons*
   e. *Bed to Chair or Wheelchair Transfers*
2. Collected:
   a. Wheelchair or armchair
   b. Bath blanket
   c. Lap blanket
   d. Robe and non-skid footwear
   e. Paper or sheet
   f. Transfer belt if needed
   g. Seat cushion if needed
3. Practiced hand hygiene.
4. Identified the person. Checked the ID bracelet against the assignment sheet. Called the person by name.
5. Provided for privacy.
6. Decided which side of the bed to use. Moved furniture for a safe transfer.

Procedure

7. Positioned the chair:
   a. The chair was near the head of the bed on the person's strong side.
   b. The chair faced the foot of the bed.
   c. The arm of the chair almost touched the bed.
8. Placed a folded bath blanket or cushion on the seat if needed.
9. Locked wheelchair wheels. Raised the footplates. Removed or swung the front rigging out of the way.
10. Lowered the bed to its lowest position. Locked the bed wheels.
11. Fan-folded top linens to the foot of the bed.
12. Placed the paper or sheet under the person's feet. Put footwear on the person.
13. Helped the person sit on the side of the bed. His or her feet touched the floor.
14. Helped the person put on a robe.
15. Applied the transfer belt if needed.

Date of Satisfactory Completion ————————————————   Instructor's Initials ————————————————

Procedure—cont'd	S	U	Comments

16. Method 1—Using a transfer belt:
   a. Stood in front of the person.
   b. Had the person hold onto the mattress.
   c. Made sure the person's feet were flat on the floor.
   d. Had the person lean forward.
   e. Grasped the transfer belt at each side. Grasped the handles or grasped the belt from underneath.
   f. Prevented the person from sliding or falling by doing one of the following:
     (1) Braced your knees against the person's knees. Blocked the person's feet with your feet.
     (2) Used the knee and foot of one leg to block the person's weak leg or foot. Placed your other foot slightly behind you for balance.
     (3) Straddled your legs around the person's weak leg.
   g. Explained the following:
     (1) You will count "1, 2, 3."
     (2) The move will be on "3."
     (3) On "3" you will push down on the mattress and stand.
   h. Asked the person to push down on the mattress and to stand on the count of "3." Pulled the person into a standing position as you straightened your knees.

17. Method 2—No transfer belt (This method was used only if directed by the nurse and the care plan.):
   a. Followed steps 16a through 16c.
   b. Placed your hands under the person's arms. Your hands were around the person's shoulder blades.
   c. Had the person lean forward.
   d. Prevented the person from sliding or falling by doing one of the following:
     (1) Braced your knees against the person's knees. Blocked the person's feet with your feet.
     (2) Used the knee and foot of one leg to block the person's weak leg or foot. Placed your other foot slightly behind you for balance.
     (3) Straddled your legs around the person's weak leg.
   e. Explained the count of "3" as in step 16g.
   f. Asked the person to push down on the mattress and to stand on the count of "3." Pulled the person up into a standing position as you straightened your knees.

18. Supported the person in the standing position. Held the transfer belt, or kept your hands around the person's shoulder blades. Continued to prevent the person from sliding or falling.

19. Turned the person so he or she could grasp the far arm of the chair. The legs touched the edge of the chair.

20. Continued to turn the person until the other armrest was grasped.

21. Lowered the person into the chair as you bent your hips and knees. The person assisted by leaning forward and bending the elbows and knees.

Date of Satisfactory Completion _____ Instructor's Initials _____

Procedure—cont'd	S	U	Comments
22. Made sure the hips were to the back of the seat. Positioned the person in good alignment.			
23. Attached the wheelchair front rigging. Positioned the person's feet on the wheelchair footplates.			
24. Covered the person's lap and legs with a lap blanket. Kept the blanket off the floor and the wheels.			
25. Removed the transfer belt if used.			
26. Positioned the chair as the person preferred. Locked the wheelchair wheels according to the care plan.			

Post-Procedure

27. Provided for comfort as noted on the inside of the front textbook cover.			
28. Placed the signal light and other needed items within reach.			
29. Unscreened the person.			
30. Completed a safety check of the room as noted on the inside of the front textbook cover.			
31. Decontaminated your hands.			
32. Reported and recorded your observations.			
33. Followed the procedure *Transferring the Person From a Chair or Wheelchair to a Bed* to return the person to bed.			

Date of Satisfactory Completion _____   Instructor's Initials _____

Transferring the Person From a Chair or Wheelchair to a Bed

Name: _____   Date: _____

Quality of Life	S	U	Comments
• Knocked before entering the person's room.	____	____	_____
• Addressed the person by name.	____	____	_____
• Introduced yourself by name and title.	____	____	_____
• Explained the procedure to the person before beginning and during the procedure.	____	____	_____
• Protected the person's rights during the procedure.	____	____	_____
• Handled the person gently during the procedure.	____	____	_____

Pre-Procedure

1. Followed *Delegation Guidelines:*   ____ ____ _____
   a. *Preventing Work-Related Injuries*
   b. *Transferring Persons*
   Reviewed *Promoting Safety and Comfort:*   ____ ____ _____
   a. *Transfer/Gait Belts*
   b. *Safely Handling, Moving, and Transferring the Person*
   c. *Preventing Work-Related Injuries*
   d. *Transferring Persons*
   e. *Bed to Chair or Wheelchair Transfers*
2. Collected a transfer belt if needed.   ____ ____ _____
3. Practiced hand hygiene.   ____ ____ _____
4. Identified the person. Checked the ID bracelet against the assignment sheet. Called the person by name.   ____ ____ _____
5. Provided for privacy.   ____ ____ _____

Procedure

6. Moved furniture for moving space.   ____ ____ _____
7. Raised the head of the bed to a sitting position. The bed was in the lowest position.   ____ ____ _____
8. Moved the signal light so it was on the strong side when the person was in bed.   ____ ____ _____
9. Positioned the chair or wheelchair so the person's strong side was next to the bed. Had a co-worker help if necessary.   ____ ____ _____
10. Locked the wheelchair and bed wheels.   ____ ____ _____
11. Removed and folded the lap blanket.   ____ ____ _____
12. Removed the person's feet from the footplates. Raised the footplates. Removed or swung the front rigging out of the way. (The person had on non-skid footwear.)   ____ ____ _____
13. Applied the transfer belt if needed.   ____ ____ _____
14. Made sure the person's feet were flat on the floor.   ____ ____ _____
15. Stood in front of the person.   ____ ____ _____
16. Asked the person to hold onto the armrests. (If the nurse directed you to do so, placed your arms under the person's arms. Your hands were around the shoulder blades.)   ____ ____ _____
17. Had the person lean forward.   ____ ____ _____
18. Grasped the transfer belt on each side if using it. Grasped underneath the belt.   ____ ____ _____

Date of Satisfactory Completion _____   Instructor's Initials _____

Procedure—cont'd	S	U	Comments

19. Prevented the person from sliding or falling by doing one of the following:
    a. Braced your knees against the person's knees. Blocked the person's feet with your feet.
    b. Used the knee and foot of one leg to block the person's weak leg or foot. Placed your other foot slightly behind you for balance.
    c. Straddled your legs around the person's weak leg.
20. Explained the count of "3" as in procedure *Transferring the Person to a Chair or Wheelchair*.
21. Asked the person to push down on the armrests on the count of "3." Pulled the person into a standing position as you straightened your knees.
22. Supported the person in the standing position. Held the transfer belt or kept your hands around the person's shoulder blades. Continued to prevent the person from sliding or falling.
23. Turned the person so he or she could reach the edge of the mattress. The person's legs touched the mattress.
24. Continued to turn the person until he or she could reach the mattress with both hands.
25. Lowered the person onto the bed as you bent your hips and knees. The person assisted by leaning forward and bending the elbows and knees.
26. Removed the transfer belt.
27. Removed the robe and footwear.
28. Helped the person lie down.

Post-Procedure
29. Provided for comfort as noted on the inside of the front textbook cover.
30. Placed the signal light and other needed items within reach.
31. Raised or lowered bed rails. Followed the care plan.
32. Arranged furniture to meet the person's needs.
33. Unscreened the person.
34. Completed a safety check of the room as noted on the inside of the front textbook cover.
35. Decontaminated your hands.
36. Reported and recorded your observations.

Date of Satisfactory Completion _____ Instructor's Initials _____

Transferring the Person Using a Mechanical Lift

View Video!

Name: _____   Date: _____

Quality of Life	S	U	Comments
• Knocked before entering the person's room.	___	___	_____
• Addressed the person by name.	___	___	_____
• Introduced yourself by name and title.	___	___	_____
• Explained the procedure to the person before beginning and during the procedure.	___	___	_____
• Protected the person's rights during the procedure.	___	___	_____
• Handled the person gently during the procedure.	___	___	_____

Pre-Procedure

1. Followed *Delegation Guidelines:*   ___ ___ _____
   a. *Preventing Work-Related Injuries*
   b. *Transferring Persons*
   c. *Using Mechanical Lifts*
   Reviewed *Promoting Safety and Comfort:*   ___ ___ _____
   a. *Safely Handling, Moving, and Transferring the Person*
   b. *Preventing Work-Related Injuries*
   c. *Transferring Persons*
   d. *Using Mechanical Lifts*
2. Asked a co-worker to help.   ___ ___ _____
3. Collected:
   a. Mechanical lift
   b. Arm chair or wheelchair
   c. Footwear
   d. Bath blanket or cushion
   e. Lap blanket
4. Practiced hand hygiene.   ___ ___ _____
5. Identified the person. Checked the ID bracelet against   ___ ___ _____
   the assignment sheet. Called the person by name.
6. Provided for privacy.   ___ ___ _____

Procedure

7. Raised the bed for body mechanics. Bed rails were up   ___ ___ _____
   if used.
8. Lowered the head of the bed to a level appropriate   ___ ___ _____
   for the person. It was as flat as possible.
9. Stood on one side of the bed. Your co-worker stood on   ___ ___ _____
   the other side.
10. Lowered the bed rails if up.   ___ ___ _____
11. Centered the sling under the person. To position the sling,   ___ ___ _____
    turned the person from side to side as if making an
    occupied bed. Positioned the sling according to the
    manufacturer's instructions.
12. Positioned the person in the semi-Fowler's position.   ___ ___ _____
13. Placed the chair at the head of the bed. It was even with   ___ ___ _____
    the headboard and about 1 foot away from the bed. Placed
    a folded bath blanket or cushion in the chair.
14. Locked the bed wheels. Lowered the bed to its   ___ ___ _____
    lowest position.
15. Raised the lift so it could be positioned over the person.   ___ ___ _____
16. Positioned the lift over the person.   ___ ___ _____
17. Locked the lift wheels in position.   ___ ___ _____

Date of Satisfactory Completion _____   Instructor's Initials _____

Procedure—cont'd	S	U	Comments
18. Attached the sling to the swivel bar.	———	———	———————
19. Raised the head of the bed to a sitting position.	———	———	———————
20. Crossed the person's arms over the chest. If needed, let the person hold onto the straps or chains, not the swivel bar.	———	———	———————
21. Raised the lift high enough until the person and sling were free of the bed.	———	———	———————
22. Had your co-worker support the person's legs as you moved the lift and the person away from the bed.	———	———	———————
23. Positioned the lift so the person's back was toward the chair.	———	———	———————
24. Positioned the chair so the person could be lowered into it.	———	———	———————
25. Lowered and guided the person into the chair.	———	———	———————
26. Lowered the swivel bar to unhook the sling. Removed the sling from under the person unless otherwise indicated.	———	———	———————
27. Put footwear on the person. Positioned the person's feet on the wheelchair footplates.	———	———	———————
28. Covered the person's lap and legs with a lap blanket. Kept it off the floor and wheels.	———	———	———————
29. Positioned the chair as the person preferred. Locked the wheelchair wheels according to the care plan.	———	———	———————

Post-Procedure

	S	U	Comments
30. Provided for comfort as noted on the inside of the front textbook cover.	———	———	———————
31. Placed the signal light and other needed items within the person's reach.	———	———	———————
32. Unscreened the person.	———	———	———————
33. Completed a safety check of the room as noted on the inside of the front textbook cover.	———	———	———————
34. Decontaminated your hands.	———	———	———————
35. Reported and recorded your observations.	———	———	———————
36. Reversed the procedure to return the person to bed.	———	———	———————

Date of Satisfactory Completion _____   Instructor's Initials _____

Transferring the Person to and From the Toilet

Name: _____   Date: _____

Quality of Life	S	U	Comments
• Knocked before entering the person's room.			
• Addressed the person by name.			
• Introduced yourself by name and title.			
• Explained the procedure to the person before beginning and during the procedure.			
• Protected the person's rights during the procedure.			
• Handled the person gently during the procedure.			

Pre-Procedure

1. Followed *Delegation Guidelines:*
   a. *Preventing Work-Related Injuries*
   b. *Transferring Persons*
   Reviewed *Promoting Safety and Comfort:*
   a. *Transfer/Gait Belts*
   b. *Safely Handling, Moving, and Transferring the Person*
   c. *Preventing Work-Related Injuries*
   d. *Transferring Persons*
   e. *Bed to Chair or Wheelchair Transfers*
   f. *Transferring the Person to and From the Toilet*
2. Practiced hand hygiene.

Procedure

3. Had the person wear non-skid footwear.
4. Positioned the wheelchair next to the toilet if there was enough room. If not, positioned the wheelchair at a right angle (90-degree angle) to the toilet. (If possible, the person's strong side was near the toilet.)
5. Locked the wheelchair wheels.
6. Raised the footplates. Removed or swung front rigging out of the way.
7. Applied the transfer belt.
8. Helped the person unfasten clothing.
9. Used the transfer belt to help the person stand and to turn to the toilet. (See procedure *Transferring the Person to a Chair or Wheelchair.*) The person used the grab bars to turn to the toilet.
10. Supported the person with the transfer belt while he or she lowered clothing, or had the person hold onto the grab bars for support. Lowered the person's pants and undergarments.
11. Used the transfer belt to lower the person onto the toilet seat. Made sure he or she was properly positioned on the toilet.
12. Removed the transfer belt.
13. Told the person you would stay nearby. Reminded the person to use the signal light or call for help when needed. Stayed with the person if required by the care plan.
14. Closed the bathroom door to provide for privacy.
15. Stayed near the bathroom. Completed other tasks in the person's room. Checked on the person every 5 minutes.

Date of Satisfactory Completion _____   Instructor's Initials _____

Procedure—cont'd	S	U	Comments
16. Knocked on the bathroom door when the person called.	___	___	_____
17. Helped with wiping, perineal care, flushing, and hand washing as needed. Wore gloves, and practiced hand hygiene after removing gloves.	___	___	_____
18. Applied the transfer belt.	___	___	_____
19. Used the transfer belt to help the person stand.	___	___	_____
20. Helped the person raise and secure clothing.	___	___	_____
21. Used the transfer belt to transfer the person to the wheelchair. (See procedure *Transferring the Person to a Chair or Wheelchair*.)	___	___	_____
22. Made sure the person's buttocks were to the back of the seat. Positioned the person in good alignment.	___	___	_____
23. Positioned the person's feet on the footplates.	___	___	_____
24. Covered the person's lap and legs with a lap blanket. Kept the blanket off the floor and wheels.	___	___	_____
25. Positioned the chair as the person preferred. Locked the wheelchair wheels according to the care plan.	___	___	_____

Post-Procedure

	S	U	Comments
26. Provided for comfort as noted on the inside of the front textbook cover.	___	___	_____
27. Placed the signal light and other needed items within the person's reach.	___	___	_____
28. Unscreened the person.	___	___	_____
29. Completed a safety check of the room as noted on the inside of the front textbook cover.	___	___	_____
30. Practiced hand hygiene.	___	___	_____
31. Reported and recorded your observations.	___	___	_____

Date of Satisfactory Completion _____ Instructor's Initials _____

Making a Closed Bed

Name: _____   Date: _____

	S	U	Comments

Quality of Life
- Knocked before entering the person's room.
- Addressed the person by name.
- Introduced yourself by name and title.
- Explained the procedure to the person before beginning and during the procedure.
- Protected the person's rights during the procedure.
- Handled the person gently during the procedure.

Pre-Procedure
1. Followed *Delegation Guidelines: Making Beds*
   Reviewed *Promoting Safety and Comfort: Making Beds*
2. Practiced hand hygiene.
3. Collected clean linen:
   - Mattress pad (if needed)
   - Bottom sheet (flat sheet or fitted sheet)
   - Plastic drawsheet or waterproof pad (if needed)
   - Cotton drawsheet (if needed)
   - Top sheet
   - Blanket
   - Bedspread
   - A pillowcase for each pillow
   - Bath towel(s)
   - Hand towel
   - Washcloth
   - Gown or pajamas
   - Bath blanket
   - Gloves
   - Laundry bag
   - Paper towels (if required as a barrier for clean linens)
4. Placed linen on a clean surface. Used paper towels as a barrier between the clean surface and clean linen if required by agency policy.
5. Raised the bed for body mechanics. Bed rails were down.

Procedure
6. Put on the gloves.
7. Removed linen. Rolled each piece away from you. Placed each piece in a laundry bag. Discarded incontinence products or disposable bed protectors in the trash. Did not put them in the laundry bag.
8. Cleaned the bedframe and mattress if this is part of your job.
9. Removed and discarded gloves. Decontaminated your hands.
10. Moved the mattress to the head of the bed.
11. Put the mattress pad on the mattress. It was even with the top of the mattress.

Date of Satisfactory Completion _____   Instructor's Initials _____

Procedure—cont'd	S	U	Comments

12. Placed the bottom sheet on the mattress pad:
    a. Unfolded it length-wise.
    b. Placed the center crease in the middle of the bed.
    c. Positioned the lower edge even with the bottom of the mattress.
    d. Placed the large hem at the top and the small hem at the bottom.
    e. Faced hem-stitching downward, away from the person.
13. Opened the sheet. Fan-folded it to the other side of the bed.
14. Tucked the top of the sheet under the mattress. The sheet was tight and smooth.
15. Made a mitered corner if using a flat sheet.
16. Placed the waterproof drawsheet on the bed. It was placed in the middle of the mattress. Or, the waterproof pad was placed on the bed.
17. Opened the waterproof drawsheet. Fan-folded it to the other side of the bed.
18. Placed a cotton drawsheet over the waterproof drawsheet so it covered the entire waterproof drawsheet.
19. Opened the cotton drawsheet. Fan-folded it to the other side of the bed.
20. Tucked both drawsheets under the mattress or tucked each in separately.
21. Went to the other side of the bed.
22. Mitered the top corner of the flat bottom sheet.
23. Pulled the bottom sheet tight so there were no wrinkles. Tucked in the sheet.
24. Pulled the drawsheets tight so there were no wrinkles. Tucked both in together or separately.
25. Went to the other side of the bed.
26. Put the top sheet on the bed:
    a. Unfolded it length-wise.
    b. Placed the center crease in the middle.
    c. Placed the large hem even with the top of the mattress.
    d. Opened the sheet. Fan-folded it to the other side.
    e. Faced hem-stitching outward, away from the person.
    f. Did not tuck the bottom in yet.
    g. Did not tuck top linens in on the sides.
27. Placed the blanket on the bed:
    a. Unfolded it so the center crease was in the middle.
    b. Put the upper hem about 6 to 8 inches from the top of the mattress.
    c. Opened the blanket. Fan-folded it to the other side.
    d. If steps 33 and 34 will be done, turned the top sheet down over the blanket. Hem-stitching was down, away from the person.
28. Placed the bedspread on the bed:
    a. Unfolded it so the center crease was in the middle.
    b. Placed the upper hem even with the top of the mattress.
    c. Opened and fan-folded the bedspread to the other side.
    d. Made sure the bedspread facing the door was even. It covered all top linens.

Date of Satisfactory Completion _____   Instructor's Initials _____

Procedure—cont'd	S	U	Comments

29. Tucked in top linens together at the foot of the bed. They were smooth and tight. Made a mitered corner.
30. Went to the other side.
31. Straightened all top linen. Worked from the head of the bed to the foot.
32. Tucked in the top linens together at the foot of the bed. Made a mitered corner.
33. Turned the top hem of the bedspread under the blanket to make a cuff.
34. Turned the top sheet down over the bedspread. Hem-stitching was down. (If steps 33 and 34 were not done, the bedspread covered the pillow and was tucked under the pillow.)
35. Put the pillowcase on the pillow. Folded extra material under the pillow at the seam end of the pillowcase.
36. Placed the pillow on the bed. The open end of the pillowcase was away from the door. The seam was toward the head of the bed.

Post-Procedure

37. Provided for comfort as noted on the inside of the front textbook cover. (Omitted this step if bed was prepared for a new patient or resident.)
38. Attached the signal light to the bed, or placed it within the person's reach.
39. Lowered the bed to its lowest position. Locked the bed wheels.
40. Put towels, washcloth, gown or pajamas, and bath blanket in the bedside stand.
41. Completed a safety check of the room as noted on the inside of the front textbook cover.
42. Followed agency policy for dirty linen.
43. Decontaminated your hands.

Date of Satisfactory Completion _____ Instructor's Initials _____

Making an Occupied Bed (NNAAP™)

Name: _____   Date: _____

	S	U	Comments

Quality of Life
- Knocked before entering the person's room.
- Addressed the person by name.
- Introduced yourself by name and title.
- Explained the procedure to the person before beginning and during the procedure.
- Protected the person's rights during the procedure.
- Handled the person gently during the procedure.

Pre-Procedure
1. Followed *Delegation Guidelines: Making Beds*
   Reviewed *Promoting Safety and Comfort:*
   a. *Making Beds*
   b. *The Occupied Bed*
2. Practiced hand hygiene.
3. Collected the following:
   - Gloves
   - Laundry bag
   - Clean linen
   - Paper towels (if required as a barrier for clean linens)
4. Placed linen on a clean surface. Used paper towels as a barrier between the clean surface and clean linen if required by agency policy.
5. Identified the person. Checked the ID bracelet against the assignment sheet. Called the person by name.
6. Provided for privacy.
7. Removed the signal light.
8. Raised the bed for body mechanics. Bed rails were up if used.
9. Lowered the head of the bed. It was as flat as possible.

Procedure
10. Decontaminated hands. Put on gloves.
11. Loosened top linens at the foot of the bed.
12. Lowered the bed rail near you if up.
13. Removed the bedspread. Then removed the blanket. Placed each over the chair.
14. Covered the person with a bath blanket. Used the blanket in the bedside stand.
    a. Unfolded a bath blanket over the top sheet.
    b. Asked the person to hold onto the bath blanket. If the person could not, tucked the top part under the person's shoulders.
    c. Grasped the top sheet under the bath blanket at the shoulders. Brought the sheet down to the foot of the bed. Removed the sheet from under the blanket.
15. Positioned the person on the side of the bed away from you. Adjusted the pillow for comfort.
16. Loosened bottom linens from the head to the foot of the bed.
17. Fan-folded bottom linens one at a time toward the person. Started with the cotton drawsheet. (If re-using the mattress pad, did not fan-fold it.)

Date of Satisfactory Completion _____   Instructor's Initials _____

Procedure—cont'd   S   U   Comments

18. Placed a clean mattress pad on the bed. Unfolded   _____ _____ _____
    it length-wise. The center crease was in the middle.
    Fan-folded the top part toward the person. (If re-using
    the mattress pad, straightened and smoothed any
    wrinkles.)
19. Placed the bottom sheet on the mattress pad.   _____ _____ _____
    Hem-stitching was away from the person. Unfolded
    the sheet so the crease was in the middle. The small
    hem was even with the bottom of the mattress.
    Fan-folded the top part toward the person.
20. Made a mitered corner at the head of the bed.   _____ _____ _____
    Tucked the sheet under the mattress from the head
    to the foot.
21. Pulled the waterproof drawsheet toward you over the
    bottom sheet. Tucked excess material under the
    mattress. Did the following for a clean waterproof
    drawsheet:
    a. Placed the waterproof drawsheet on the bed. It was in _____ _____ _____
       the middle of the mattress.
    b. Fan-folded the top part toward the person.   _____ _____ _____
    c. Tucked in the excess fabric.   _____ _____ _____
22. Placed the cotton drawsheet over the waterproof drawsheet _____ _____ _____
    so it covered the entire waterproof drawsheet. Fan-folded
    the top part toward the person. Tucked in excess fabric.
23. Explained to the person that he or she would roll over _____ _____ _____
    a bump. Assured the person that he or she would
    not fall.
24. Helped the person turn to the other side. Adjusted the _____ _____ _____
    pillow for comfort.
25. Raised the bed rail. Went to the other side, and lowered _____ _____ _____
    the bed rail.
26. Loosened bottom linens. Removed one piece at a time. _____ _____ _____
    Placed each piece in the laundry bag. Discarded
    disposable bed protectors and incontinence products
    in the trash. (Did not put them in the laundry bag.)
27. Removed and discarded the gloves. Decontaminated   _____ _____ _____
    your hands.
28. Straightened and smoothed the mattress pad.   _____ _____ _____
29. Pulled the clean bottom sheet toward you. Made a   _____ _____ _____
    mitered corner at the top. Tucked the sheet under the
    mattress from the head to the foot of the bed.
30. Pulled the drawsheets tightly toward you. Tucked both _____ _____ _____
    under together or separately.
31. Positioned the person supine in the center of the bed. _____ _____ _____
    Adjusted the pillow for comfort.
32. Put the top sheet on the bed. Unfolded it length-wise. _____ _____ _____
    The crease was in the middle. The large hem was even
    with the top of the mattress. Hem-stitching was on
    the outside.
33. Asked the person to hold onto the top sheet so you _____ _____ _____
    could remove the bath blanket. Or tucked the top
    sheet under the person's shoulders. Removed the
    bath blanket.

Date of Satisfactory Completion _____   Instructor's Initials _____

Procedure—cont'd	S	U	Comments
34. Placed the blanket on the bed. Unfolded it so the crease was in the middle and it covered the person. The upper hem was 6 to 8 inches from the top of the mattress.	___	___	_____
35. Placed the bedspread on the bed. Unfolded it so the center crease was in the middle and it covered the person. The top hem was even with the mattress top.	___	___	_____
36. Turned the top hem of the bedspread under the blanket to make a cuff.	___	___	_____
37. Brought the top sheet down over the bedspread to form a cuff.	___	___	_____
38. Went to the foot of the bed.	___	___	_____
39. Made a 2-inch toe pleat across the foot of the bed. It was 6 to 8 inches from the foot of the bed.	___	___	_____
40. Lifted the mattress corner with one arm. Tucked all top linens under the mattress. Made a mitered corner.	___	___	_____
41. Raised the bed rail. Went to the other side and lowered the bed rail.	___	___	_____
42. Straightened and smoothed top linens.	___	___	_____
43. Tucked all top linens under the mattress. Made a mitered corner.	___	___	_____
44. Changed the pillowcase(s).	___	___	_____

Post-Procedure

	S	U	Comments
45. Provided for comfort as noted on the inside of the front textbook cover.	___	___	_____
46. Placed the signal light within reach.	___	___	_____
47. Lowered the bed to its lowest position. Locked the bed wheels.	___	___	_____
48. Raised or lowered bed rails. Followed the care plan.	___	___	_____
49. Put the towels, washcloth, gown or pajamas, and bath blanket in the bedside stand.	___	___	_____
50. Unscreened the person.	___	___	_____
51. Completed a safety check of the room as noted on the inside of the front textbook cover.	___	___	_____
52. Followed agency policy for dirty linen.	___	___	_____
53. Decontaminated hands.	___	___	_____

Date of Satisfactory Completion _____   Instructor's Initials _____

Making a Surgical Bed

Name:———————————————————— Date: ————————————————

Procedure	S	U	Comments
1. Followed *Delegation Guidelines: Making Beds* Reviewed *Promoting Safety and Comfort:* a. *Making Beds* b. *The Surgical Bed*	_____	_____	_____
2. Practiced hand hygiene.	_____	_____	_____
3. Collected the following:	_____	_____	_____
• Clean linen as for procedure Making a Closed Bed	_____	_____	_____
• Gloves	_____	_____	_____
• Laundry bag	_____	_____	_____
• Equipment requested by the nurse	_____	_____	_____
• Paper towels (if required as a barrier for clean linens)	_____	_____	_____
4. Placed linen on a clean surface. Used paper towels as a barrier between the clean surface and clean linen if required by agency policy.	_____	_____	_____
5. Removed the signal light.	_____	_____	_____
6. Raised the bed for body mechanics.	_____	_____	_____
7. Removed all linen from the bed. Wore gloves. Decontaminated your hands after removing gloves.	_____	_____	_____
8. Made a closed bed. (See procedure *Making a Closed Bed*.) Did not tuck the top linens under the mattress.	_____	_____	_____
9. Folded all top linens at the foot of the bed back onto the bed. The fold was even with the edge of the mattress.	_____	_____	_____
10. Fan-folded linen length-wise to the side of the bed farthest from the door.	_____	_____	_____
11. Put the pillowcase(s) on the pillow(s).	_____	_____	_____
12. Placed the pillow(s) on a clean surface.	_____	_____	_____
13. Left the bed in its highest position.	_____	_____	_____
14. Left both bed rails down.	_____	_____	_____
15. Put the towels, washcloth, gown or pajamas, and bath blanket in the bedside stand.	_____	_____	_____
16. Moved furniture away from the bed. Allowed room for the stretcher and for the staff.	_____	_____	_____
17. Did not attach the signal light to the bed.	_____	_____	_____
18. Completed a safety check of the room as noted on the inside of the front textbook cover.	_____	_____	_____
19. Followed agency policy for soiled linen.	_____	_____	_____
20. Decontaminated your hands.	_____	_____	_____

Date of Satisfactory Completion ——————————— Instructor's Initials ——————————

Brushing and Flossing the Person's Teeth (NNAAP™)

Name: _____ Date: _____

	S	U	Comments
Quality of Life			
• Knocked before entering the person's room.			
• Addressed the person by name.			
• Introduced yourself by name and title.			
• Explained the procedure to the person before beginning and during the procedure.			
• Protected the person's rights during the procedure.			
• Handled the person gently during the procedure.			
Pre-Procedure			
1. Followed *Delegation Guidelines: Oral Hygiene.* Reviewed *Promoting Safety and Comfort: Oral Hygiene.*			
2. Practiced hand hygiene.			
3. Collected the following:			
• Toothbrush with soft bristles			
• Toothpaste			
• Mouthwash (or other solution noted on the care plan)			
• Dental floss (if used)			
• Water glass with cool water			
• Straw			
• Kidney basin			
• Hand towel			
• Paper towels			
• Gloves			
4. Placed the paper towels on the overbed table. Arranged items on top of them.			
5. Identified the person. Checked the ID bracelet against the assignment sheet. Called the person by name.			
6. Provided for privacy.			
7. Raised the bed for body mechanics. Bed rails were up if used.			
Procedure			
8. Lowered the bed rail near you if up.			
9. Assisted the person to a sitting position or to a side-lying position near you.			
10. Placed the towel across the person's chest.			
11. Adjusted the overbed table so you could reach it with ease.			
12. Decontaminated your hands. Put on the gloves.			
13. Held the toothbrush over the kidney basin. Poured some water over the brush.			
14. Applied toothpaste to the toothbrush.			
15. Brushed the teeth gently.			
16. Brushed the tongue gently.			
17. Let the person rinse the mouth with water. Held the kidney basin under the person's chin. Repeated this step as needed.			
18. Flossed the person's teeth (optional):			
a. Broke off an 18-inch piece of floss from the dispenser.			
b. Held the floss between the middle fingers of each hand.			
c. Stretched the floss with your thumbs.			
d. Started at the upper back tooth on the right side. Worked around to the left side.			

Date of Satisfactory Completion _____   Instructor's Initials _____

Procedure—cont'd   S   U   Comments

    e. Moved the floss gently up and down between the teeth. _____ _____ _____
       Moved floss up and down against the sides of
       each tooth. Worked from the top of the crown to the
       gum line.

    f. Moved to a new section of floss after every _____ _____ _____
       second tooth.

    g. Flossed the lower teeth. Used up and down motions _____ _____ _____
       as for the upper teeth. Started on the right side.
       Worked around to the left side.

19. Let the person use mouthwash or other solution. Held the _____ _____ _____
    kidney basin under the chin.

20. Wiped the person's mouth and removed the towel. _____ _____ _____

21. Removed and discarded the gloves. Decontaminated _____ _____ _____
    your hands.

Post-Procedure

22. Provided for comfort as noted on the inside of the front _____ _____ _____
    textbook cover.

23. Placed the signal light within reach. _____ _____ _____

24. Lowered the bed to its lowest position. _____ _____ _____

25. Raised or lowered bed rails. Followed the care plan. _____ _____ _____

26. Cleaned and returned equipment to its proper place. _____ _____ _____
    Wore gloves.

27. Wiped off the overbed table with the paper towels. _____ _____ _____
    Discarded the paper towels.

28. Unscreened the person. _____ _____ _____

29. Completed a safety check of the room as noted on the _____ _____ _____
    inside of the front textbook cover.

30. Followed agency policy for dirty linen. _____ _____ _____

31. Removed the gloves. Decontaminated your hands. _____ _____ _____

32. Reported and recorded your observations. _____ _____ _____

Date of Satisfactory Completion _____ Instructor's Initials _____

Providing Mouth Care for the Unconscious Person

View Video! **Video CLIP** Name: _____ Date: _____

	S	U	Comments
Quality of Life			
• Knocked before entering the person's room.	___	___	_____
• Addressed the person by name.	___	___	_____
• Introduced yourself by name and title.	___	___	_____
• Explained the procedure to the person before beginning and during the procedure.	___	___	_____
• Protected the person's rights during the procedure.	___	___	_____
• Handled the person gently during the procedure.	___	___	_____

Pre-Procedure

1. Followed *Delegation Guidelines: Oral Hygiene.* Reviewed *Promoting Safety and Comfort:*
   a. *Oral Hygiene*
   b. *Mouth Care for the Unconscious Person*
2. Practiced hand hygiene.
3. Collected the following:
   • Cleaning agent according to the care plan
   • Sponge swabs
   • Padded tongue blade
   • Water glass or cup with cool water
   • Hand towel
   • Kidney basin
   • Lip lubricant
   • Paper towels
   • Gloves
4. Placed the paper towels on the overbed table. Arranged items on top of them.
5. Identified the person. Checked the ID bracelet against the assignment sheet. Called the person by name.
6. Provided for privacy.
7. Raised the bed for body mechanics. Bed rails were up if used.

Procedure

8. Lowered the bed rail near you if up.
9. Decontaminated your hands. Put on the gloves.
10. Positioned the person in a side-lying position near you. Turned the person's head well to the side.
11. Placed the towel under the person's face.
12. Placed the kidney basin under the chin.
13. Separated the upper and lower teeth. Used the padded tongue blade. Was gentle. Never used force. Asked the nurse for help as needed.
14. Cleaned the mouth using sponge swabs moistened with the cleaning agent.
    a. Cleaned the chewing and inner surfaces of the teeth.
    b. Cleaned the gums and outer surfaces of the teeth.
    c. Swabbed the roof of the mouth, inside of the cheeks, and the lips.
    d. Swabbed the tongue.
    e. Moistened a clean swab with water. Swabbed the mouth to rinse.
    f. Placed used swabs in the kidney basin.

Date of Satisfactory Completion _____ Instructor's Initials _____

Procedure—cont'd

	S	U	Comments
15. Applied lubricant to the lips.			
16. Removed the kidney basin and supplies.			
17. Wiped the person's mouth. Removed the towel.			
18. Removed and discarded the gloves. Decontaminated your hands.			

Post-Procedure

	S	U	Comments
19. Provided for comfort as noted on the inside of the front textbook cover.			
20. Placed the signal light within reach.			
21. Lowered the bed to its lowest position.			
22. Raised or lower bed rails. Followed the care plan.			
23. Cleaned and returned equipment to its proper place. Discarded disposable items. (Wore gloves.)			
24. Wiped off the overbed table with paper towels. Discarded the paper towels.			
25. Unscreened the person.			
26. Completed a safety check of the room as noted on the inside of the front textbook cover.			
27. Told the person that you were leaving the room. Told him or her when you would return.			
28. Followed agency policy for dirty linen.			
29. Removed the gloves. Decontaminated your hands.			
30. Reported and recorded your observations.			

Date of Satisfactory Completion _____   Instructor's Initials _____

Providing Denture Care (NNAAP™)

Name: _____   Date: _____

	S	U	Comments

Quality of Life
- Knocked before entering the person's room.
- Addressed the person by name.
- Introduced yourself by name and title.
- Explained the procedure to the person before beginning and during the procedure.
- Protected the person's rights during the procedure.
- Handled the person gently during the procedure.

Pre-Procedure
1. Followed *Delegation Guidelines: Oral Hygiene.*
   Reviewed *Promoting Safety and Comfort:*
   a. *Oral Hygiene*
   b. *Denture Care*
2. Practiced hand hygiene.
3. Collected the following:
   - Denture brush or toothbrush
   - Denture cup labeled with the person's name and room and bed number
   - Denture cleaning agent
   - Soft-bristled toothbrush or sponge swabs
   - Toothpaste
   - Water glass with cool water
   - Straw
   - Mouthwash or other noted solution
   - Kidney basin
   - Two hand towels
   - Gauze squares
   - Paper towels
   - Gloves
4. Placed the paper towels on the overbed table. Arranged items on top of them.
5. Identified the person. Checked the ID bracelet against the assignment sheet. Called the person by name.
6. Provided for privacy.
7. Raised the bed for body mechanics.

Procedure
8. Lowered the bed rail near you if used.
9. Decontaminated your hands. Put on the gloves.
10. Placed a towel over the person's chest.
11. Asked the person to remove the dentures. Carefully placed them in the kidney basin.
12. Removed the dentures if the person could not do so. Used gauze squares to get a good grip on the dentures.
    a. Grasped the upper denture with your thumb and index finger. Moved it up and down slightly to break the seal. Gently removed the denture. Placed it in the kidney basin.
    b. Grasped and removed the lower denture with your thumb and index finger. Turned it slightly and lifted it out of the person's mouth. Placed it in the kidney basin.

Date of Satisfactory Completion _____   Instructor's Initials _____

Procedure—cont'd	S	U	Comments
13. Followed the care plan for raising bed rails.	___	___	_____
14. Took the kidney basin, denture cup, denture brush, and denture cleaning agent to the sink.	___	___	_____
15. Lined the sink with a towel. Filled the sink half-way with water.	___	___	_____
16. Rinsed each denture under cool or warm running water. Followed agency policy for water temperature.	___	___	_____
17. Returned dentures to the kidney basin or denture cup.	___	___	_____
18. Applied denture cleaning agent to the brush.	___	___	_____
19. Brushed the dentures.	___	___	_____
20. Rinsed dentures under running water. Used warm or cool water as directed by the cleaning agent manufacturer. (Some states require cool water.)	___	___	_____
21. Rinsed the denture cup and lid. Placed dentures in the denture cup. Covered the dentures with cool or warm water. Followed agency policy for water temperature.	___	___	_____
22. Cleaned the kidney basin.	___	___	_____
23. Took the denture cup and kidney basin to the overbed table.	___	___	_____
24. Lowered the bed rail if up.	___	___	_____
25. Positioned the person for oral hygiene.	___	___	_____
26. Cleaned the person's gums and tongue, using toothpaste and the toothbrush (or sponge swabs).	___	___	_____
27. Had the person use mouthwash or noted solution. Held the kidney basin under the chin.	___	___	_____
28. Asked the person to insert the dentures. Inserted them if the person could not.			
a. Held the upper denture firmly with your thumb and index finger. Raised the upper lip with the other hand. Inserted the denture. Gently pressed on the denture with your index fingers to make sure it was in place.	___	___	_____
b. Held the lower denture with your thumb and index finger. Pulled the lower lip down slightly. Inserted the denture. Gently pressed down on it to make sure it was in place.	___	___	_____
29. Placed the denture cup in the top drawer of the bedside stand if the dentures were not worn. The dentures were in water or in a denture soaking solution.	___	___	_____
30. Wiped the person's mouth. Removed the towel.	___	___	_____
31. Removed the gloves. Decontaminated your hands.	___	___	_____

Post-Procedure

	S	U	Comments
32. Assisted with hand washing.	___	___	_____
33. Provided for comfort as noted on the inside of the front textbook cover.	___	___	_____
34. Placed the signal light within reach.	___	___	_____
35. Lowered the bed to its lowest position.	___	___	_____
36. Raised or lowered bed rails. Followed the care plan.	___	___	_____
37. Removed the towel from the sink. Drained the sink.	___	___	_____
38. Cleaned and returned equipment to its proper place. Discarded disposable items. Wore gloves for this step.	___	___	_____

Date of Satisfactory Completion _____ Instructor's Initials _____

Post-Procedure—cont'd	S	U	Comments
39. Wiped off the overbed table with paper towels. Discarded the paper towels.	_____	_____	_____
40. Unscreened the person.	_____	_____	_____
41. Completed a safety check of the room as noted on the inside of the front textbook cover.	_____	_____	_____
42. Followed agency policy for dirty linen.	_____	_____	_____
43. Removed gloves. Decontaminated your hands.	_____	_____	_____
44. Reported and recorded your observations.	_____	_____	_____

Date of Satisfactory Completion _____ Instructor's Initials _____

Giving a Complete Bed Bath (NNAAP™)

Name: ————————————   Date: ————————————

Quality of Life	S	U	Comments
• Knocked before entering the person's room.			
• Addressed the person by name.			
• Introduced yourself by name and title.			
• Explained the procedure to the person before beginning and during the procedure.			
• Protected the person's rights during the procedure.			
• Handled the person gently during the procedure.			

Pre-Procedure

1. Followed *Delegation Guidelines: Bathing*. Reviewed *Promoting Safety and Comfort: Bathing*.
2. Practiced hand hygiene.
3. Identified the person. Checked the ID bracelet against the assignment sheet. Called the person by name.
4. Collected clean linen for a closed bed. (See procedure *Making a Closed Bed* in Chapter 14.) Placed linen on a clean surface.
5. Collected the following:
   Wash basin
   • Soap
   • Bath thermometer
   • Orange stick or nail file
   • Washcloth
   • Two bath towels and two hand towels
   • Bath blanket
   • Clothing or sleepwear
   • Lotion
   • Powder
   • Deodorant or antiperspirant
   • Brush and comb
   • Other grooming items as requested
   • Paper towels
   • Gloves
6. Covered the overbed table with paper towels. Arranged items on the overbed table. Adjusted the height as needed.
7. Provided for privacy.
8. Raised the bed for body mechanics. Bed rails were up if used.

Procedure

9. Removed the signal light.
10. Decontaminated your hands. Put on gloves.
11. Covered the person with a bath blanket. Removed top linens. (See procedure *Making an Occupied Bed* in Chapter 14.)
12. Lowered the head of the bed. It was as flat as possible. The person had at least one pillow.
13. Filled the wash basin two-thirds full with water. (Water temperature was 110° to 115° F [43.3° to 46.1° C] for adults or as directed by the nurse.) Measured water temperature. Used a bath thermometer or tested the water by dipping your elbow or inner wrist into the basin.

Date of Satisfactory Completion ————————————   Instructor's Initials ————————————

Procedure—cont'd	**S**	**U**	**Comments**
14. Lowered the bed rail near you if up.	_____	_____	_____
15. Asked the person to check the water temperature. Adjusted temperature if too hot or too cold. Raised the bed rail before leaving the bedside. Lowered it when you returned.	_____	_____	_____
16. Placed the basin on the overbed table.	_____	_____	_____
17. Removed the sleepwear. Did not expose the person.	_____	_____	_____
18. Placed a hand towel over the person's chest.	_____	_____	_____
19. Made a mitt with the washcloth. Used a mitt for the entire bath.	_____	_____	_____

20. Washed around the person's eyes with water. Did not use soap.
   a. Cleaned the far eye. Gently wiped from the inner to the outer aspect of the eye with a corner of the mitt.
   b. Cleaned around the near eye. Used a clean part of the washcloth for each stroke.
	_____	_____	_____

21. Asked the person if you should use soap to wash the face.	_____	_____	_____
22. Washed the face, ears, and neck. Rinsed and patted dry with the towel on the chest.	_____	_____	_____
23. Helped the person move to the side of the bed near you.	_____	_____	_____
24. Exposed the far arm. Placed a bath towel length-wise under the arm. Applied soap to the washcloth.	_____	_____	_____
25. Supported the arm with your palm under the person's elbow. The person's forearm rested on your forearm.	_____	_____	_____
26. Washed the arm, shoulder, and underarm. Used long, firm strokes. Rinsed and patted dry.	_____	_____	_____
27. Placed the basin on the towel. Put the person's hand into the water. Washed it well. Cleaned under the fingernails with an orange stick or nail file.	_____	_____	_____
28. Had the person exercise the hand and fingers.	_____	_____	_____
29. Removed the basin. Dried the hand well. Covered the arm with the bath blanket.	_____	_____	_____
30. Repeated steps 24 to 29 for the near arm.	_____	_____	_____
31. Placed a bath towel over the chest cross-wise. Held the towel in place. Pulled the bath blanket from under the towel to the waist. Applied soap to the washcloth.	_____	_____	_____
32. Lifted the towel slightly and washed the chest. Did not expose the person. Rinsed and patted dry, especially under breasts.	_____	_____	_____
33. Moved the towel length-wise over the chest and abdomen. Did not expose the person. Pulled the bath blanket down to the pubic area. Applied soap to the washcloth.	_____	_____	_____
34. Lifted the towel slightly and washed the abdomen. Rinsed and patted dry.	_____	_____	_____
35. Pulled the bath blanket up to the shoulders, covering both arms. Removed the towel.	_____	_____	_____
36. Changed soapy or cool water. Measured bath water temperature as in step 13. If bed rails were used, raised the bed rail near you before leaving the bedside. Lowered it when you returned.	_____	_____	_____

Date of Satisfactory Completion _____   Instructor's Initials _____

Procedure—cont'd	S	U	Comments
37. Uncovered the far leg. Did not expose the genital area. Placed a towel length-wise under the foot and leg. Applied soap to the washcloth.	___	___	_____
38. Bent the knee and supported the leg with your arm. Washed it with long, firm strokes. Rinsed and patted dry.	___	___	_____
39. Placed the basin on the towel near the foot.	___	___	_____
40. Lifted the leg slightly. Slid the basin under the foot.	___	___	_____
41. Placed the foot in the basin. Used an orange stick or nail file to clean under toenails if necessary. If the person could not bend the knees:	___	___	_____
a. Washed the foot. Carefully separated the toes. Rinsed and patted dry.	___	___	_____
b. Cleaned under the toenails with an orange stick or nail file if necessary.	___	___	_____
42. Removed the basin. Dried the leg and foot. Applied lotion to the foot if directed by the nurse and the care plan. Covered the leg with the bath blanket. Removed the towel.	___	___	_____
43. Repeated steps 37 to 42 for the near leg.	___	___	_____
44. Changed the water. Measured water temperature as in step 13. If bed rails were used, raised the bed rail near you before leaving the bedside. Lowered it when you returned.	___	___	_____
45. Turned the person onto the side away from you. The person was covered with the bath blanket.	___	___	_____
46. Uncovered the back and buttocks. Did not expose the person. Placed a towel length-wise on the bed along the back. Applied soap to the washcloth.	___	___	_____
47. Washed the back. Worked from the back of the neck to the lower end of the buttocks. Used long, firm, continuous strokes. Rinsed and dried well.	___	___	_____
48. Gave a back massage (unless the person preferred a back massage after the bath).	___	___	_____
49. Turned the person onto his or her back.	___	___	_____
50. Changed the water for perineal care. Measured water temperature as in step 13. Changed gloves and performed hand hygiene if required by the state competency test. If bed rails were used, raised the bed rail near you before leaving the bedside. Lowered it when you returned.	___	___	_____
51. Let the person wash the genital area. Adjusted the overbed table so the person could reach the wash basin, soap, and towels with ease. Placed the signal light within reach. Asked the person to signal when finished. Made sure the person understood what to do.	___	___	_____
52. Removed the gloves. Decontaminated your hands.	___	___	_____
53. Answered the signal light promptly. Knocked before entering the room. Provided perineal care if the person could not do so. (Decontaminated your hands and wore gloves for perineal care.)	___	___	_____
54. Gave a back massage if you had not already done so.	___	___	_____
55. Applied deodorant or antiperspirant. Applied lotion and powder as requested.	___	___	_____
56. Put clean garments on the person.	___	___	_____

Date of Satisfactory Completion _____ Instructor's Initials _____

Procedure—cont'd	S	U	Comments
57. Combed and brushed the hair.	_____	_____	_____
58. Made the bed.	_____	_____	_____
Post-Procedure			
59. Provided for comfort as noted on the inside of the front textbook cover.	_____	_____	_____
60. Placed the signal light within reach.	_____	_____	_____
61. Lowered the bed to its lowest position.	_____	_____	_____
62. Raised or lowered bed rails. Followed the care plan.	_____	_____	_____
63. Put on clean gloves.	_____	_____	_____
64. Emptied, cleaned, and dried the wash basin. Returned it and other supplies to their proper place.	_____	_____	_____
65. Wiped off the overbed table with paper towels. Discarded the paper towels.	_____	_____	_____
66. Unscreened the person.	_____	_____	_____
67. Completed a safety check of the room as noted on the inside of the front textbook cover.	_____	_____	_____
68. Followed agency policy for dirty linen.	_____	_____	_____
69. Removed gloves. Decontaminated your hands.	_____	_____	_____
70. Reported and recorded your observations.	_____	_____	_____

Date of Satisfactory Completion _____   Instructor's Initials _____

Assisting With the Partial Bath

Name: _____   Date: _____

	S	U	Comments
Quality of Life			
• Knocked before entering the person's room.	___	___	_____
• Addressed the person by name.	___	___	_____
• Introduced yourself by name and title.	___	___	_____
• Explained the procedure to the person before beginning and during the procedure.	___	___	_____
• Protected the person's rights during the procedure.	___	___	_____
• Handled the person gently during the procedure.	___	___	_____

Pre-Procedure
1. Followed *Delegation Guidelines: Bathing*. Reviewed *Promoting Safety and Comfort: Bathing*.
2. Followed steps 2 through 7 in procedure *Giving a Complete Bed Bath*.

Procedure
3. Made sure the bed was in the lowest position.
4. Decontaminated your hands. Put on gloves.
5. Covered the person with a bath blanket. Removed top linens.
6. Filled the wash basin two-thirds full with water. (Water temperature was 110° to 115° F [43.3° to 46.1° C] or as directed by the nurse.) Measured water temperature with the bath thermometer, or tested bath water by dipping your elbow or inner wrist into the basin.
7. Asked the person to check the water temperature. Adjusted temperature if too hot or too cold.
8. Placed the basin on the overbed table.
9. Positioned the person in Fowler's position or assisted the person to sit at the bedside.
10. Adjusted the overbed table so the person could reach the basin and supplies.
11. Helped the person undress. Provided for privacy and warmth with the bath blanket.
12. Asked the person to wash easy to reach body parts. Explained that you would wash the back and areas the person could not reach.
13. Placed the signal light within reach. Asked the person to signal when help was needed or bathing was complete.
14. Left the room after decontaminating your hands.
15. Returned when the signal light was on. Knocked before entering. Decontaminated your hands.
16. Changed the bath water. Measured bath water temperature as in step 6.
17. Raised the bed for body mechanics. The far bed rail was up if used.
18. Asked what was washed. Put on gloves. Washed and dried areas the person could not reach. Made sure that the face, hands, underarms, back, buttocks, and perineal area were washed.
19. Removed the gloves. Decontaminated your hands.

Date of Satisfactory Completion _____   Instructor's Initials _____

Procedure—cont'd	S	U	Comments
20. Gave a back massage. (See procedure *Giving a Back Massage*.)	_____	_____	_____
21. Applied lotion, powder, and deodorant or antiperspirant as requested.	_____	_____	_____
22. Helped the person put on clean garments.	_____	_____	_____
23. Assisted with hair care and other grooming needs.	_____	_____	_____
24. Assisted the person to a chair. (Lowered the bed if the person transferred to a chair.) Otherwise, turned the person onto the side away from you.	_____	_____	_____
25. Made the bed. (Raised the bed for body mechanics.)	_____	_____	_____

Post-Procedure

	S	U	Comments
26. Provided for comfort as noted on the inside of the front textbook cover.	_____	_____	_____
27. Placed the signal light within reach.	_____	_____	_____
28. Lowered the bed to its lowest position.	_____	_____	_____
29. Raised or lowered bed rails. Followed the care plan.	_____	_____	_____
30. Put on clean gloves.	_____	_____	_____
31. Emptied, cleaned, and dried the bath basin. Returned the basin and supplies to their proper place.	_____	_____	_____
32. Wiped off the overbed table with the paper towels. Discarded the paper towels.	_____	_____	_____
33. Unscreened the person.	_____	_____	_____
34. Completed a safety check of the room as noted on the inside of the front textbook cover.	_____	_____	_____
35. Followed agency policy for dirty linen.	_____	_____	_____
36. Removed the gloves. Decontaminated your hands.	_____	_____	_____
37. Reported and recorded your observations.	_____	_____	_____

Date of Satisfactory Completion _____   Instructor's Initials _____

Assisting With a Tub Bath or Shower

Name:_____ Date:_____

Quality of Life	S	U	Comments
• Knocked before entering the person's room.	___	___	_____
• Addressed the person by name.	___	___	_____
• Introduced yourself by name and title.	___	___	_____
• Explained the procedure to the person before beginning and during the procedure.	___	___	_____
• Protected the person's rights during the procedure.	___	___	_____
• Handled the person gently during the procedure.	___	___	_____

Pre-Procedure

1. Followed *Delegation Guidelines:*
   a. *Bathing*
   b. *Tub Baths and Showers*
   Reviewed *Promoting Safety and Comfort:*
   a. *Bathing*
   b. *Tub Baths and Showers*
2. Reserved the bathtub or shower.
3. Practiced hand hygiene.
4. Identified the person. Checked the ID bracelet against the assignment sheet. Called the person by name.
5. Collected the following:
   • Washcloth and two bath towels
   • Soap
   • Bath thermometer (for a tub bath)
   • Clothing or sleepwear
   • Grooming items as requested
   • Robe and non-skid footwear
   • Rubber bath mat if needed
   • Disposable bath mat
   • Gloves
   • Wheelchair, shower chair, transfer bench, and so on as needed

Procedure

6. Placed items in the tub or shower room. Used the space provided or a chair.
7. Cleaned and disinfected the tub or shower.
8. Placed a rubber bath mat in the tub or on the shower floor. Did not block the drain.
9. Placed the disposable bath mat on the floor in front of the tub or shower.
10. Put the OCCUPIED sign on the door.
11. Returned to the person's room. Provided for privacy. Decontaminated your hands.
12. Helped the person sit on the side of the bed.
13. Helped the person put on a robe and non-skid footwear. (Or the person left clothing on.)
14. Assisted or transported the person to the tub or shower room.
15. Had the person sit on a chair if he or she walked to the tub or shower room.
16. Provided for privacy.

Date of Satisfactory Completion _____ Instructor's Initials _____

Procedure—cont'd	S	U	Comments

17. For a tub bath:
  a. Filled the tub half-way with warm water (105° F; 40.5° C). ____ ____ _____
  b. Measured water temperature with the bath thermometer or checked the digital display. ____ ____ _____
  c. Asked the person to check the water temperature. Adjusted temperature if it was too hot or too cold. ____ ____ _____
18. For a shower:
  a. Turned on the shower. ____ ____ _____
  b. Adjusted water temperature and pressure. Checked the digital display. ____ ____ _____
  c. Asked the person to check the water temperature. Adjusted water temperature if it was too hot or too cold. ____ ____ _____
19. Helped the person undress and remove footwear. ____ ____ _____
20. Helped the person into the tub or shower. Positioned the shower chair, and locked the wheels. ____ ____ _____
21. Assisted with washing if necessary. Wore gloves. ____ ____ _____
22. Asked the person to use the signal light when done or when help was needed. Reminded the person that a tub bath lasts no longer than 20 minutes. ____ ____ _____
23. Placed a towel across the chair. ____ ____ _____
24. Left the room if the person could bathe alone. If not, stayed in the room or nearby. Removed the gloves and decontaminated your hands if you left the room. ____ ____ _____
25. Checked the person at least every 5 minutes. ____ ____ _____
26. Returned when the person signaled. Knocked before entering. Decontaminated your hands. ____ ____ _____
27. Turned off the shower or drained the tub. Covered the person while the tub drained. ____ ____ _____
28. Helped the person out of the shower or tub and onto the chair. ____ ____ _____
29. Helped the person dry off. Patted gently. Dried under breasts, between skin folds, in the perineal area, and between the toes. ____ ____ _____
30. Assisted with lotion and other grooming items as needed. ____ ____ _____
31. Helped the person dress and put on footwear. ____ ____ _____
32. Helped the person return to the room. Provided for privacy. ____ ____ _____
33. Assisted the person to a chair or into bed. ____ ____ _____
34. Provided a back massage if the person returned to bed. ____ ____ _____
35. Assisted with hair care and other grooming needs. ____ ____ _____

Post-Procedure

36. Provided for comfort as noted on the inside of the front textbook cover. ____ ____ _____
37. Placed the signal light within reach. ____ ____ _____
38. Raised or lowered bed rails. Followed the care plan. ____ ____ _____
39. Unscreened the person ____ ____ _____
40. Completed a safety check of the room as noted on the inside of the front textbook cover. ____ ____ _____

Date of Satisfactory Completion _____   Instructor's Initials _____

Post-Procedure—cont'd

	S	U	Comments
41. Cleaned and disinfected the tub or shower. Removed soiled linen. Wore gloves.	_____	_____	_____
42. Discarded disposable items. Put the UNOCCUPIED sign on the door. Returned supplies to their proper place.	_____	_____	_____
43. Followed agency policy for dirty linen.	_____	_____	_____
44. Removed the gloves. Decontaminated your hands.	_____	_____	_____
45. Reported and recorded your observations.	_____	_____	_____

Date of Satisfactory Completion _____   Instructor's Initials _____

Giving a Back Massage

Name: _____   Date: _____

Quality of Life	S	U	Comments
• Knocked before entering the person's room.	___	___	_____
• Addressed the person by name.	___	___	_____
• Introduced yourself by name and title.	___	___	_____
• Explained the procedure to the person before beginning and during the procedure.	___	___	_____
• Protected the person's rights during the procedure.	___	___	_____
• Handled the person gently during the procedure.	___	___	_____

Pre-Procedure

	S	U	Comments
1. Followed *Delegation Guidelines: Back Massage.* Reviewed *Promoting Safety and Comfort: Back Massage.*	___	___	_____
2. Practiced hand hygiene.	___	___	_____
3. Identified the person. Checked the ID bracelet against the assignment sheet. Called the person by name.	___	___	_____
4. Collected the following:			
• Bath blanket	___	___	_____
• Bath towel	___	___	_____
• Lotion	___	___	_____
5. Provided for privacy.	___	___	_____
6. Raised the bed for body mechanics. Bed rails were up if used.	___	___	_____

Procedure

	S	U	Comments
7. Lowered the bed rail near you if up.	___	___	_____
8. Positioned the person in the prone or side-lying position with the back toward you.	___	___	_____
9. Exposed the back, shoulders, upper arms, and buttocks. Covered the rest of the body with the bath blanket.	___	___	_____
10. Laid the towel on the bed along the back (if the person was in a side-lying position).	___	___	_____
11. Warmed the lotion.	___	___	_____
12. Explained that the lotion may feel cool and wet.	___	___	_____
13. Applied lotion to the lower back area.	___	___	_____
14. Stroked up from the buttocks to the shoulders. Then stroked down over the upper arms. Stroked up the upper arms, across the shoulders, and down the back to the buttocks. Used firm strokes. Kept your hands in contact with the person's skin.			
15. Repeated step 14 for at least 3 minutes.	___	___	_____
16. Kneaded the back:			
a. Grasped the skin between your thumb and fingers.	___	___	_____
b. Kneaded half of the back. Started at the buttocks and moved up to the shoulder. Then kneaded down from the shoulder to the buttocks.	___	___	_____
c. Repeated on the other half of the back.	___	___	_____
17. Applied lotion to bony areas. Used circular motions with the tips of your index and middle fingers. (Did not massage reddened bony areas.)	___	___	_____
18. Used fast movements to stimulate. Used slow movements to relax the person.	___	___	_____

Date of Satisfactory Completion _____   Instructor's Initials _____

Procedure—cont'd	S	U	Comments
19. Stroked with long, firm movements to end the massage. Told the person you were finishing.	_____	_____	_____
20. Straightened and secured clothing or sleepwear.	_____	_____	_____
21. Covered the person. Removed the towel and bath blanket.	_____	_____	_____

Post-Procedure

	S	U	Comments
22. Provided for comfort as noted on the inside of the front textbook cover.	_____	_____	_____
23. Placed the signal light within reach.	_____	_____	_____
24. Lowered the bed to its lowest position.	_____	_____	_____
25. Raised or lowered bed rails. Followed the care plan.	_____	_____	_____
26. Returned lotion to its proper place.	_____	_____	_____
27. Unscreened the person.	_____	_____	_____
28. Completed a safety check of the room as noted on the inside of the front textbook cover.	_____	_____	_____
29. Followed agency policy for dirty linen.	_____	_____	_____
30. Decontaminated your hands.	_____	_____	_____
31. Reported and recorded your observations.	_____	_____	_____

Date of Satisfactory Completion _____   Instructor's Initials _____

Giving Female Perineal Care (NNAAP™)

View Video! Video CLIP

Name: _____   Date: _____

	S	U	Comments

Quality of Life
- Knocked before entering the person's room.
- Addressed the person by name.
- Introduced yourself by name and title.
- Explained the procedure to the person before beginning and during the procedure.
- Protected the person's rights during the procedure.
- Handled the person gently during the procedure.

Pre-Procedure
1. Followed *Delegation Guidelines: Perineal Care.* Reviewed *Promoting Safety and Comfort: Perineal Care.*
2. Practiced hand hygiene.
3. Collected the following:
   - Soap or other cleaning agent as directed
   - At least 4 washcloths
   - Bath towel
   - Bath blanket
   - Bath thermometer
   - Wash basin
   - Waterproof pad
   - Gloves
   - Paper towels
4. Covered the overbed table with paper towels. Arranged items on top of them.
5. Identified the person. Checked the ID bracelet against the assignment sheet. Called the person by name.
6. Provided for privacy.
7. Raised the bed for body mechanics. Bed rails were up if used.

Procedure
8. Lowered the bed rail near you if up.
9. Decontaminated your hands. Put on gloves.
10. Covered the person with a bath blanket. Moved top linens to the foot of the bed.
11. Positioned the person on the back.
12. Draped the person. (See Figure 15-24 in the textbook.)
13. Raised the bed rail if used.
14. Filled the wash basin. (Water temperature was 105° F to 109° F [40.5° C to 42.7° C]). Measured water temperature according to agency policy.
15. Asked the person to check the water temperature. Adjusted water temperature if too hot or too cold. Raised the bed rail before leaving the bedside. Lowered it when you returned.
16. Placed the basin on the overbed table.
17. Lowered the bed rail if up.
18. Helped the person flex her knees and spread her legs, or helped her spread her legs as much as possible with the knees straight.
19. Placed a waterproof pad under her buttocks. Protected the person and dry linen from wet or soiled incontinence product.

Date of Satisfactory Completion _____   Instructor's Initials _____

Procedure—cont'd	S	U	Comments
20. Folded the corner of the bath blanket between her legs onto her abdomen.	___	___	_____
21. Wet the washcloths.	___	___	_____
22. Squeezed out excess water from the washcloth. Made a mitted washcloth. Applied soap.	___	___	_____
23. Separated the labia. Cleaned downward from front to back with one stroke.	___	___	_____
24. Repeated steps 22 and 23 until the area was clean. Used a clean part of the washcloth for each stroke. Used more than one washcloth if needed.	___	___	_____
25. Rinsed the perineum with a clean washcloth. Separated the labia. Stroked downward from front to back. Repeated as necessary. Used a clean part of the washcloth for each stroke. Used more than one washcloth if needed.	___	___	_____
26. Patted the area dry with the towel. Dried from front to back.	___	___	_____
27. Folded the blanket back between her legs.	___	___	_____
28. Helped the person lower her legs and turn onto her side away from you.	___	___	_____
29. Applied soap to a mitted washcloth.	___	___	_____
30. Cleaned the rectal area. Cleaned from the vagina to the anus with one stroke.	___	___	_____
31. Repeated steps 29 and 30 until the area was clean. Used a clean part of the washcloth for each stroke. Used more than one washcloth if needed.	___	___	_____
32. Rinsed the rectal area with a washcloth. Stroked from the vagina to the anus. Repeated as necessary. Used a clean part of the washcloth for each stroke. Used more than one washcloth if needed.	___	___	_____
33. Patted the area dry with the towel. Dried from front to back.	___	___	_____
34. Removed any wet or soiled incontinence product. Removed the waterproof pad.	___	___	_____
35. Removed and discarded the gloves. Decontaminated your hands. Put on clean gloves.	___	___	_____
36. Provided clean and dry linens and incontinence products as needed.	___	___	_____

Post-Procedure

	S	U	Comments
37. Covered the person. Removed the bath blanket.	___	___	_____
38. Provided for comfort as noted on the inside of the front textbook cover.	___	___	_____
39. Placed the signal light within reach.	___	___	_____
40. Lowered the bed to its lowest position.	___	___	_____
41. Raised or lowered bed rails. Followed the care plan.	___	___	_____
42. Emptied, cleaned, and dried the wash basin.	___	___	_____
43. Returned the basin and supplies to their proper place.	___	___	_____
44. Wiped off the overbed table with the paper towels. Discarded the paper towels.	___	___	_____
45. Unscreened the person.	___	___	_____
46. Completed a safety check of the room as noted on the inside of the front textbook cover.	___	___	_____
47. Followed agency policy for dirty linen.	___	___	_____
48. Removed the gloves. Decontaminated your hands.	___	___	_____
49. Reported and recorded your observations.	___	___	_____

Date of Satisfactory Completion _____   Instructor's Initials _____

Giving Male Perineal Care (NNAAP™)

Name: _____   Date: _____

Quality of Life	S	U	Comments
• Knocked before entering the person's room.	___	___	_____
• Addressed the person by name.	___	___	_____
• Introduced yourself by name and title.	___	___	_____
• Explained the procedure to the person before beginning and during the procedure.	___	___	_____
• Protected the person's rights during the procedure.	___	___	_____
• Handled the person gently during the procedure.	___	___	_____

Procedure

1. Followed steps 1 through 17 in procedure *Giving Female Perineal Care*. Draped the person as in Figure 15-24 in the textbook.
2. Placed a waterproof pad under his buttocks. Protected the person and dry linen from the wet or soiled incontinence product.
3. Retracted the foreskin if the person was uncircumcised.
4. Grasped the penis.
5. Cleaned the tip. Used a circular motion. Started at the meatus of the urethra, and worked outward. Repeated as needed. Used a clean part of the washcloth each time.
6. Rinsed the area with another washcloth.
7. Returned the foreskin to its natural position immediately after rinsing.
8. Cleaned the shaft of the penis. Used firm downward strokes. Rinsed the area.
9. Helped the person flex his knees and spread his legs, or helped him spread his legs as much as possible with his knees straight.
10. Cleaned the scrotum. Rinsed well. Observed for redness and irritation in the skin folds.
11. Patted dry the penis and scrotum with the towel.
12. Folded the bath blanket back between his legs.
13. Helped him lower his legs and turn onto his side away from you.
14. Cleaned the rectal area. See procedure *Giving Female Perineal Care*. Rinsed and dried well.
15. Removed any wet or soiled incontinence product. Removed the waterproof pad.
16. Removed and discarded the gloves. Decontaminated your hands. Put on clean gloves.
17. Provided clean and dry linens and incontinence products.

Post-Procedure

18. Followed steps 37 through 49 in procedure *Giving Female Perineal Care*.

Date of Satisfactory Completion _____   Instructor's Initials _____

Brushing and Combing the Person's Hair

Name: _____   Date: _____

Quality of Life

	S	U	Comments

- Knocked before entering the person's room.
- Addressed the person by name.
- Introduced yourself by name and title.
- Explained the procedure to the person before beginning and during the procedure.
- Protected the person's rights during the procedure.
- Handled the person gently during the procedure.

Pre-Procedure

1. Followed *Delegation Guidelines: Brushing and Combing Hair*.
   Reviewed *Promoting Safety and Comfort: Brushing and Combing Hair*.
2. Practiced hand hygiene.
3. Identified the person. Checked the ID bracelet against the assignment sheet. Called the person by name.
4. Asked the person how to style hair.
5. Collected the following:
   - Comb and brush
   - Bath towel
   - Other hair care items as requested
6. Arranged items on the bedside stand.
7. Provided for privacy.

Procedure

8. Lowered the bed rail if up.
9. Helped the person to the chair. The person put on a robe and non-skid footwear. (If the person was in bed, raised the bed for body mechanics. Bed rails were up if used. Lowered the bed rail near you. Assisted the person to a semi-Fowler's position if allowed.)
10. Placed a towel across the person's back and shoulders or across the pillow.
11. Asked the person to remove eyeglasses. Put them in the eyeglass case. Put the case inside the bedside stand.
12. Brushed and combed hair that was not matted or tangled:
    a. Used the comb to part the hair.
       (1) Parted hair down the middle into 2 sides.
       (2) Divided one side into 2 smaller sections.
    b. Brushed one of the small sections of hair. Started at the scalp and brushed toward the hair ends. Did the same for the other small sections of hair.
    c. Repeated steps 12a(2) and 12b for the other side.
13. Brushed and combed matted or tangled hair:
    a. Took a small section of hair near the ends.
    b. Combed or brushed through to the hair ends.
    c. Added small sections of hair as you worked up to the scalp.
    d. Combed or brushed through each longer section to the hair ends.
    e. Brushed or combed from the scalp to the hair ends.

Date of Satisfactory Completion _____   Instructor's Initials _____

Procedure—cont'd	S	U	Comments
14. Styled the hair as the person preferred.	____	____	_____
15. Removed the towel.	____	____	_____
16. Let the person put on the eyeglasses.	____	____	_____

Post-Procedure

17. Provided for comfort as noted on the inside of the front textbook cover.	____	____	_____
18. Placed the signal light within reach.	____	____	_____
19. Lowered the bed to its lowest position.	____	____	_____
20. Raised or lowered bed rails. Followed the care plan.	____	____	_____
21. Cleaned and returned hair care items to their proper place.	____	____	_____
22. Unscreened the person.	____	____	_____
23. Completed a safety check of the room as noted on the inside of the front textbook cover.	____	____	_____
24. Followed agency policy for dirty linen.	____	____	_____
25. Decontaminated your hands.	____	____	_____

Date of Satisfactory Completion _____   Instructor's Initials _____

Shampooing the Person's Hair

Name: _____   Date: _____

Quality of Life	S	U	Comments
• Knocked before entering the person's room.	___	___	_____
• Addressed the person by name.	___	___	_____
• Introduced yourself by name and title.	___	___	_____
• Explained the procedure to the person before beginning and during the procedure.	___	___	_____
• Protected the person's rights during the procedure.	___	___	_____
• Handled the person gently during the procedure.	___	___	_____

Pre-Procedure

	S	U	Comments
1. Followed *Delegation Guidelines: Shampooing.* Reviewed *Promoting Safety and Comfort: Shampooing.*	___	___	_____
2. Practiced hand hygiene.	___	___	_____
3. Collected the following:			
• Two bath towels	___	___	_____
• Washcloth	___	___	_____
• Shampoo	___	___	_____
• Hair conditioner (if requested)	___	___	_____
• Bath thermometer	___	___	_____
• Pitcher or hand-held nozzle (if needed)	___	___	_____
• Shampoo tray (if needed)	___	___	_____
• Basin or pan (if needed)	___	___	_____
• Waterproof pad (if needed)	___	___	_____
• Gloves (if needed)	___	___	_____
• Comb and brush	___	___	_____
• Hair dryer	___	___	_____
4. Arranged items nearby.	___	___	_____
5. Identified the person. Checked the ID bracelet against the assignment sheet. Called the person by name.	___	___	_____
6. Provided for privacy.	___	___	_____
7. Raised the bed for body mechanics for a shampoo in bed. Bed rails were up if used.	___	___	_____
8. Decontaminated your hands.	___	___	_____

Procedure

	S	U	Comments
9. Lowered the bed rail near you if up.	___	___	_____
10. Covered the person's chest with a bath towel.	___	___	_____
11. Brushed and combed the hair to remove snarls and tangles.	___	___	_____
12. Positioned the person for the method used. To shampoo the person in bed:			
a. Lowered the head of the bed and removed the pillow.	___	___	_____
b. Placed the waterproof pad and shampoo tray under the head and shoulders.	___	___	_____
c. Supported the head and neck with a folded towel if necessary.	___	___	_____
13. Raised the bed rail if used.	___	___	_____
14. Obtained water. Water temperature was 105° F (40.5° C). Tested water temperature according to agency policy. Asked the person to check the water temperature. Adjusted water temperature as needed. Raised bed rail before leaving the bedside.	___	___	_____

Date of Satisfactory Completion _____   Instructor's Initials _____

Procedure—cont'd	S	U	Comments
15. Lowered the bed rail near you if up.	___	___	_____
16. Put on gloves (if needed).	___	___	_____
17. Asked the person to hold a washcloth over the eyes. It did not cover the nose and mouth. (Some state competency tests require a dry washcloth.)	___	___	_____
18. Used the pitcher or nozzle to wet the hair.	___	___	_____
19. Applied a small amount of shampoo.	___	___	_____
20. Worked up a lather with both hands. Started at the hairline. Worked toward the back of the head.	___	___	_____
21. Massaged the scalp with your fingertips. Did not scratch the scalp.	___	___	_____
22. Rinsed the hair until the water ran clear.	___	___	_____
23. Repeated steps 19 through 22.	___	___	_____
24. Applied conditioner. Followed directions on the container.	___	___	_____
25. Squeezed water from the person's hair.	___	___	_____
26. Covered the hair with a bath towel.	___	___	_____
27. Removed the shampoo tray, basin, and waterproof pad.	___	___	_____
28. Dried the person's face with the towel. Used the towel on the person's chest.	___	___	_____
29. Helped the person raise the head if appropriate. For the person in bed, raised the head of the bed.	___	___	_____
30. Rubbed the hair and scalp with the towel. Used the second towel if the first was wet.	___	___	_____
31. Combed the hair to remove snarls and tangles.	___	___	_____
32. Dried and styled hair as quickly as possible.	___	___	_____
33. Removed and discarded the gloves (if used). Decontaminated your hands.			

Post-Procedure

	S	U	Comments
34. Provided for comfort as noted on the inside of the front textbook cover.	___	___	_____
35. Placed the signal light within reach.	___	___	_____
36. Lowered the bed to its lowest position.	___	___	_____
37. Raised or lowered bed rails. Followed the care plan.	___	___	_____
38. Unscreened the person.	___	___	_____
39. Completed a safety check of the room as noted on the inside of the front textbook cover.	___	___	_____
40. Cleaned, dried, and returned equipment to its proper place. Cleaned the brush and comb. Discarded disposable items.	___	___	_____
41. Followed agency policy for dirty linen.	___	___	_____
42. Decontaminated your hands.	___	___	_____
43. Reported and recorded your observations.	___	___	_____

Date of Satisfactory Completion _____   Instructor's Initials _____

Shaving the Person's Face With a Safety Razor

Name: _____   Date: _____

	S	U	Comments

Quality of Life
- Knocked before entering the person's room.
- Addressed the person by name.
- Introduced yourself by name and title.
- Explained the procedure to the person before beginning and during the procedure.
- Protected the person's rights during the procedure.
- Handled the person gently during the procedure.

Pre-Procedure
1. Followed *Delegation Guidelines: Shaving.* Reviewed *Promoting Safety and Comfort: Shaving.*
2. Practiced hand hygiene.
3. Collected the following:
   - Wash basin
   - Bath towel
   - Hand towel
   - Washcloth
   - Safety razor
   - Mirror
   - Shaving cream, soap, or lotion
   - Shaving brush
   - After-shave or lotion
   - Tissues or paper towels
   - Paper towels
   - Gloves
4. Arranged paper towels and supplies on the overbed table.
5. Identified the person. Checked the ID bracelet against the assignment sheet. Called the person by name.
6. Provided for privacy.
7. Raised the bed for body mechanics. Bed rails were up if used.

Procedure
8. Filled the wash basin with warm water.
9. Placed the basin on the overbed table.
10. Lowered the bed rail near you if up.
11. Decontaminated your hands. Put on gloves.
12. Assisted the person to semi-Fowler's position if allowed or to the supine position.
13. Adjusted lighting to clearly see the person's face.
14. Placed the bath towel over the person's chest and shoulders.
15. Adjusted the overbed table for easy reach.
16. Tightened the razor blade to the shaver.
17. Washed the person's face. Did not dry.
18. Wet the washcloth or towel. Wrung it out.
19. Applied the washcloth or towel to the face for a few minutes.
20. Applied shaving cream with your hands, or used a shaving brush to apply lather.
21. Held the skin taut with one hand.

Date of Satisfactory Completion _____ Instructor's Initials _____

Procedure—cont'd   S   U   **Comments**

22. Shaved in the direction of hair growth. Used shorter
    strokes around the chin and lips.

23. Rinsed the razor often. Wiped it with tissues or paper
    towels.

24. Applied direct pressure to any bleeding areas.

25. Washed off any remaining shaving cream or soap.
    Patted dry with a towel.

26. Applied after-shave or lotion if requested. (If there
    were nicks or cuts, did not apply after-shave or lotion.)

27. Removed the towel and gloves. Decontaminated your
    hands.

Post-Procedure

28. Provided for comfort as noted on the inside of the
    front textbook cover.

29. Placed the signal light within reach.

30. Lowered the bed to its lowest position.

31. Raised or lowered bed rails. Followed the care plan.

32. Cleaned and returned equipment and supplies to
    their proper place. Discarded a razor blade or a
    disposable razor into the sharps container. Discarded
    other disposable items. Wore gloves.

33. Wiped off the overbed table with paper towels.
    Discarded the paper towels.

34. Unscreened the person.

35. Completed a safety check of the room as noted on the
    inside of the front textbook cover.

36. Followed agency policy for dirty linen.

37. Removed the gloves. Decontaminated your hands.

38. Reported nicks, cuts, irritation, or bleeding to
    the nurse at once. Reported and recorded other
    observations.

Date of Satisfactory Completion _____   Instructor's Initials _____

Giving Nail and Foot Care (NNAAP™)

Name: _____ Date: _____

Quality of Life	S	U	Comments
• Knocked before entering the person's room.			
• Addressed the person by name.			
• Introduced yourself by name and title.			
• Explained the procedure to the person before beginning and during the procedure.			
• Protected the person's rights during the procedure.			
• Handled the person gently during the procedure.			

Pre-Procedure

	S	U	Comments
1. Followed *Delegation Guidelines: Nail and Foot Care.* Reviewed *Promoting Safety and Comfort: Nail and Foot Care.*			
2. Practiced hand hygiene.			
3. Collected the following:			
• Wash basin or whirlpool foot bath			
• Soap			
• Bath thermometer			
• Bath towel			
• Hand towel			
• Washcloth			
• Kidney basin			
• Nail clippers			
• Orangewood stick			
• Emery board or nail file			
• Lotion for the hands			
• Lotion or petroleum jelly for the feet			
• Paper towels			
• Bath mat			
• Gloves			
4. Arranged paper towels and other items on the overbed table.			
5. Identified the person. Checked the ID bracelet against the assignment sheet. Called the person by name.			
6. Provided for privacy.			
7. Assisted the person to the bedside chair. Placed the signal light within reach.			

Procedure

	S	U	Comments
8. Placed the bath mat under the feet.			
9. Filled the wash basin or whirlpool foot bath two-thirds full with water. Followed the nurse's directions for water temperature. (Measured water temperature with a bath thermometer or tested it by dipping your elbow or inner wrist into the basin. Followed agency policy.) Asked the person to check the water temperature. Adjusted water temperature as needed.			
10. Placed the basin or foot bath on the bath mat.			
11. Put on gloves.			
12. Helped the person put the feet into the basin or foot bath. Made sure both feet were completely covered by water.			
13. Adjusted the overbed table in front of the person.			

Date of Satisfactory Completion _____ Instructor's Initials _____

Procedure—cont'd

	S	U	Comments
14. Filled the kidney basin two-thirds full with water. Measured water temperature (see step 9).	___	___	_____
15. Placed the kidney basin on the overbed table.	___	___	_____
16. Placed the person's fingers into the basin. Positioned the arms for comfort.	___	___	_____
17. Let the fingers soak for 5 to 10 minutes. Let the feet soak for 15 to 20 minutes. Re-warmed water as needed.	___	___	_____
18. Removed the kidney basin.	___	___	_____
19. Cleaned under the fingernails with the orangewood stick. Used a towel to wipe the orangewood stick after each nail.	___	___	_____
20. Dried the hands and between the fingers thoroughly.	___	___	_____
21. Clipped fingernails straight across with the nail clippers.	___	___	_____
22. Shaped nails with an emery board or nail file. Nails were smooth with no rough edges. Checked each nail for smoothness. Filed as needed.	___	___	_____
23. Pushed cuticles back with the orangewood stick or a washcloth.	___	___	_____
24. Applied lotion to the hands. Warmed lotion before applying it.	___	___	_____
25. Moved the overbed table to the side.	___	___	_____
26. Lifted a foot out of the water. Supported the foot and ankle with one hand. With your other hand, washed the foot and between the toes with soap and a washcloth. Returned the foot to the water for rinsing. Made sure to rinse between the toes.	___	___	_____
27. Repeated step 26 for the other foot.	___	___	_____
28. Removed the feet from the basin or foot bath. Dried thoroughly, especially between the toes.	___	___	_____
29. Applied lotion or petroleum jelly to the tops and soles of the feet. Did not apply between the toes. Warmed lotion or petroleum jelly before applying it. Removed excess lotion or petroleum jelly with a towel.	___	___	_____
30. Removed and discarded the gloves. Decontaminated your hands.	___	___	_____
31. Helped the person put on non-skid footwear.	___	___	_____

Post-Procedure

	S	U	Comments
32. Provided for comfort as noted on the inside of the front textbook cover.	___	___	_____
33. Placed the signal light within reach.	___	___	_____
34. Raised or lowered bed rails. Followed the care plan.	___	___	_____
35. Cleaned, dried, and returned equipment and supplies to their proper place. Discarded disposable items. Wore gloves for this step.	___	___	_____
36. Unscreened the person.	___	___	_____
37. Completed a safety check of the room as noted on the inside of the front textbook cover.	___	___	_____
38. Followed agency policy for dirty linen.	___	___	_____
39. Removed the gloves. Decontaminated your hands.	___	___	_____
40. Reported and recorded your observations.	___	___	_____

Date of Satisfactory Completion _____   Instructor's Initials _____

Undressing the Person

Name: _____   Date: _____

Quality of Life	S	U	Comments
• Knocked before entering the person's room.	___	___	_____
• Addressed the person by name.	___	___	_____
• Introduced yourself by name and title.	___	___	_____
• Explained the procedure to the person before beginning and during the procedure.	___	___	_____
• Protected the person's rights during the procedure.	___	___	_____
• Handled the person gently during the procedure.	___	___	_____

Pre-Procedure

1. Followed *Delegation Guidelines: Dressing and Undressing*.
2. Practiced hand hygiene.
3. Collected a bath blanket and clothing requested by the person.
4. Identified the person. Checked the ID bracelet against the assignment sheet. Called the person by name.
5. Provided for privacy.
6. Raised the bed for body mechanics. Bed rails were up if used.
7. Lowered the bed rail on the person's weak side.
8. Positioned the person supine.
9. Covered the person with a bath blanket. Fan-folded linens to the foot of the bed.

Procedure

10. To remove garments that opened in the back:
    a. Raised the head and shoulders, or turned the person onto the side away from you.
    b. Undid buttons, zippers, ties, or snaps.
    c. Brought the sides of the garment to the sides of the person. If the person was in a side-lying position, tucked the far side under the person. Folded the near side onto the chest.
    d. Positioned the person supine.
    e. Slid the garment off the shoulder on the strong side. Removed it from the arm.
    f. Removed the garment from the weak side.
11. To remove garments that opened in the front:
    a. Undid buttons, zippers, ties, or snaps.
    b. Slid the garment off the shoulder and arm on the strong side.
    c. Assisted the person to sit up or raised the head and shoulders. Brought the garment over to the weak side.
    d. Lowered the head and shoulders. Removed the garment from the weak side.
    e. If you could not raise the head and shoulders:
       (1) Turned the person toward you. Tucked the removed part under the person.
       (2) Turned the person onto the side away from you.
       (3) Pulled the side of the garment out from under the person. Made sure he or she would not lie on it when supine.
       (4) Returned the person to the supine position.
       (5) Removed the garment from the weak side.

Date of Satisfactory Completion _____   Instructor's Initials _____

Procedure—cont'd	S	U	Comments

Procedure—cont'd

12. To remove pullover garments:
    a. Undid buttons, zippers, ties, or snaps.
    b. Removed the garment from the strong side.
    c. Raised the head and shoulders, or turned the person onto the side away from you. Brought the garment up to the person's neck.
    d. Removed the garment from the weak side.
    e. Brought the garment over the person's head.
    f. Positioned the person in the supine position.
13. To remove pants or slacks:
    a. Removed footwear and socks.
    b. Positioned the person supine.
    c. Undid buttons, zippers, ties, snaps, or buckles.
    d. Removed the belt.
    e. Asked the person to lift the buttocks off the bed. Slid the pants down over the hips and buttocks. Had the person lower the hips and buttocks.
    f. If the person could not raise the hips off the bed:
       (1) Turned the person toward you.
       (2) Slid the pants off the hip and buttock on the strong side.
       (3) Turned the person away from you.
       (4) Slid the pants off the hip and buttock on the weak side.
    g. Slid the pants down the legs and over the feet.
14. Dressed the person. See procedure *Dressing the Person*.

Post-Procedure

15. Provided for comfort as noted on the inside of the front textbook cover.
16. Placed the signal light within reach.
17. Lowered the bed to its lowest level.
18. Raised or lowered bed rails. Followed the care plan.
19. Unscreened the person.
20. Completed a safety check of the room as noted on the inside of the front textbook cover.
21. Followed agency policy for soiled clothing.
22. Decontaminated your hands.
23. Reported and recorded your observations.

Date of Satisfactory Completion _____   Instructor's Initials _____

Dressing the Person (NNAAP™)

Name: _____ Date: _____

	S	U	Comments

Quality of Life
- Knocked before entering the person's room.
- Addressed the person by name.
- Introduced yourself by name and title.
- Explained the procedure to the person before beginning and during the procedure.
- Protected the person's rights during the procedure.
- Handled the person gently during the procedure.

Pre-Procedure
1. Followed *Delegation Guidelines: Dressing and Undressing*.
2. Practiced hand hygiene.
3. Asked the person what he or she would like to wear.
4. Got a bath blanket and clothing requested by the person.
5. Identified the person. Checked the ID bracelet against the assignment sheet. Called the person by name.
6. Provided for privacy.
7. Raised the bed for body mechanics. Bed rails were up if used.
8. Lowered the bed rail (if up) on the person's strong side.
9. Positioned the person supine.
10. Covered the person with the bath blanket. Fan-folded linens to the foot of the bed.
11. Undressed the person. (See procedure *Undressing the Person*.)

Procedure
12. To put on garments that opened in the back:
    a. Slid the garment onto the arm and shoulder of the weak side.
    b. Slid the garment onto the arm and shoulder of the strong side.
    c. Raised the person's head and shoulders.
    d. Brought the sides to the back.
    e. If you could not raise the person's head and shoulders:
       (1) Turned the person toward you.
       (2) Brought one side of the garment to the person's back.
       (3) Turned the person away from you.
       (4) Brought the other side to the person's back.
    f. Fastened buttons, zippers, snaps, or other closures.
    g. Positioned the person supine.
13. To put on garments that opened in the front:
    a. Slid the garment onto the arm and shoulder on the weak side.
    b. Raised the head and shoulders. Brought the side of the garment around to the back. Lowered the person down. Slid the garment onto the arm and shoulder of the strong arm.

Date of Satisfactory Completion _____ Instructor's Initials _____

Procedure—cont'd   S   U   **Comments**

   c. If the person could not raise the head and
      shoulders:
     (1) Turned the person away from you.   ____ ____ _____
     (2) Tucked the garment under the person.   ____ ____ _____
     (3) Turned the person toward you.   ____ ____ _____
     (4) Pulled the garment out from under him or her. ____ ____ _____
     (5) Turned the person back to the supine position. ____ ____ _____
     (6) Slid the garment over the arm and shoulder of ____ ____ _____
        the strong arm.
   d. Fastened buttons, zippers, ties, snaps, or other ____ ____ _____
     closures.

14. To put on pullover garments:
   a. Positioned the person supine.   ____ ____ _____
   b. Brought the neck of the garment over the head. ____ ____ _____
   c. Slid the arm and shoulder of the garment onto the ____ ____ _____
     weak side.
   d. Raised the person's head and shoulders.   ____ ____ _____
   e. Brought the garment down.   ____ ____ _____
   f. Slid the arm and shoulder of the garment onto the ____ ____ _____
     strong side.
   g. If the person could not assume a semi-sitting
     position:
     (1) Turned the person away from you.   ____ ____ _____
     (2) Tucked the garment under the person.   ____ ____ _____
     (3) Turned the person toward you.   ____ ____ _____
     (4) Pulled the garment out from under him or her. ____ ____ _____
     (5) Positioned the person supine.   ____ ____ _____
     (6) Slid the arm and shoulder of the garment onto ____ ____ _____
        the strong side.
   h. Fastened buttons, zippers, ties, snaps, or other ____ ____ _____
     closures.

15. To put on pants or slacks:
   a. Slid the pants over the feet and up the legs. ____ ____ _____
   b. Asked the person to raise the hips and buttocks off ____ ____ _____
     the bed.
   c. Brought the pants up over the buttocks and hips. ____ ____ _____
   d. Asked the person to lower the hips and buttocks. ____ ____ _____
   e. If the person could not raise the hips and buttocks:
     (1) Turned the person onto the strong side.   ____ ____ _____
     (2) Pulled the pants over the buttock and hip on the ____ ____ _____
        weak side.
     (3) Turned the person onto the weak side.   ____ ____ _____
     (4) Pulled the pants over the buttock and hip on the ____ ____ _____
        strong side.
     (5) Positioned the person supine.   ____ ____ _____
   f. Fastened buttons, zippers, ties, snaps, a belt buckle, ____ ____ _____
     or other closures.

16. Put socks and non-skid footwear on the person. Made ____ ____ _____
    sure socks were up all the way and were smooth.
17. Helped the person get out of bed. If the person stayed ____ ____ _____
    in bed, covered the person. Removed the bath blanket.

Date of Satisfactory Completion _____   Instructor's Initials _____

Post-Procedure	**S**	**U**	**Comments**
18. Provided for comfort as noted on the inside of the front textbook cover.	_____	_____	_____
19. Placed the signal light within reach.	_____	_____	_____
20. Lowered the bed to its lowest position.	_____	_____	_____
21. Raised or lowered bed rails. Followed the care plan.	_____	_____	_____
22. Unscreened the person.	_____	_____	_____
23. Completed a safety check of the room as noted on the inside of the front textbook cover.	_____	_____	_____
24. Followed agency policy for soiled clothing.	_____	_____	_____
25. Decontaminated your hands.	_____	_____	_____
26. Reported and recorded your observations.	_____	_____	_____

Date of Satisfactory Completion _____   Instructor's Initials _____

Changing the Gown of the Person With an IV

View Video!

Name: _____   Date: _____

	S	U	Comments

Quality of Life
- Knocked before entering the person's room.
- Addressed the person by name.
- Introduced yourself by name and title.
- Explained the procedure to the person before beginning and during the procedure.
- Protected the person's rights during the procedure.
- Handled the person gently during the procedure.

Pre-Procedure
1. Followed *Delegation Guidelines: Changing Hospital Gowns*.
   Reviewed *Promoting Safety and Comfort: Changing Hospital Gowns*.
2. Practiced hand hygiene.
3. Got a clean gown and a bath blanket.
4. Identified the person. Checked the ID bracelet against the assignment sheet. Called the person by name.
5. Provided for privacy.
6. Raised the bed for body mechanics. Bed rails were up if used.

Procedure
7. Lowered the bed rail near you if up.
8. Covered the person with a bath blanket. Fan-folded linens to the foot of the bed.
9. Untied the gown. Freed parts that the person was lying on.
10. Removed the gown from the arm with no IV.
11. Gathered up the sleeve of the arm with the IV. Slid it over the IV site and tubing. Removed the arm and hand from the sleeve.
12. Kept the sleeve gathered. Slid your arm along the tubing to the bag.
13. Removed the bag from the pole. Slid the bag and tubing through the sleeve. Did not pull on the tubing. Kept the bag above the person.
14. Hung the IV bag on the pole.
15. Gathered the sleeve of the clean gown that would go on the arm with the IV infusion.
16. Removed the bag from the pole. Slipped the sleeve over the bag at the shoulder part of the gown. Hung the bag.
17. Slid the gathered sleeve over the tubing, hand, arm, and IV site. Then slid it onto the shoulder.
18. Put the other side of the gown on the person. Fastened the gown.
19. Covered the person. Removed the bath blanket.

Post-Procedure
20. Provided for comfort as noted on the inside of the front textbook cover.
21. Placed the signal light within reach.
22. Lowered the bed to its lowest position.

Date of Satisfactory Completion _____   Instructor's Initials _____

Post-Procedure—cont'd   **S**   **U**   **Comments**

23. Raised or lowered bed rails. Followed the care plan.
24. Unscreened the person.
25. Completed a safety check of the room as noted on the inside of the front textbook cover.
26. Followed agency policy for dirty linen.
27. Decontaminated your hands.
28. Asked the nurse to check the flow rate.
29. Reported and recorded your observations.

Date of Satisfactory Completion _____ Instructor's Initials _____

Giving the Bedpan

View Video! Video CLIP

Name: _____   Date: _____

Quality of Life	S	U	Comments
• Knocked before entering the person's room.			
• Addressed the person by name.			
• Introduced yourself by name and title.			
• Explained the procedure to the person before beginning and during the procedure.			
• Protected the person's rights during the procedure.			
• Handled the person gently during the procedure.			

Pre-Procedure

	S	U	Comments
1. Followed *Delegation Guidelines: Bedpans*. Reviewed *Promoting Safety and Comfort: Bedpans*.			
2. Provided for privacy.			
3. Practiced hand hygiene.			
4. Put on gloves.			
5. Collected the following:			
• Bedpan			
• Bedpan cover			
• Toilet tissue			
• Waterproof pad if required			
6. Arranged equipment on the chair or bed.			

Procedure

	S	U	Comments
7. Lowered the bed rail near you if up.			
8. Positioned the person supine. Raised the head of the bed slightly.			
9. Folded the top linens and gown out of the way. Kept the lower body covered.			
10. Asked the person to flex the knees and raise the buttocks by pushing against the mattress with his or her feet.			
11. Slid your hand under the lower back. Helped raise the buttocks. If using a waterproof pad, placed it under the person's buttocks.			
12. Slid the bedpan under the person.			
13. If the person could not assist in getting on the bedpan:			
a. Placed the waterproof pad under the person's buttocks if using one.			
b. Turned the person onto the side away from you.			
c. Placed the bedpan firmly against the buttocks.			
d. Pushed the bedpan down and toward the person.			
e. Held the bedpan securely. Turned the person onto his or her back.			
f. Made sure the bedpan was centered under the person.			
14. Covered the person.			
15. Raised the head of the bed so the person was in a sitting position (if the person used a standard bedpan). (If required by state competency tests, removed the gloves and washed your hands before raising the head of the bed.)			
16. Made sure the person was correctly positioned on the bedpan.			

Date of Satisfactory Completion _____   Instructor's Initials _____

Procedure—cont'd   S   U   **Comments**

17. Raised the bed rail if used.
18. Placed the toilet tissue and signal light within reach.
19. Asked the person to signal when done or when help was needed.
20. Removed the gloves. Practiced hand hygiene.
21. Left the room and closed the door.
22. Returned when the person signaled. Or checked on the person every 5 minutes. Knocked before entering.
23. Practiced hand hygiene. Put on gloves.
24. Raised the bed for body mechanics. Lowered the bed rail (if used) and lowered the head of the bed.
25. Asked the person to raise the buttocks. Removed the bedpan. Or held the bedpan and turned the person onto the side away from you.
26. Cleaned the genital area if the person could not do so. Cleaned from front (urethra) to back (anus) with toilet tissue. Used fresh tissue for each wipe. Provided perineal care if needed. Removed and discarded the waterproof pad if using one.
27. Covered the bedpan. Took it to the bathroom. Raised the bed rail (if used) before leaving the bedside.
28. Noted the color, amount, and character of urine or feces.
29. Emptied the bedpan contents into the toilet and flushed.
30. Rinsed the bedpan. Poured the rinse into the toilet and flushed.
31. Cleaned the bedpan with a disinfectant.
32. Removed soiled gloves. Practiced hand hygiene, and put on clean gloves.
33. Returned the bedpan and clean cover to the bedside stand.
34. Helped the person with hand washing. Wore gloves.
35. Removed the gloves. Practiced hand hygiene.

Post-Procedure

36. Provided for comfort as noted on the inside of the front textbook cover.
37. Placed the signal light within reach.
38. Lowered the bed to its lowest position.
39. Raised or lowered bed rails. Followed the care plan.
40. Unscreened the person.
41. Completed a safety check of the room as noted on the inside of the front textbook cover.
42. Followed agency policy for soiled linen.
43. Practiced hand hygiene.
44. Reported and recorded your observations.

Date of Satisfactory Completion _____   Instructor's Initials _____

Giving the Urinal

Name:———————————————   Date: ————————————————

	S	U	Comments
Quality of Life			
• Knocked before entering the person's room.			
• Addressed the person by name.			
• Introduced yourself by name and title.			
• Explained the procedure to the person before beginning and during the procedure.			
• Protected the person's rights during the procedure.			
• Handled the person gently during the procedure.			
Pre-Procedure			
1. Followed *Delegation Guidelines: Urinals.* Reviewed *Promoting Safety and Comfort: Urinals.*			
2. Provided for privacy.			
3. Determined if the man would stand, sit, or lie in bed.			
4. Practiced hand hygiene.			
5. Put on gloves.			
6. Collected the following:			
• Urinal			
• Non-skid footwear if the person would stand to void			
Procedure			
7. Gave him the urinal if he was in bed. Reminded him to tilt the bottom down to prevent spills.			
8. If he was going to stand:			
a. Helped him sit on the side of the bed.			
b. Put non-skid footwear on him.			
c. Helped him stand. Provided support if he was unsteady.			
d. Gave him the urinal.			
9. Positioned the urinal if necessary. Positioned his penis in the urinal if he could not do so.			
10. Placed the signal light within reach. Asked him to signal when done or if he needed help.			
11. Provided for privacy.			
12. Removed the gloves. Practiced hand hygiene.			
13. Left the room and closed the door.			
14. Returned when he signaled. Or checked on him every 5 minutes. Knocked before entering.			
15. Practiced hand hygiene. Put on gloves.			
16. Closed the cap on the urinal. Took it to the bathroom.			
17. Noted the color, amount, and character of the urine.			
18. Emptied the urinal into the toilet and flushed.			
19. Rinsed the urinal with cold water. Poured the rinse into the toilet and flushed.			
20. Cleaned the urinal with a disinfectant.			
21. Returned the urinal to its proper place.			
22. Removed soiled gloves. Practiced hand hygiene, and put on clean gloves.			
23. Assisted with hand washing.			
24. Removed the gloves. Practiced hand hygiene.			

Date of Satisfactory Completion ————————————   Instructor's Initials ————————————————

Post-Procedure

	S	U	Comments
25. Provided for comfort as noted on the inside of the front textbook cover.	___	___	_____
26. Placed the signal light within reach.	___	___	_____
27. Raised or lower bed rails. Followed the care plan.	___	___	_____
28. Unscreened him.	___	___	_____
29. Completed a safety check of the room as noted on the inside of the front textbook cover.	___	___	_____
30. Followed agency policy for soiled linen.	___	___	_____
31. Practiced hand hygiene.	___	___	_____
32. Reported and recorded your observations.	___	___	_____

Date of Satisfactory Completion _____ Instructor's Initials _____

Helping the Person to the Commode

View Video!

Name:_____   Date: _____

	S	U	Comments

Quality of Life
- Knocked before entering the person's room.
- Addressed the person by name.
- Introduced yourself by name and title.
- Explained the procedure to the person before beginning and during the procedure.
- Protected the person's rights during the procedure.
- Handled the person gently during the procedure.

Pre-Procedure
1. Followed *Delegation Guidelines: Commodes.* Reviewed *Promoting Safety and Comfort: Commodes.*
2. Provided for privacy.
3. Practiced hand hygiene.
4. Put on gloves.
5. Collected the following:
   - Commode
   - Toilet tissue
   - Bath blanket
   - Transfer belt
   - Robe and non-skid footwear

Procedure
6. Brought the commode next to the bed. Removed the chair seat and container lid.
7. Helped the person sit on the side of the bed. Lowered bed rail if used.
8. Helped the person put on a robe and non-skid footwear.
9. Assisted the person to the commode. Used the transfer belt.
10. Removed the transfer belt. Covered the person with a bath blanket for warmth.
11. Placed the toilet tissue and signal light within reach.
12. Asked the person to signal when done or when help was needed. (Stayed with the person if necessary. Was respectful and provided as much privacy as possible.)
13. Removed the gloves. Practiced hand hygiene.
14. Left the room. Closed the door.
15. Returned when the person signaled. Or checked on the person every 5 minutes. Knocked before entering.
16. Decontaminated your hands. Put on the gloves.
17. Helped the person clean the genital area as needed. Removed the gloves, and practiced hand hygiene.
18. Applied the transfer belt. Helped the person back to bed using the transfer belt. Removed the transfer belt, robe, and footwear. Raised the bed rail if used.
19. Put on clean gloves. Removed and covered the commode container. Cleaned the commode.
20. Took the container to the bathroom.
21. Observed urine and feces for color, amount, and character.
22. Emptied the container contents into the toilet and flushed.
23. Rinsed the container. Poured the rinse into the toilet and flushed.

Date of Satisfactory Completion _____   Instructor's Initials _____

Procedure—cont'd	S	U	Comments
24. Cleaned and disinfected the container.	_____	_____	_____
25. Returned the container to the commode. Returned other supplies to their proper place.	_____	_____	_____
26. Removed soiled gloves. Practiced hand hygiene, and put on clean gloves.	_____	_____	_____
27. Assisted with hand washing.	_____	_____	_____
28. Removed the gloves. Practiced hand hygiene.	_____	_____	_____

Post-Procedure

	S	U	Comments
29. Provided for comfort as noted on the inside of the front textbook cover.	_____	_____	_____
30. Placed the signal light within reach.	_____	_____	_____
31. Raised or lowered bed rails. Followed the care plan.	_____	_____	_____
32. Unscreened the person.	_____	_____	_____
33. Completed a safety check of the room as noted on the inside of the front textbook cover.	_____	_____	_____
34. Followed agency policy for dirty linen.	_____	_____	_____
35. Practiced hand hygiene.	_____	_____	_____
36. Reported and recorded your observations.	_____	_____	_____

Date of Satisfactory Completion _____ Instructor's Initials _____

Giving Catheter Care (NNAAP™)

Name: _____   Date: _____

	S	U	Comments

Quality of Life
- Knocked before entering the person's room.
- Addressed the person by name.
- Introduced yourself by name and title.
- Explained the procedure to the person before beginning and during the procedure.
- Protected the person's rights during the procedure.
- Handled the person gently during the procedure.

Pre-Procedure
1. Followed *Delegation Guidelines:*
   a. *Perineal Care*
   b. *Catheters*
   Reviewed *Promoting Safety and Comfort:*
   a. *Perineal Care*
   b. *Catheters*
2. Practiced hand hygiene.
3. Collected the following:
   - Items for perineal care (Chapter 15)
   - Gloves
   - Bath blanket
4. Covered the overbed table with paper towels. Arranged items on top of them.
5. Identified the person. Checked the ID bracelet against the assignment sheet. Called the person by name.
6. Provided for privacy.
7. Filled the wash basin. Water temperature was about 105° F (40.5° C). Measured water temperature according to agency policy. Asked the person to check the water temperature. Adjusted water temperature as needed.
8. Raised the bed for body mechanics. Bed rails were up if used.

Procedure
9. Lowered the bed rail near you if up.
10. Decontaminated your hands. Put on gloves.
11. Covered the person with a bath blanket. Fan-folded top linens to the foot of the bed.
12. Draped the person for perineal care (Chapter 15).
13. Folded back the bath blanket to expose the genital area.
14. Placed the waterproof pad under the buttocks. Asked the person to flex the knees and raise the buttocks off the bed.
15. Separated the labia (female). In an uncircumcised male, retracted the foreskin. Checked for crusts, abnormal drainage, or secretions.
16. Gave perineal care. (See procedure *Giving Female Perineal Care* or *Giving Male Perineal Care* in Chapter 15.)
17. Applied soap to a clean, wet washcloth.
18. Held the catheter near the meatus.

Date of Satisfactory Completion _____   Instructor's Initials _____

Procedure—cont'd	S	U	Comments
19. Cleaned the catheter from the meatus down the catheter about 4 inches. Cleaned downward, away from the meatus with 1 stroke. Did not tug or pull on the catheter. Repeated as needed with a clean area of the washcloth. Used a clean washcloth if needed.	_____	_____	_____
20. Rinsed the catheter with a clean washcloth. Rinsed from the meatus down the catheter about 4 inches. Rinsed downward, away from the meatus with 1 stroke. Did not tug or pull on the catheter. Repeated as needed with a clean area of the washcloth. Used a clean washcloth if needed.	_____	_____	_____
21. Dried the catheter with a towel. Dried from the meatus down the catheter about 4 inches. Did not tug or pull on the catheter.	_____	_____	_____
22. Patted dry the perineal area. Dried from front to back.	_____	_____	_____
23. Returned the foreskin to its natural position.	_____	_____	_____
24. Secured the catheter. Coiled and secured tubing.	_____	_____	_____
25. Removed the waterproof pad.	_____	_____	_____
26. Covered the person. Removed the bath blanket.	_____	_____	_____
27. Removed the gloves. Practiced hand hygiene.	_____	_____	_____

Post-Procedure

	S	U	Comments
28. Provided for comfort as noted on the inside of the front textbook cover.	_____	_____	_____
29. Placed the signal light within reach.	_____	_____	_____
30. Lowered the bed to its lowest position.	_____	_____	_____
31. Raised or lowered bed rails. Followed the care plan.	_____	_____	_____
32. Cleaned, dried, and returned equipment to its proper place. Discarded disposable items. Wore gloves for this step.	_____	_____	_____
33. Unscreened the person.	_____	_____	_____
34. Completed a safety check of the room as noted on the inside of the front textbook cover.	_____	_____	_____
35. Followed agency policy for soiled linen.	_____	_____	_____
36. Removed the gloves. Practiced hand hygiene.	_____	_____	_____
37. Reported and recorded your observations.	_____	_____	_____

Date of Satisfactory Completion _____ Instructor's Initials _____

Emptying a Urinary Drainage Bag

View Video!

Name: _____   Date: _____

Quality of Life	S	U	Comments
• Knocked before entering the person's room.	___	___	_____
• Addressed the person by name.	___	___	_____
• Introduced yourself by name and title.	___	___	_____
• Explained the procedure to the person before beginning and during the procedure.	___	___	_____
• Protected the person's rights during the procedure.	___	___	_____
• Handled the person gently during the procedure.	___	___	_____

Pre-Procedure

	S	U	Comments
1. Followed *Delegation Guidelines: Drainage Systems*. Reviewed *Promoting Safety and Comfort: Drainage Systems*.	___	___	_____
2. Collected the following:			
• Graduate (measuring container)	___	___	_____
• Gloves	___	___	_____
• Paper towels	___	___	_____
3. Practiced hand hygiene.	___	___	_____
4. Identified the person. Checked the ID bracelet against the assignment sheet. Called the person by name.	___	___	_____
5. Provided for privacy.	___	___	_____

Procedure

	S	U	Comments
6. Put on the gloves.	___	___	_____
7. Placed a paper towel on the floor. Placed the graduate on top of it.	___	___	_____
8. Positioned the graduate under the collection bag.	___	___	_____
9. Opened the clamp on the drain.	___	___	_____
10. Let all urine drain into the graduate. Did not let the drain touch the graduate.	___	___	_____
11. Closed and positioned the clamp.	___	___	_____
12. Measured urine.	___	___	_____
13. Removed and discarded the paper towel.	___	___	_____
14. Emptied the contents of the graduate into the toilet and flushed.	___	___	_____
15. Rinsed the graduate. Emptied the rinse into the toilet and flushed.	___	___	_____
16. Cleaned and disinfected the graduate.	___	___	_____
17. Returned the graduate to its proper place.	___	___	_____
18. Removed the gloves. Practiced hand hygiene.	___	___	_____
19. Recorded the time and amount on the intake and output (I&O) record (Chapter 20).	___	___	_____

Post-Procedure

	S	U	Comments
20. Provided for comfort as noted on the inside of the front textbook cover.	___	___	_____
21. Placed the signal light within reach.	___	___	_____
22. Unscreened the person.	___	___	_____
23. Completed a safety check of the room as noted on the inside of the front textbook cover.	___	___	_____
24. Reported and recorded the amount and other observations.	___	___	_____

Date of Satisfactory Completion _____   Instructor's Initials _____

Applying a Condom Catheter

View Video!

Name: _____   Date: _____

	S	U	Comments

Quality of Life
- Knocked before entering the person's room.
- Addressed the person by name.
- Introduced yourself by name and title.
- Explained the procedure to the person before beginning and during the procedure.
- Protected the person's rights during the procedure.
- Handled the person gently during the procedure.

Pre-Procedure
1. Followed *Delegation Guidelines:*
   a. *Perineal Care* (Chapter 15)
   b. *Condom Catheters*
   Reviewed *Promoting Safety and Comfort:*
   a. *Perineal Care* (Chapter 15)
   b. *Condom Catheters*
2. Practiced hand hygiene.
3. Collected the following:
   - Condom catheter
   - Elastic tape
   - Drainage bag or leg bag
   - Cap for the drainage bag
   - Basin of warm water
   - Soap
   - Towel and washcloths
   - Bath blanket
   - Gloves
   - Waterproof pad
   - Paper towels
4. Arranged paper towels and equipment on the overbed table.
5. Identified the person. Checked the ID bracelet against the assignment sheet. Called the person by name.
6. Provided for privacy.
7. Raised the bed for body mechanics. Bed rails were up if used.

Procedure
8. Lowered the bed rail near you if up.
9. Practiced hand hygiene. Put on the gloves.
10. Covered the person with a bath blanket. Lowered top linens to the knees.
11. Asked the person to raise his buttocks off the bed or turned him onto his side away from you.
12. Slid the waterproof pad under his buttocks.
13. Had the person lower his buttocks or turned him onto his back.
14. Secured the drainage bag to the bed frame or had a leg bag ready. Closed the drain.
15. Exposed the genital area.

Date of Satisfactory Completion _____   Instructor's Initials _____

Procedure—cont'd	**S**	**U**	**Comments**
16. Removed the condom catheter.			
a. Removed the tape. Rolled the sheath off the penis.	_____	_____	_____
b. Disconnected the drainage tubing from the condom. Capped the drainage tube.	_____	_____	_____
c. Discarded the tape and condom.	_____	_____	_____
17. Provided perineal care (Chapter 15). Observed the penis for reddened areas, skin breakdown, and irritation.	_____	_____	_____
18. Removed the gloves, and practiced hand hygiene. Put on clean gloves.	_____	_____	_____
19. Removed the protective backing from the condom to expose the adhesive strip.	_____	_____	_____
20. Held the penis firmly. Rolled the condom onto the penis. Left a 1-inch space between the penis and the end of the catheter.	_____	_____	_____
21. Secured the condom.			
a. For a self-adhering condom, pressed the condom to the penis.	_____	_____	_____
b. For a condom secured with elastic tape, applied elastic tape in a spiral. Did not apply the tape completely around the penis.	_____	_____	_____
22. Made sure the penis tip did not touch the condom. Made sure the condom was not twisted.	_____	_____	_____
23. Connected the condom to the drainage tubing. Coiled and secured excess tubing on the bed or attached a leg bag.	_____	_____	_____
24. Removed the waterproof pad and gloves. Discarded them. Practiced hand hygiene.	_____	_____	_____
25. Covered the person. Removed the bath blanket.	_____	_____	_____
Post-Procedure			
26. Provided for comfort as noted on the inside of the front textbook cover.	_____	_____	_____
27. Placed the signal light within reach.	_____	_____	_____
28. Lowered the bed to its lowest position.	_____	_____	_____
29. Raised or lowered bed rails. Followed the care plan.	_____	_____	_____
30. Unscreened the person.	_____	_____	_____
31. Practiced hand hygiene. Put on clean gloves.	_____	_____	_____
32. Measured and recorded the amount of urine in the bag. Cleaned or discarded the collection bag.	_____	_____	_____
33. Cleaned, dried, and returned the wash basin and other equipment. Returned items to their proper place.	_____	_____	_____
34. Removed the gloves. Practiced hand hygiene.	_____	_____	_____
35. Completed a safety check of the room as noted on the inside of the front textbook cover.	_____	_____	_____
36. Reported and recorded your observations.	_____	_____	_____

Date of Satisfactory Completion _____ Instructor's Initials _____

Giving a Cleansing Enema

Name: _____   Date: _____

Quality of Life	S	U	Comments
• Knocked before entering the person's room.	___	___	_____
• Addressed the person by name.	___	___	_____
• Introduced yourself by name and title.	___	___	_____
• Explained the procedure to the person before beginning and during the procedure.	___	___	_____
• Protected the person's rights during the procedure.	___	___	_____
• Handled the person gently during the procedure.	___	___	_____

Pre-Procedure

	S	U	Comments
1. Followed *Delegation Guidelines: Enemas.* Reviewed *Promoting Safety and Comfort: Enemas.*	___	___	_____
2. Practiced hand hygiene.	___	___	_____
3. Collected the following before going to the person's room:			
• Disposable enema kit as directed by the nurse (enema bag, tube, clamp, and waterproof pad)	___	___	_____
• Bath thermometer	___	___	_____
• Waterproof pad (if not in the enema kit)	___	___	_____
• Water soluble lubricant	___	___	_____
• 3 to 5 mL (1 teaspoon) of castile soap or 1 to 2 teaspoons of salt	___	___	_____
• IV (intravenous) pole	___	___	_____
• Gloves	___	___	_____
4. Arranged items in the person's room and bathroom.	___	___	_____
5. Decontaminated your hands.	___	___	_____
6. Identified the person. Checked the ID bracelet against the assignment sheet. Called the person by name.	___	___	_____
7. Put on gloves.	___	___	_____
8. Collected the following:			
• Commode or bedpan and cover	___	___	_____
• Toilet tissue	___	___	_____
• Bath blanket	___	___	_____
• Robe and non-skid footwear	___	___	_____
• Paper towels	___	___	_____
9. Provided for privacy.	___	___	_____
10. Raised the bed for body mechanics. Bed rails were up if used.	___	___	_____

Procedure

	S	U	Comments
11. Lowered the bed rail near you if up.	___	___	_____
12. Removed gloves, and decontaminated your hands. Put on clean gloves.	___	___	_____
13. Covered the person with a bath blanket. Fan-folded top linens to the foot of the bed.	___	___	_____
14. Positioned the IV pole so the enema bag was 12 inches above the anus, or it was at a height directed by the nurse.	___	___	_____
15. Raised the bed rail if used.	___	___	_____

Date of Satisfactory Completion _____   Instructor's Initials _____

Procedure—cont'd   **S**   **U**   **Comments**

16. Prepared the enema:
   a. Closed the clamp on the tube.   _____   _____   _____
   b. Adjusted water flow until it was lukewarm.   _____   _____   _____
   c. Filled the enema bag for the amount ordered.   _____   _____   _____
   d. Measured water temperature with the bath
      thermometer as directed by the nurse.   _____   _____   _____
   e. Prepared the solution as directed by the nurse:
      (1) Tap water enema: added nothing   _____   _____   _____
      (2) Saline enema: added salt as directed   _____   _____   _____
      (3) Soapsuds enema: added castile soap as directed _____   _____   _____
   f. Stirred the solution with the bath thermometer.
      Scooped off any suds (SSE).   _____   _____   _____
   g. Sealed the bag.   _____   _____   _____
   h. Hung the bag on the IV pole.   _____   _____   _____
17. Lowered the bed rail near you if up.   _____   _____   _____
18. Positioned the person in Sims' position or in a
    left side-lying position.   _____   _____   _____
19. Placed a waterproof pad under the buttocks.   _____   _____   _____
20. Exposed the anal area.   _____   _____   _____
21. Placed the bedpan behind the person.   _____   _____   _____
22. Positioned the enema tube in the bedpan. Removed the
    cap from the tubing.   _____   _____   _____
23. Opened the clamp. Let solution flow through the tube to
    remove air. Clamped the tube.   _____   _____   _____
24. Lubricated the tube 2 to 4 inches from the tip.   _____   _____   _____
25. Separated the buttocks to see the anus.   _____   _____   _____
26. Asked the person to take a deep breath through
    the mouth.   _____   _____   _____
27. Inserted the tube gently 2 to 4 inches into the adult's
    rectum. Did this when the person was exhaling. Stopped
    if the person complained of pain, you felt resistance,
    or bleeding occurred.   _____   _____   _____
28. Checked the amount of solution in the bag.   _____   _____   _____
29. Unclamped the tube. Gave the solution slowly.   _____   _____   _____
30. Asked the person to take slow deep breaths.   _____   _____   _____
31. Clamped the tube if the person needed to defecate,
    had cramping, or started to expel solution. Clamped the
    tube if the person was sweating or complained of nausea
    or weakness. Unclamped when symptoms subsided.   _____   _____   _____
32. Gave the amount of solution ordered. Stopped if the
    person could not tolerate the procedure.   _____   _____   _____
33. Clamped the tube before it was empty.   _____   _____   _____
34. Held toilet tissue around the tube and against the anus.
    Removed the tube.   _____   _____   _____
35. Discarded the toilet tissue into the bedpan.   _____   _____   _____
36. Wrapped the tubing tip with paper towels. Placed it
    inside the enema bag.   _____   _____   _____
37. Assisted the person to the bathroom or commode.   _____   _____   _____
    The person wore a robe and non-skid footwear when up.
    The bed was in the lowest position. Or, helped the person
    onto the bedpan. Raised the head of the bed. Raised or
    lowered bed rails according to the care plan.

Date of Satisfactory Completion _____   Instructor's Initials _____

Procedure—cont'd	S	U	Comments
38. Placed the signal light and toilet tissue within reach. Reminded the person not to flush the toilet.	_____	_____	_____
39. Discarded disposable items.	_____	_____	_____
40. Removed the gloves. Practiced hand hygiene.	_____	_____	_____
41. Left the room if the person could be left alone.	_____	_____	_____
42. Returned when the person signaled. Or checked on the person every 5 minutes. Knocked before entering the room or bathroom.	_____	_____	_____
43. Decontaminated your hands, and put on gloves. Lowered the bed rail if up.	_____	_____	_____
44. Observed enema results for amount, color, consistency, shape, and odor. Called for the nurse to observe the results.	_____	_____	_____
45. Provided perineal care as needed.	_____	_____	_____
46. Removed the waterproof pad.	_____	_____	_____
47. Emptied, cleaned, and disinfected equipment. Flushed the toilet after the nurse observed the results.	_____	_____	_____
48. Returned equipment to its proper place.	_____	_____	_____
49. Removed the gloves. Practiced hand hygiene.	_____	_____	_____
50. Assisted with hand washing. Wore gloves.	_____	_____	_____
51. Covered the person. Removed the bath blanket.	_____	_____	_____

Post-Procedure

	S	U	Comments
52. Provided for comfort as noted on the inside of the front textbook cover.	_____	_____	_____
53. Placed the signal light within reach.	_____	_____	_____
54. Lowered the bed to its lowest position.	_____	_____	_____
55. Raised or lowered bed rails. Followed the care plan.	_____	_____	_____
56. Unscreened the person.	_____	_____	_____
57. Completed a safety check of the room as noted on the inside of the front textbook cover.	_____	_____	_____
58. Followed agency policy for dirty linen and used supplies.	_____	_____	_____
59. Practiced hand hygiene.	_____	_____	_____
60. Reported and recorded your observations.	_____	_____	_____

Date of Satisfactory Completion _____   Instructor's Initials _____

Giving a Small-Volume Enema

View Video!

Name: _____   Date: _____

	S	U	Comments

Quality of Life
- Knocked before entering the person's room.
- Addressed the person by name.
- Introduced yourself by name and title.
- Explained the procedure to the person before beginning and during the procedure.
- Protected the person's rights during the procedure.
- Handled the person gently during the procedure.

Pre-Procedure
1. Followed *Delegation Guidelines: Enemas.* Reviewed *Promoting Safety and Comfort: Enemas.*
2. Practiced hand hygiene.
3. Collected the following before going to the person's room:
   - Small-volume enema
   - Waterproof pad
   - Gloves
4. Arranged items in the person's room.
5. Practiced hand hygiene.
6. Identified the person. Checked the ID bracelet against the assignment sheet. Called the person by name.
7. Put on gloves.
8. Collected the following:
   - Commode or bedpan
   - Waterproof pad
   - Toilet tissue
   - Robe and non-skid footwear
   - Bath blanket
9. Provided for privacy.
10. Raised the bed for body mechanics. Bed rails were up if used.

Procedure
11. Lowered the bed rail near you if up.
12. Removed the gloves, and practiced hand hygiene. Put on clean gloves.
13. Covered the person with a bath blanket. Fan-folded top linens to the foot of the bed.
14. Positioned the person in Sims' or a left side-lying position.
15. Placed the waterproof pad under the buttocks.
16. Exposed the anal area.
17. Positioned the bedpan near the person.
18. Removed the cap from the enema tip.
19. Separated the buttocks to see the anus.
20. Asked the person to take a deep breath through the mouth.
21. Inserted the enema tip 2 inches into the adult's rectum. Did this when the person was exhaling. Inserted the tip gently. Stopped if the person complained of pain, you felt resistance, or bleeding occurred.
22. Squeezed and rolled the bottle gently. Released pressure on the bottle after you removed the tip from the rectum.

Date of Satisfactory Completion _____   Instructor's Initials _____

Procedure—cont'd	S	U	Comments
23. Put the bottle into the box, tip first.	___	___	_____
24. Assisted the person to the bathroom or commode when he or she had the urge to have a BM. The person wore a robe and non-skid footwear when up. The bed was in the lowest position. Or helped the person onto the bedpan and raised the head of the bed. Raised or lowered bed rails according to the care plan.	___	___	_____
25. Placed the signal light and toilet tissue within reach. Reminded the person not to flush the toilet.	___	___	_____
26. Discarded disposable items.	___	___	_____
27. Removed the gloves. Practiced hand hygiene.	___	___	_____
28. Left the room if the person could be left alone.	___	___	_____
29. Returned when the person signaled. Or checked on the person every 5 minutes. Knocked before entering the room or bathroom.	___	___	_____
30. Practiced hand hygiene. Put on gloves.	___	___	_____
31. Lowered the bed rail if up.	___	___	_____
32. Observed enema results for amount, color, consistency, shape, and odor. Called for the nurse to observe the results.	___	___	_____
33. Provided perineal care as needed.	___	___	_____
34. Removed the waterproof pad.	___	___	_____
35. Emptied, cleaned, and disinfected the equipment. Flushed the toilet after the nurse observed the results.	___	___	_____
36. Returned equipment to its proper place.	___	___	_____
37. Removed the gloves, and practiced hand hygiene.	___	___	_____
38. Assisted the person with hand washing. Wore gloves.	___	___	_____
39. Covered the person. Removed the bath blanket.	___	___	_____

Post-Procedure

	S	U	Comments
40. Provided for comfort as noted on the inside of the front textbook cover.	___	___	_____
41. Placed the signal light within reach.	___	___	_____
42. Lowered the bed to its lowest position.	___	___	_____
43. Raised or lowered bed rails. Followed the care plan.	___	___	_____
44. Unscreened the person.	___	___	_____
45. Completed a safety check of the room as noted on the inside of the front textbook cover.	___	___	_____
46. Followed agency policy for dirty linen and used supplies.	___	___	_____
47. Practiced hand hygiene.	___	___	_____
48. Reported and recorded your observations.	___	___	_____

Date of Satisfactory Completion _____ Instructor's Initials _____

Preparing the Person for a Meal

Name: _____   Date: _____

Quality of Life	S	U	Comments
• Knocked before entering the person's room.	____	____	_____
• Addressed the person by name.	____	____	_____
• Introduced yourself by name and title.	____	____	_____
• Explained the procedure to the person before beginning and during the procedure.	____	____	_____
• Protected the person's rights during the procedure.	____	____	_____
• Handled the person gently during the procedure.	____	____	_____

Pre-Procedure

	S	U	Comments
1. Followed *Delegation Guidelines: Preparing for Meals.* Reviewed *Promoting Safety and Comfort: Preparing for Meals.*	____	____	_____
2. Practiced hand hygiene.	____	____	_____
3. Collected the following:			
• Equipment for oral hygiene	____	____	_____
• Bedpan and cover, urinal, commode, or specimen pan	____	____	_____
• Toilet tissue	____	____	_____
• Wash basin	____	____	_____
• Soap	____	____	_____
• Washcloth	____	____	_____
• Towel	____	____	_____
• Gloves	____	____	_____
4. Provided for privacy.	____	____	_____

Procedure

	S	U	Comments
5. Made sure eyeglasses and hearing aids were in place.	____	____	_____
6. Assisted with oral hygiene. Made sure dentures were in place. Wore gloves, and decontaminated your hands after removing them.	____	____	_____
7. Assisted with elimination. Made sure the incontinent person was clean and dry. Wore gloves, and practiced hand hygiene after removing them.	____	____	_____
8. Assisted the person with hand washing. Wore gloves, and practiced hand hygiene after removing them.	____	____	_____
9. Did the following if the person would eat in bed:			
a. Raised the head of the bed to a comfortable position.	____	____	_____
b. Removed items from the overbed table. Cleaned the overbed table.	____	____	_____
c. Adjusted the overbed table in front of the person.	____	____	_____
10. Did the following if the person would sit in a chair.			
a. Positioned the person in a chair or wheelchair.	____	____	_____
b. Removed items from the overbed table. Cleaned the table.	____	____	_____
c. Adjusted the overbed table in front of the person.	____	____	_____
11. Assisted the person to the dining area (if the person would eat in the dining area).	____	____	_____

Post-Procedure

	S	U	Comments
12. Provided for comfort as noted on the inside of the front textbook cover.	____	____	_____
13. Placed the signal light within reach.	____	____	_____

Date of Satisfactory Completion _____   Instructor's Initials _____

Post-Procedure—cont'd	S	U	Comments
14. Emptied, cleaned, and disinfected equipment. Returned equipment to its proper place. Wore gloves, and practiced hand hygiene after removing them.	_____	_____	_____
15. Straightened the room. Eliminated unpleasant noise, odors, or equipment.	_____	_____	_____
16. Unscreened the person.	_____	_____	_____
17. Completed a safety check of the room as noted on the inside of the front textbook cover.	_____	_____	_____
18. Decontaminated your hands.	_____	_____	_____

Date of Satisfactory Completion _____ Instructor's Initials _____

Serving Meal Trays

View Video!

Name: _____   Date: _____

	S	U	Comments

Quality of Life
- Knocked before entering the person's room.
- Addressed the person by name.
- Introduced yourself by name and title.
- Explained the procedure to the person before beginning and during the procedure.
- Protected the person's rights during the procedure.
- Handled the person gently during the procedure.

Pre-Procedure
1. Followed *Delegation Guidelines: Serving Meal Trays.* Reviewed *Promoting Safety and Comfort: Serving Meal Trays.*
2. Practiced hand hygiene.

Procedure
3. Made sure the tray was complete. Checked items on the tray with the dietary card. Made sure assistive devices were included.
4. Identified the person. Checked the ID bracelet against the dietary card. Called the person by name.
5. Placed the tray within the person's reach. Adjusted the overbed table as needed.
6. Removed food covers. Opened cartons, cut food into bite-size pieces, buttered bread, and so on as needed. Seasoned food as the person preferred and as allowed on the care plan.
7. Placed the napkin, clothes protector, assistive devices, and eating utensils within reach.
8. Placed the signal light within reach.
9. Did the following when the person was done eating:
   a. Measured and recorded intake if ordered (Chapter 20).
   b. Noted the amount and type of foods eaten.
   c. Checked for and removed any food in the mouth (pocketing). Wore gloves. Decontaminated your hands after removing them.
   d. Removed the tray.
   e. Cleaned spills. Changed soiled linen and clothing.
   f. Helped the person return to bed if needed.
   g. Assisted the person with oral hygiene and hand washing. Wore gloves. Decontaminated your hands after removing the gloves.

Post-Procedure
10. Provided for comfort as noted on the inside of the front textbook cover.
11. Placed the signal light within reach.
12. Raised or lowered bed rails. Followed the care plan.
13. Completed a safety check of the room as noted on the inside of the front textbook cover.
14. Followed agency policy for soiled linen.
15. Decontaminated your hands.
16. Reported and recorded your observations.

Date of Satisfactory Completion _____   Instructor's Initials _____

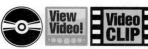

Feeding the Person (NNAAP™)

Name: _____   Date: _____

Quality of Life	S	U	Comments
• Knocked before entering the person's room.			
• Addressed the person by name.			
• Introduced yourself by name and title.			
• Explained the procedure to the person before beginning and during the procedure.			
• Protected the person's rights during the procedure.			
• Handled the person gently during the procedure.			

Pre-Procedure

	S	U	Comments
1. Followed *Delegation Guidelines: Feeding the Person.* Reviewed *Promoting Safety and Comfort: Feeding the Person.*			
2. Practiced hand hygiene.			
3. Positioned the person in a comfortable position for eating.			
4. Got the tray. Placed it on the overbed table or dining table.			

Procedure

	S	U	Comments
5. Identified the person. Checked the ID bracelet against the dietary card. Called the person by name.			
6. Draped a napkin across the person's chest and underneath the chin.			
7. Told the person what foods and fluids were on the tray.			
8. Prepared food for eating. Cut food into bite-size pieces. Seasoned food as the person preferred and as allowed on the care plan.			
9. Placed the chair where you could sit comfortably. Sat facing the person.			
10. Served foods in the order the person preferred. Identified foods as you served them. Alternated between solid and liquid foods. Used a spoon for safety. Allowed enough time for chewing and swallowing. Did not rush the person. Offered water, coffee, tea, or other beverage on the tray.			
11. Checked the person's mouth before offering more food or fluids. Made sure the person's mouth was empty between bites and swallows.			
12. Used straws for liquids if the person could not drink out of a glass or cup. Had one straw for each liquid. Provided short straws for weak persons.			
13. Wiped the person's hands, face, and mouth as needed during the meal. Used the napkin.			
14. Followed the care plan if the person had dysphagia. Gave thickened liquid with a spoon.			
15. Conversed with the person in a pleasant manner.			
16. Encouraged the person to eat as much as possible.			
17. Wiped the person's mouth with a napkin. Discarded the napkin.			
18. Noted how much and which foods were eaten.			
19. Measured and recorded intake if ordered (Chapter 20).			
20. Removed the tray.			
21. Took the person back to his or her room (if in a dining area).			
22. Assisted with oral hygiene and hand washing. Provided for privacy, and put on gloves. Decontaminated your hands after removing the gloves.			

Date of Satisfactory Completion _____   Instructor's Initials _____

Post-Procedure   S   U   Comments

23. Provided for comfort as noted on the inside of the front
    textbook cover.   _____   _____   _____
24. Placed the signal light within reach.   _____   _____   _____
25. Raised or lowered bed rails. Followed the care plan. _____   _____   _____
26. Completed a safety check of the room as noted on the
    inside of the front textbook cover.   _____   _____   _____
27. Returned the food tray to the food cart.   _____   _____   _____
28. Decontaminated your hands.   _____   _____   _____
29. Reported and recorded your observations.   _____   _____   _____

Date of Satisfactory Completion _____   Instructor's Initials _____

Providing Drinking Water

Name: _____ Date: _____

	S	U	C...

Quality of Life

- Knocked before entering the person's room.
- Addressed the person by name.
- Introduced yourself by name and title.
- Explained the procedure to the person before beginning and during the procedure.
- Protected the person's rights during the procedure.
- Handled the person gently during the procedure.

Pre-Procedure

1. Followed *Delegation Guidelines: Providing Drinking Water*. Reviewed *Promoting Safety and Comfort: Providing Drinking Water*.
2. Obtained a list of persons with special fluid orders from the nurse or used your assignment sheet.
3. Practiced hand hygiene.
4. Collected the following:
   - Cart
   - Ice chest filled with ice
   - Cover for the ice chest
   - Scoop
   - Disposable cups
   - Straws
   - Paper towels
   - Water pitchers for patient and resident use
   - Large water pitcher filled with cold water (depending on agency procedure)
   - Towel for the scoop
5. Covered the cart with paper towels. Arranged equipment on top of the paper towels.

Procedure

6. Took the cart to the person's room door. Did not take the cart into the room.
7. Checked the person's fluid orders. Used the list from the nurse.
8. Identified the person. Checked the ID bracelet against the fluid orders sheet or your assignment sheet. Called the person by name.
9. Took the pitcher from the person's overbed table. Emptied it into the bathroom sink.
10. Determined if a new water pitcher was needed.
11. Used the scoop to fill the pitcher with ice. Did not let the scoop touch the rim or inside of the pitcher.
12. Placed the ice scoop on the towel.
13. Filled the water pitcher with water. Got water from the bathroom or used the larger water pitcher on the cart.
14. Placed the pitcher, disposable cup, and straw (if used) on the overbed table. Filled the cup with water. Did not let the water pitcher touch the rim or inside of the cup.
15. Made sure the water pitcher, cup, and straw (if used) were within the person's reach.

Date of Satisfactory Completion _____ Instructor's Initials _____

	S	U	Comments

292   Chapter 19

...e of the front

Post-Procedure

16. Provided fo... ...reach.
    ...eck of the room as noted on the
    textbook ...nt textbook cover.
17. Plac... ...nated your hands.
18. C...
    ...peated steps 6 through 19 for each person.

Taking a Temperature With a Glass Thermometer

Name: _____   Date: _____

Quality of Life	S	U	Comments
• Knocked before entering the person's room.	___	___	_____
• Addressed the person by name.	___	___	_____
• Introduced yourself by name and title.	___	___	_____
• Explained the procedure to the person before beginning and during the procedure.	___	___	_____
• Protected the person's rights during the procedure.	___	___	_____
• Handled the person gently during the procedure.	___	___	_____

Pre-Procedure

	S	U	Comments
1. Followed *Delegation Guidelines: Taking Temperatures*. Reviewed *Promoting Safety and Comfort:* a. *Glass Thermometers* b. *Taking Temperatures*	___ ___	___ ___	_____ _____
2. For an oral temperature, asked the person not to eat, drink, smoke, or chew gum for at least 15 to 20 minutes before the measurement or as required by agency policy.	___	___	_____
3. Practiced hand hygiene.	___	___	_____
4. Collected the following: • Oral or rectal thermometer and holder • Tissues • Plastic covers if used • Gloves • Toilet tissue (rectal temperature) • Water-soluble lubricant (rectal temperature) • Towel (axillary temperature)	___ ___ ___ ___ ___ ___ ___	___ ___ ___ ___ ___ ___ ___	_____ _____ _____ _____ _____ _____ _____
5. Decontaminated your hands.	___	___	_____
6. Identified the person. Checked the ID bracelet against the assignment sheet. Called the person by name.	___	___	_____
7. Provided for privacy.	___	___	_____

Procedure

	S	U	Comments
8. Put on the gloves.	___	___	_____
9. Rinsed the thermometer in cold water if it was soaking in a disinfectant. Dried it with tissues.	___	___	_____
10. Checked for breaks, cracks, or chips.	___	___	_____
11. Shook down the thermometer below the lowest number. Held the thermometer by the stem.	___	___	_____
12. Inserted it into a plastic cover if used.	___	___	_____
13. For an oral temperature: a. Asked the person to moisten his or her lips. b. Placed the bulb end of the thermometer under the tongue and to one side. c. Asked the person to close the lips around the thermometer to hold it in place. d. Asked the person not to talk. Reminded the person not to bite down on the thermometer. e. Left it in place for 2 to 3 minutes or as required by agency policy.	___ ___ ___ ___ ___	___ ___ ___ ___ ___	_____ _____ _____ _____ _____
14. For a rectal temperature: a. Positioned the person in Sims' position. b. Put a small amount of lubricant on a tissue. c. Lubricated the bulb end of the thermometer. d. Folded back top linens to expose the anal area.	___ ___ ___ ___	___ ___ ___ ___	_____ _____ _____ _____

Date of Satisfactory Completion _____   Instructor's Initials _____

Procedure—cont'd	S	U	Comments
e. Raised the upper buttock to expose the anus.	____	____	_____
f. Inserted the thermometer 1 inch into the rectum. Did not force the thermometer.	____	____	_____
g. Held the thermometer in place for 2 minutes or as required by agency policy. Did not let go of it while it was in the rectum.	____	____	_____
15. For an axillary temperature:			
a. Helped the person remove an arm from the gown. Did not expose the person.	____	____	_____
b. Dried the axilla with the towel.	____	____	_____
c. Placed the bulb end of the thermometer in the center of the axilla.	____	____	_____
d. Asked the person to place the arm over the chest to hold the thermometer in place. Held it and the arm in place if he or she could not help.	____	____	_____
e. Left the thermometer in place for 5 to 10 minutes or as required by agency policy.	____	____	_____
16. Removed the thermometer.	____	____	_____
17. Used tissues to remove the plastic cover. Discarded the cover and tissues. Wiped the thermometer with a tissue if no cover was used. Wiped from the stem to the bulb end. Discarded the tissue.	____	____	_____
18. Read the thermometer.	____	____	_____
19. Noted the person's name and temperature on your notepad or assignment sheet. Wrote R for a rectal temperature. Wrote A for an axillary temperature.	____	____	_____
20. For a rectal temperature:			
a. Placed used toilet tissue on several thicknesses of toilet tissue.	____	____	_____
b. Placed the thermometer on clean toilet tissue.	____	____	_____
c. Wiped the anal area to remove excess lubricant and any feces.	____	____	_____
d. Covered the person.	____	____	_____
21. For an axillary temperature: Helped the person put the gown back on.	____	____	_____
22. Shook down the thermometer.	____	____	_____
23. Cleaned the thermometer according to agency policy. Returned it to the holder.	____	____	_____
24. Discarded tissues and disposed of toilet tissue.	____	____	_____
25. Removed the gloves. Decontaminated your hands.	____	____	_____
Post-Procedure			
26. Provided for comfort as noted on the inside of the front textbook cover.	____	____	_____
27. Placed the signal light within reach.	____	____	_____
28. Unscreened the person.	____	____	_____
29. Completed a safety check of the room as noted on the inside of the front textbook cover.	____	____	_____
30. Decontaminated your hands.	____	____	_____
31. Reported and recorded the temperature. Noted the temperature site. Reported an abnormal temperature at once.	____	____	_____

Date of Satisfactory Completion _____   Instructor's Initials _____

Taking a Temperature With an Electronic Thermometer

Name: _____ Date: _____

	S	U	Comments

Quality of Life
- Knocked before entering the person's room.
- Addressed the person by name.
- Introduced yourself by name and title.
- Explained the procedure to the person before beginning and during the procedure.
- Protected the person's rights during the procedure.
- Handled the person gently during the procedure.

Pre-Procedure
1. Followed *Delegation Guidelines: Taking Temperatures*. Reviewed *Promoting Safety and Comfort: Taking Temperatures*.
2. For an oral temperature, asked the person not to eat, drink, smoke, or chew gum for at least 15 to 20 minutes before the measurement or as required by agency policy.
3. Practiced hand hygiene.
4. Collected the following:
   - Thermometer—electronic, tympanic membrane, or temporal artery
   - Probe (Blue for an oral or axillary temperature. Red for a rectal temperature.)
   - Probe covers
   - Toilet tissue (rectal temperature)
   - Water-soluble lubricant (rectal temperature)
   - Gloves
   - Towel (axillary temperature)
5. Plugged the probe into the thermometer. (This was not done for a tympanic membrane or temporal artery thermometer.)
6. Decontaminated your hands.
7. Identified the person. Checked the ID bracelet against the assignment sheet. Called the person by name.

Procedure
8. Provided for privacy. Positioned the person for an oral, rectal, axillary, or tympanic membrane temperature.
9. Put on gloves if contact with blood, body fluids, secretions, or excretions was likely.
10. Inserted the probe into a probe cover.
11. For an oral temperature:
    a. Asked the person to open the mouth and raise the tongue.
    b. Placed the covered probe at the base of the tongue and to one side.
    c. Asked the person to lower the tongue and close the mouth.
12. For a rectal temperature:
    a. Placed some lubricant on toilet tissue.
    b. Lubricated the end of the covered probe.
    c. Exposed the anal area.
    d. Raised the upper buttock.
    e. Inserted the probe ½ inch into the rectum.
    f. Held the probe in place.

Date of Satisfactory Completion _____   Instructor's Initials _____

Procedure—cont'd	S	U	Comments
13. For an axillary temperature:			
a. Helped the person remove an arm from the gown. Did not expose the person.	___	___	_____
b. Dried the axilla with the towel.	___	___	_____
c. Placed the covered probe in the center of the axilla.	___	___	_____
d. Placed the person's arm over the chest.	___	___	_____
e. Held the probe in place.	___	___	_____
14. For a tympanic membrane temperature:			
a. Asked the person to turn his or her head so the ear was in front of you.	___	___	_____
b. Pulled back on the adult's ear to straighten the ear canal.	___	___	_____
c. Inserted the covered probe gently.	___	___	_____
15. Started the thermometer.	___	___	_____
16. Held the probe in place until you heard a tone or you saw a flashing or steady light.	___	___	_____
17. Read the temperature on the display.	___	___	_____
18. Removed the probe. Pressed the eject button to discard the cover.	___	___	_____
19. Noted the person's name and temperature on your notepad or assignment sheet. Noted the temperature site. Wrote R for a rectal temperature. Wrote A for an axillary temperature.	___	___	_____
20. Returned the probe to the holder.	___	___	_____
21. Helped the person put the gown back on (axillary temperature). For a rectal temperature:			
a. Wiped the anal area with toilet tissue to remove lubricant.	___	___	_____
b. Covered the person.	___	___	_____
c. Disposed of used toilet tissue.	___	___	_____
d. Removed the gloves. Decontaminated your hands.	___	___	_____

Post-Procedure

	S	U	Comments
22. Provided for comfort as noted on the inside of the front textbook cover.	___	___	_____
23. Placed the signal light within reach.	___	___	_____
24. Unscreened the person.	___	___	_____
25. Completed a safety check of the room as noted on the inside of the front textbook cover.	___	___	_____
26. Returned the thermometer to the charging unit.	___	___	_____
27. Decontaminated your hands.	___	___	_____
28. Reported and recorded the temperature. Noted the temperature site. Reported an abnormal temperature at once.	___	___	_____

Date of Satisfactory Completion _____ Instructor's Initials _____

Taking a Radial Pulse (NNAAP™)

Name: _____   Date: _____

Quality of Life	S	U	Comments
• Knocked before entering the person's room.			
• Addressed the person by name.			
• Introduced yourself by name and title.			
• Explained the procedure to the person before beginning and during the procedure.			
• Protected the person's rights during the procedure.			
• Handled the person gently during the procedure.			

Pre-Procedure

	S	U	Comments
1. Followed *Delegation Guidelines: Taking Pulses.* Reviewed *Promoting Safety and Comfort: Taking Pulses.*			
2. Practiced hand hygiene.			
3. Identified the person. Checked the ID bracelet against the assignment sheet. Called the person by name.			
4. Provided for privacy.			

Procedure

	S	U	Comments
5. Had the person sit or lie down.			
6. Located the radial pulse on the thumb side of the person's wrist. Used your first 2 or 3 middle fingertips.			
7. Noted if the pulse was strong or weak, and regular or irregular.			
8. Counted the pulse for 30 seconds. Multiplied the number of beats by 2. Or counted the pulse for 1 minute if:			
a. Directed by the nurse and care plan			
b. Required by agency policy			
c. The pulse was irregular			
d. Required for your state competency test			
9. Noted the person's name and pulse on your notepad or assignment sheet. Noted the strength of the pulse. Noted if it was regular or irregular.			

Post-Procedure

	S	U	Comments
10. Provided for comfort as noted on the inside of the front textbook cover.			
11. Placed the signal light within reach.			
12. Unscreened the person.			
13. Completed a safety check of the room as noted on the inside of the front textbook cover.			
14. Decontaminated your hands.			
15. Reported and recorded the pulse rate and your observations. Reported an abnormal pulse at once.			

Date of Satisfactory Completion _____   Instructor's Initials _____

Taking an Apical Pulse

View Video!

Name: _____   Date: _____

Quality of Life	S	U	Comments
• Knocked before entering the person's room.	____	____	_____
• Addressed the person by name.	____	____	_____
• Introduced yourself by name and title.	____	____	_____
• Explained the procedure to the person before beginning and during the procedure.	____	____	_____
• Protected the person's rights during the procedure.	____	____	_____
• Handled the person gently during the procedure.	____	____	_____

Pre-Procedure

	S	U	Comments
1. Followed *Delegation Guidelines: Taking Pulses.* Reviewed *Promoting Safety and Comfort: Using a Stethoscope.*	____	____	_____
2. Practiced hand hygiene.	____	____	_____
3. Collected a stethoscope and antiseptic wipes.	____	____	_____
4. Decontaminated your hands.	____	____	_____
5. Identified the person. Checked the ID bracelet against the assignment sheet. Called the person by name.	____	____	_____
6. Provided for privacy.	____	____	_____

Procedure

	S	U	Comments
7. Cleaned the earpieces and diaphragm with the wipes.	____	____	_____
8. Had the person sit or lie down.	____	____	_____
9. Exposed the nipple area of the left chest. Limited exposure of a woman's breasts to the extent necessary.	____	____	_____
10. Warmed the diaphragm in your palm.	____	____	_____
11. Placed the earpieces in your ears.	____	____	_____
12. Found the apical pulse. Placed the diaphragm 2 to 3 inches to the left of the breastbone and below the left nipple.	____	____	_____
13. Counted the pulse for 1 minute. Noted if it was regular or irregular.	____	____	_____
14. Covered the person. Removed the earpieces.	____	____	_____
15. Noted the person's name and pulse on your notepad or assignment sheet. Noted if the pulse was regular or irregular.	____	____	_____

Post-Procedure

	S	U	Comments
16. Provided for comfort as noted on the inside of the front textbook cover.	____	____	_____
17. Placed the signal light within reach.	____	____	_____
18. Unscreened the person.	____	____	_____
19. Completed a safety check of the room as noted on the inside of the front textbook cover.	____	____	_____
20. Cleaned the earpieces and diaphragm with the wipes.	____	____	_____
21. Returned the stethoscope to its proper place.	____	____	_____
22. Decontaminated your hands.	____	____	_____
23. Reported and recorded your observations. Recorded the pulse rate with *Ap* for apical pulse. Reported an abnormal pulse rate at once.	____	____	_____

Date of Satisfactory Completion _____   Instructor's Initials _____

Counting Respirations (NNAAP™)

Name: ———————————   Date: ———————————

Procedure	S	U	Comments
1. Followed *Delegation Guidelines: Respirations*.	———	———	———————
2. Kept your fingers or the stethoscope over the pulse site.	———	———	———————
3. Did not tell the person you were counting respirations.	———	———	———————
4. Began counting when the chest rose. Counted each rise and fall of the chest as 1 respiration.	———	———	———————
5. Noted the following:			
a. If respirations were regular	———	———	———————
b. If both sides of the chest rose equally	———	———	———————
c. The depth of respirations	———	———	———————
d. If the person had any pain or difficulty breathing	———	———	———————
e. An abnormal respiratory pattern	———	———	———————
6. Counted respirations for 30 seconds. Multiplied the number by 2. Counted respirations for 1 minute if:	———	———	———————
a. Directed by the nurse and care plan	———	———	———————
b. Required by agency policy	———	———	———————
c. They were abnormal or irregular	———	———	———————
d. Required for your state competency test	———	———	———————
7. Noted the person's name, respiratory rate, and other observations on your notepad or assignment sheet.	———	———	———————

Post-Procedure

	S	U	Comments
8. Provided for comfort as noted on the inside of the front textbook cover.	———	———	———————
9. Placed the signal light within reach.	———	———	———————
10. Unscreened the person.	———	———	———————
11. Completed a safety check of the room as noted on the inside of the front textbook cover.	———	———	———————
12. Decontaminated your hands.	———	———	———————
13. Reported and recorded the respiratory rate and your observations. Reported abnormal respirations at once.	———	———	———————

Date of Satisfactory Completion ———————————   Instructor's Initials ———————————

Measuring Blood Pressure (NNAAP™)

Name: ———————————————   Date: ———————————————

	S	**U**	**Comments**

Quality of Life
- Knocked before entering the person's room.
- Addressed the person by name.
- Introduced yourself by name and title.
- Explained the procedure to the person before beginning and during the procedure.
- Protected the person's rights during the procedure.
- Handled the person gently during the procedure.

Pre-Procedure
1. Followed *Delegation Guidelines: Measuring Blood Pressure.* Reviewed *Promoting Safety and Comfort:*
   a. *Using a Stethoscope*
   b. *Equipment*
2. Practiced hand hygiene.
3. Collected the following:
   - Sphygmomanometer
   - Stethoscope
   - Antiseptic wipes
4. Decontaminated your hands.
5. Identified the person. Checked the ID bracelet against the assignment sheet. Called the person by name.
6. Provided for privacy.

Procedure
7. Wiped the stethoscope earpieces and diaphragm with the wipes. Warmed the diaphragm in your palm.
8. Had the person sit or lie down.
9. Positioned the person's arm level with the heart. The palm was up.
10. Stood no more than 3 feet away from the manometer. The mercury type was vertical, on a flat surface, and at eye level. The aneroid type was directly in front of you.
11. Exposed the upper arm.
12. Squeezed the cuff to expel any remaining air. Closed the valve on the bulb.
13. Found the brachial artery at the inner aspect of the elbow (on the little finger side of the arm). Used your fingertips.
14. Located the arrow on the cuff. Placed the arrow over the brachial artery. Wrapped the cuff around the upper arm at least 1 inch above the elbow. It was even and snug.
15. Placed the stethoscope earpieces in your ears.
16. Found the radial or brachial pulse.
17. Method one:
    a. Inflated the cuff until you could no longer feel the pulse. Noted this point.
    b. Inflated the cuff 30 mm Hg beyond the point where you last felt the pulse.

Date of Satisfactory Completion ———————————————   Instructor's Initials ———————————————

Procedure—cont'd   S   U   Comments

18. Method two:
    a. Inflated the cuff until you could no longer feel the pulse. Noted this point.   _____ _____ _____
    b. Inflated the cuff 30 mm Hg beyond the point where you last felt the pulse.   _____ _____ _____
    c. Deflated the cuff slowly. Noted the point when you felt the pulse.   _____ _____ _____
    d. Waited 30 seconds.   _____ _____ _____
    e. Inflated the cuff again, 30 mm Hg beyond the point where you felt the pulse return.   _____ _____ _____
19. Placed the diaphragm of the stethoscope over the brachial artery. Did not place it under the cuff.   _____ _____ _____
20. Deflated the cuff at an even rate of 2 to 4 millimeters per second. Turned the valve counter-clockwise to deflate the cuff.   _____ _____ _____
21. Noted the point where you heard the first sound. This was the systolic reading.   _____ _____ _____
22. Continued to deflate the cuff. Noted the point where the sound disappeared. This was the diastolic reading.   _____ _____ _____
23. Deflated the cuff completely. Removed it from the person's arm. Removed the stethoscope earpieces from your ears.   _____ _____ _____
24. Noted the person's name and blood pressure on the notepad or assignment sheet.   _____ _____ _____
25. Returned the cuff to the case or wall holder.   _____ _____ _____

Post-Procedure

26. Provided for comfort as noted on the inside of the front textbook cover.   _____ _____ _____
27. Placed the signal light within reach.   _____ _____ _____
28. Unscreened the person.   _____ _____ _____
29. Completed a safety check of the room as noted on the inside of the front textbook cover.   _____ _____ _____
30. Cleaned the earpieces and diaphragm with the wipes.   _____ _____ _____
31. Returned the equipment to its proper place.   _____ _____ _____
32. Decontaminated your hands.   _____ _____ _____
33. Reported and recorded the blood pressure. Noted which arm was used. Reported an abnormal blood pressure at once.   _____ _____ _____

Date of Satisfactory Completion _____ Instructor's Initials _____

View Video! Video CLIP Measuring Intake and Output (NNAAP™)

Name: ————————————   Date: ————————————

Quality of Life	S	U	Comments
• Knocked before entering the person's room.			
• Addressed the person by name.			
• Introduced yourself by name and title.			
• Explained the procedure to the person before beginning and during the procedure.			
• Protected the person's rights during the procedure.			
• Handled the person gently during the procedure.			

Pre-Procedure

1. Followed *Delegation Guidelines: Intake and Output.* Reviewed *Promoting Safety and Comfort: Intake and Output.*
2. Practiced hand hygiene.
3. Collected the following:
   • I&O record
   • Graduates
   • Gloves

Procedure

4. Put on gloves.
5. Measured intake as follows:
   a. Poured liquid remaining in a container into the graduate.
   b. Measured the amount at eye level or on a flat surface. Kept the container level.
   c. Checked the serving amount on the I&O record.
   d. Subtracted the remaining amount from the full serving amount. Noted the amount.
   e. Poured the fluid in the graduate back into the container.
   f. Repeated steps 5a through 5e for each liquid.
   g. Added the amounts from each liquid together.
   h. Recorded the time and amount on the I&O record.
6. Measured output as follows:
   a. Poured the fluid into the graduate used to measure output.
   b. Measured the amount at eye level or on a flat surface. Kept the container level.
   c. Disposed of fluid in the toilet. Avoided splashes.
7. Cleaned and rinsed the graduates. Disposed of rinse into the toilet. Returned the graduates to their proper place.
8. Cleaned and rinsed the bedpan, urinal, commode container, specimen pan, kidney basin, or other drainage container. Disposed of the rinse into the toilet. Returned the item to its proper place.
9. Removed the gloves. Practiced hand hygiene.
10. Recorded the amount on the I&O record.

Post-Procedure

11. Provided for comfort as noted on the inside of the front textbook cover.
12. Made sure the signal light was within reach.
13. Completed a safety check of the room as noted on the inside of the front textbook cover.
14. Reported and recorded your observations.

Date of Satisfactory Completion ————————————   Instructor's Initials ————————————

Measuring Weight and Height (NNAAP™)

Name: _____   Date: _____

Quality of Life	S	U	Comments
• Knocked before entering the person's room.	___	___	_____
• Addressed the person by name.	___	___	_____
• Introduced yourself by name and title.	___	___	_____
• Explained the procedure to the person before beginning and during the procedure.	___	___	_____
• Protected the person's rights during the procedure.	___	___	_____
• Handled the person gently during the procedure.	___	___	_____

Pre-Procedure

	S	U	Comments
1. Followed *Delegation Guidelines: Measuring Weight and Height.*	___	___	_____
Reviewed *Promoting Safety and Comfort: Measuring Weight and Height.*	___	___	_____
2. Asked the person to void.	___	___	_____
3. Practiced hand hygiene.	___	___	_____
4. Brought the scale and paper towels (for a standing scale) to the person's room.	___	___	_____
5. Decontaminated your hands.	___	___	_____
6. Identified the person. Checked the ID bracelet against the assignment sheet. Called the person by name.	___	___	_____
7. Provided for privacy.	___	___	_____

Procedure

	S	U	Comments
8. Placed the paper towels on the scale platform.	___	___	_____
9. Raised the height rod.	___	___	_____
10. Moved the weights to zero (0). The pointer was in the middle.	___	___	_____
11. Had the person remove the robe and footwear. Assisted as needed.	___	___	_____
12. Helped the person stand on the scale. The person stood in the center of the scale. Arms were at the sides.	___	___	_____
13. Moved the weights until the balance pointer was in the middle.	___	___	_____
14. Noted the weight on your notepad or assignment sheet.	___	___	_____
15. Asked the person to stand very straight.	___	___	_____
16. Lowered the height rod until it rested on the person's head.	___	___	_____
17. Noted the height on your notepad or assignment sheet.	___	___	_____
18. Raised the height rod. Helped the person step off of the scale.	___	___	_____
19. Helped the person put on a robe and non-skid footwear if he or she would be up. Or helped the person back to bed.	___	___	_____
20. Lowered the height rod. Adjusted the weights to zero (0) according to agency policy.	___	___	_____

Post-Procedure

	S	U	Comments
21. Provided for comfort as noted on the inside of the front textbook cover.	___	___	_____
22. Placed the signal light within reach.	___	___	_____
23. Raised or lowered bed rails. Followed the care plan.	___	___	_____

Date of Satisfactory Completion _____   Instructor's Initials _____

Post-Procedure—cont'd   **S**   **U**   **Comments**

24. Unscreened the person.

25. Completed a safety check of the room as noted on the inside of the front textbook cover.

26. Discarded the paper towels.

27. Returned the scale to its proper place.

28. Decontaminated your hands.

29. Reported and recorded the measurements.

Date of Satisfactory Completion _____   Instructor's Initials _____

Collecting a Random Urine Specimen

View Video!

Name: _____   Date: _____

Quality of Life	S	U	Comments
• Knocked before entering the person's room.			
• Addressed the person by name.			
• Introduced yourself by name and title.			
• Explained the procedure to the person before beginning and during the procedure.			
• Protected the person's rights during the procedure.			
• Handled the person gently during the procedure.			

Pre-Procedure

1. Followed *Delegation Guidelines: Urine Specimens.* Reviewed *Promoting Safety and Comfort: Urine Specimens.*
2. Practiced hand hygiene.
3. Collected the following before going to the person's room:
   • Laboratory requisition slip
   • Specimen container and lid
   • Specimen label
   • Plastic bag
   • biohazard label if needed
   • Gloves
4. Arranged collected items in the person's bathroom.
5. Decontaminated your hands.
6. Identified the person. Checked the ID bracelet against the requisition slip. Called the person by name.
7. Labeled the container in the person's presence.
8. Put on gloves.
9. Collected the following:
   • Voiding receptacle—bedpan and cover, urinal, commode, or specimen pan
   • Graduate to measure output
10. Provided for privacy.

Procedure

11. Asked the person to void into the receptacle. Reminded him or her to put toilet tissue into the wastebasket or toilet (not in the bedpan or specimen pan).
12. Took the receptacle to the bathroom.
13. Poured about 120 mL (4 oz) of urine into the specimen container.
14. Placed the lid on the specimen container. Put the container in the plastic bag. Did not let the container touch the outside of the bag. Applied a BIOHAZARD label according to agency policy.
15. Measured urine if I&O was ordered. Included the amount in the specimen container.
16. Emptied, cleaned, and disinfected equipment. Returned equipment to its proper place.
17. Removed the gloves, and practiced hand hygiene. Put on clean gloves.
18. Assisted with hand washing.
19. Removed the gloves. Practiced hand hygiene.

Date of Satisfactory Completion _____   Instructor's Initials _____

Post-procedure   **S**   **U**   **Comments**

20. Provided for comfort as noted on the inside of the
    front textbook cover.   _____   _____   _____
21. Placed the signal light within reach.   _____   _____   _____
22. Raised or lowered bed rails. Followed the care plan.   _____   _____   _____
23. Unscreened the person.   _____   _____   _____
24. Completed a safety check of the room as noted on the
    inside of the front textbook cover.   _____   _____   _____
25. Decontaminated your hands.   _____   _____   _____
26. Delivered the specimen and the requisition slip to the   _____   _____   _____
    laboratory or storage area. Followed agency policy.
    Wore gloves.
27. Reported and recorded your observations.   _____   _____   _____

Date of Satisfactory Completion _____   Instructor's Initials _____

Collecting a Midstream Specimen

Name: _____   Date: _____

	S	U	Comments

Quality of Life
- Knocked before entering the person's room.
- Addressed the person by name.
- Introduced yourself by name and title.
- Explained the procedure to the person before beginning and during the procedure.
- Protected the person's rights during the procedure.
- Handled the person gently during the procedure.

Pre-Procedure
1. Followed *Delegation Guidelines: Urine Specimens*. Reviewed *Promoting Safety and Comfort: Urine Specimens*.
2. Practiced hand hygiene.
3. Collected the following before going to the person's room:
   - Laboratory requisition slip
   - Midstream specimen kit—includes specimen container, label, and towelettes; may include sterile gloves
   - Plastic bag
   - Sterile gloves (if not part of the kit)
   - Disposable gloves
   - BIOHAZARD label (if needed)
4. Arranged work area.
5. Decontaminated your hands.
6. Identified the person. Checked the ID bracelet against the requisition slip. Called the person by name.
7. Put on disposable gloves.
8. Collected the following:
   - Voiding receptacle—bedpan and cover, urinal, commode, or specimen pan if needed
   - Supplies for perineal care
   - Graduate to measure output
   - Paper towel
9. Provided for privacy.

Procedure
10. Provided perineal care. (Wore gloves. Decontaminated your hands after removing them.)
11. Opened the sterile kit.
12. Put on the sterile gloves.
13. Opened the packet of towelettes inside the kit.
14. Opened the sterile specimen container. Did not touch the inside of the container or lid. Set the lid down so the inside was up.
15. For a female: cleaned the perineal area with towelettes.
    a. Spread the labia with your thumb and index finger. Used your non-dominant hand (now this hand did not touch anything sterile).
    b. Cleaned down the urethral area from front to back. Used a clean towelette for each stroke.
    c. Kept the labia separated to collect the urine specimen (steps 17 through 20).

Date of Satisfactory Completion _____   Instructor's Initials _____

Procedure—cont'd	**S**	**U**	**Comments**
16. For a male: cleaned the penis with the towelettes.			
a. Held the penis with your non-dominant hand (now this hand did not touch anything sterile).	——	——	————————
b. Cleaned the penis starting at the meatus. Cleaned in a circular motion. Started at the center and worked outward.	——	——	————————
c. Kept holding the penis until the specimen was collected (steps 17 through 20).	——	——	————————
17. Asked the person to void into the receptacle.	——	——	————————
18. Passed the specimen container into the stream of urine. Kept the labia separated.	——	——	————————
19. Collected about 30 to 60 mL (1 to 2 oz) of urine.	——	——	————————
20. Removed the specimen container before the person stopped voiding.	——	——	————————
21. Released the labia or penis. Let the person finish voiding into the receptacle.	——	——	————————
22. Put the lid on the specimen container. Touched only the outside of the container and lid. Wiped the outside of the container. Set the container on a paper towel.	——	——	————————
23. Provided toilet tissue after the person was done voiding.	——	——	————————
24. Took the receptacle to the bathroom.	——	——	————————
25. Measured urine if I&O was ordered. Included the amount in the specimen container.	——	——	————————
26. Emptied, cleaned, and disinfected equipment. Returned equipment to its proper place.	——	——	————————
27. Removed the gloves, and practiced hand hygiene. Put on clean disposable gloves.	——	——	————————
28. Labeled the specimen container in the person's presence. Placed the container in a plastic bag. Did not let the container touch the outside of the bag. Applied a BIOHAZARD label according to agency policy.	——	——	————————
29. Assisted with hand washing	——	——	————————
30. Removed the gloves. Practiced hand hygiene.	——	——	————————
Post-Procedure			
31. Provided for comfort as noted on the inside of the front textbook cover.	——	——	————————
32. Placed the signal light within reach.	——	——	————————
33. Raised or lowered bed rails. Followed the care plan.	——	——	————————
34. Unscreened the person.	——	——	————————
35. Completed a safety check of the room as noted on the inside of the front textbook cover.	——	——	————————
36. Decontaminated your hands.	——	——	————————
37. Delivered the specimen and the requisition slip to the laboratory or storage area. Followed agency policy. Wore gloves.	——	——	————————
38. Reported and recorded your observations.	——	——	————————

Date of Satisfactory Completion _____   Instructor's Initials _____

Collecting a Double-Voided Specimen

Name: _____ Date: _____

Quality of Life	S	U	Comments
• Knocked before entering the person's room.			
• Addressed the person by name.			
• Introduced yourself by name and title.			
• Explained the procedure to the person before beginning and during the procedure.			
• Protected the person's rights during the procedure.			
• Handled the person gently during the procedure.			

Pre-Procedure

	S	U	Comments
1. Followed *Delegation Guidelines: Urine Specimens*. Reviewed *Promoting Safety and Comfort: Urine Specimens*.			
2. Practiced hand hygiene. Put on gloves.			
3. Collected the following:			
• Voiding receptacle—bedpan and cover, urinal, commode, or specimen pan			
• Two specimen containers			
• Urine testing equipment			
• Graduate to measure output			
• Gloves			
4. Removed the gloves. Decontaminated your hands.			
5. Identified the person. Checked the ID bracelet against the assignment sheet. Called the person by name.			
6. Provided for privacy.			

Procedure

	S	U	Comments
7. Put on the gloves.			
8. Asked the person to void into the receptacle. Reminded the person not to put toilet tissue in the receptacle.			
9. Took the receptacle to the bathroom.			
10. Measured urine if I&O was ordered.			
11. Poured some urine into a specimen container.			
12. Tested the specimen in case the person could not provide a second specimen. Discarded the urine. Noted the result on your assignment sheet.			
13. Emptied, cleaned, and disinfected equipment. Returned equipment to its proper place.			
14. Removed the gloves, and practiced hand hygiene. Put on clean gloves.			
15. Assisted with hand washing.			
16. Removed the gloves. Practiced hand hygiene.			
17. Asked the person to drink an 8-ounce glass of water.			
18. Did the following before leaving the room:			
a. Provided for comfort as noted on the inside of the front textbook cover.			
b. Placed the signal light within reach.			
c. Raised or lowered the bed rails. Followed the care plan.			
d. Unscreened the person.			
e. Completed a safety check of the room as noted on the inside of the front textbook cover.			
f. Decontaminated your hands.			

Date of Satisfactory Completion _____ Instructor's Initials _____

Procedure—cont'd	S	U	Comments
19. Returned to the room in 20 to 30 minutes. Decontaminated your hands.	_____	_____	_____
20. Repeated steps 2 through 16.	_____	_____	_____
Post-Procedure			
21. Provided for comfort as noted on the inside of the front textbook cover.	_____	_____	_____
22. Placed the signal light within reach.	_____	_____	_____
23. Raised or lowered the bed rails. Followed the care plan.	_____	_____	_____
24. Unscreened the person.	_____	_____	_____
25. Completed a safety check of the room as noted on the inside of the front textbook cover.	_____	_____	_____
26. Decontaminated your hands.	_____	_____	_____
27. Reported and recorded the results of the second test and any other observations.	_____	_____	_____

Date of Satisfactory Completion _____   Instructor's Initials _____

Testing Urine With Reagent Strips

Name: —————————————————   Date: —————————————————

Quality of Life	S	U	Comments
• Knocked before entering the person's room.			
• Addressed the person by name.			
• Introduced yourself by name and title.			
• Explained the procedure to the person before beginning and during the procedure.			
• Protected the person's rights during the procedure.			
• Handled the person gently during the procedure.			

Pre-Procedure

	S	U	Comments

1. Followed *Delegation Guidelines: Testing Urine.* Reviewed *Promoting Safety and Comfort:*
  a. *Testing Urine*
  b. *Using Reagent Strips*			

2. Practiced hand hygiene.			
3. Collected gloves and the reagent strips ordered.			
4. Decontaminated your hands.			
5. Identified the person. Checked the ID bracelet against the assignment sheet. Called the person by name.			
6. Put on gloves.			
7. Collected equipment for collecting the urine specimen needed. (See procedure *Collecting a Random Urine Specimen* or *Collecting a Double-Voided Specimen*.)			
8. Provided for privacy.			

Procedure

	S	U	Comments
9. Collected the urine specimen. (See procedure *Collecting a Random Urine Specimen* or *Collecting a Double-Voided Specimen*.)			
10. Removed the strip from the bottle. Put the cap on the bottle at once. The cap was on tight.			
11. Dipped the strip test areas into the urine.			
12. Removed the strip after the correct amount of time. Followed the manufacturer's instructions.			
13. Tapped the strip gently against the container to remove excess urine.			
14. Waited the required amount of time. Followed the manufacturer's instructions.			
15. Compared the strip with the color chart on the bottle. Read the results.			
16. Discarded disposable items and the specimen.			
17. Emptied, cleaned, and disinfected equipment. Returned equipment to its proper place.			
18. Removed the gloves. Practiced hand hygiene.			

Post-Procedure

	S	U	Comments
19. Provided for comfort as noted on the inside of the front textbook cover.			
20. Placed the signal light within reach.			
21. Raised or lowered the bed rails. Followed the care plan.			
22. Unscreened the person.			
23. Completed a safety check of the room as noted on the inside of the front textbook cover.			
24. Decontaminated your hands.			
25. Reported and recorded the results and other observations.			

Date of Satisfactory Completion ——————————   Instructor's Initials ——————————

Collecting a Stool Specimen

Name: _____   Date: _____

	S	U	Comments

Quality of Life
- Knocked before entering the person's room.
- Addressed the person by name.
- Introduced yourself by name and title.
- Explained the procedure to the person before beginning and during the procedure.
- Protected the person's rights during the procedure.
- Handled the person gently during the procedure.

Pre-Procedure
1. Followed *Delegation Guidelines: Stool Specimens*. Reviewed *Promoting Safety and Comfort: Stool Specimens*.
2. Practiced hand hygiene.
3. Collected the following before going to the person's room:
   - Laboratory requisition slip
   - Specimen pan for the toilet
   - Specimen container and lid
   - Specimen label
   - Tongue blade
   - Disposable bag
   - Plastic bag
   - BIOHAZARD label (if needed)
   - Gloves
4. Arranged collected items in the person's bathroom.
5. Decontaminated your hands.
6. Identified the person. Checked the ID bracelet against the requisition slip. Called the person by name.
7. Labeled the specimen container in the person's presence.
8. Put on gloves.
9. Collected the following:
   - Receptacle for voiding—bedpan and cover, urinal, commode, or specimen pan
   - Toilet tissue
10. Provided for privacy.

Procedure
11. Asked the person to void. Provided the receptacle for voiding if the person did not use the bathroom. Emptied, cleaned, and disinfected the device. Returned it to its proper place.
12. Put the specimen pan on the toilet if the person would use the bathroom. Placed it at the back of the toilet. Or provided a bedpan or commode.
13. Asked the person not to put toilet tissue into the bedpan, commode, or specimen pan. Provided a bag for toilet tissue.
14. Placed the signal light and toilet tissue within reach. Raised or lowered bed rails. Followed the care plan.
15. Removed the gloves. Decontaminated your hands. Left the room.
16. Returned when the person signaled. Or checked on the person every 5 minutes. Knocked before entering.

Date of Satisfactory Completion _____   Instructor's Initials _____

Procedure—cont'd   S   U   Comments

17. Decontaminated your hands. Put on clean gloves.   _____   _____   _____
18. Lowered the bed rail near you if up.   _____   _____   _____
19. Removed the bedpan. Noted the color, amount,   _____   _____   _____
    consistency, and odor of stools.
20. Provided perineal care if needed.   _____   _____   _____
21. Collected the specimen:
    a. Used a tongue blade to take about 2 tablespoons of   _____   _____   _____
       formed or liquid stool to the specimen container.
       Took the sample from the middle of a formed stool.
    b. Included pus, mucus, or blood present in the stool. _____   _____   _____
    c. Took stool from 2 different places on the bowel   _____   _____   _____
       movement if required by agency policy.
    d. Put the lid on the specimen container.   _____   _____   _____
    e. Placed the container in the plastic bag. Did not let _____   _____   _____
       the container touch the outside of the bag. Applied
       a BIOHAZARD label according to agency policy.
22. Wrapped the tongue blade in toilet tissue. Discarded   _____   _____   _____
    it into the disposable bag.
23. Emptied, cleaned, and disinfected equipment.   _____   _____   _____
    Returned equipment to its proper place.
24. Removed the gloves, and practiced hand hygiene. Put   _____   _____   _____
    on clean gloves.
25. Assisted with hand washing.   _____   _____   _____
26. Removed the gloves. Practiced hand hygiene.   _____   _____   _____

Post-Procedure
27. Provided for comfort as noted on the inside of the   _____   _____   _____
    front textbook cover.
28. Placed the signal light within reach.   _____   _____   _____
29. Raised or lowered bed rails. Followed the care plan.   _____   _____   _____
30. Unscreened the person.   _____   _____   _____
31. Completed a safety check of the room as noted on the   _____   _____   _____
    inside of the front textbook cover.
32. Delivered the specimen and requisition slip to the   _____   _____   _____
    laboratory or storage area. Followed agency policy.
    Wore gloves.
33. Reported and recorded your observations.   _____   _____   _____

Date of Satisfactory Completion _____   Instructor's Initials _____

Collecting a Sputum Specimen

View Video!

Name: _____   Date: _____

	S	U	Comments

Quality of Life
- Knocked before entering the person's room.
- Addressed the person by name.
- Introduced yourself by name and title.
- Explained the procedure to the person before beginning and during the procedure.
- Protected the person's rights during the procedure.
- Handled the person gently during the procedure.

Pre-Procedure
1. Followed *Delegation Guidelines: Sputum Specimens.* Reviewed *Promoting Safety and Comfort: Sputum Specimens.*
2. Practiced hand hygiene.
3. Collected the following before going to the person's room:
   - Laboratory requisition slip
   - Sputum specimen container and lid
   - Specimen label
   - Plastic bag
   - BIOHAZARD label (if needed)
4. Arranged collected items in the person's bathroom.
5. Decontaminated your hands.
6. Identified the person. Checked the ID bracelet against the requisition slip. Called the person by name.
7. Labeled the specimen container in the person's presence.
8. Collected gloves and tissues.
9. Provided for privacy. If able, the person used the bathroom for the procedure.

Procedure
10. Put on gloves.
11. Asked the person to rinse the mouth out with clear water.
12. Had the person hold the container. Only the outside was touched.
13. Asked the person to cover the mouth and nose with tissues when coughing. Followed agency policy for used tissues.
14. Asked the person to take 2 or 3 deep breaths and cough up the sputum.
15. Had the person expectorate directly into the container. Sputum did not touch the outside of the container.
16. Collected 1 to 2 teaspoons of sputum unless told to collect more.
17. Put the lid on the container.
18. Placed the container in the plastic bag. Did not let the container touch the outside of the bag. Applied a BIOHAZARD label according to agency policy.
19. Removed the gloves, and decontaminated your hands. Put on clean gloves.
20. Assisted with hand washing.
21. Removed the gloves. Decontaminated your hands.

Date of Satisfactory Completion _____   Instructor's Initials _____

Post-Procedure

	S	U	Comments
22. Provided for comfort as noted on the inside of the front textbook cover.	_____	_____	_____
23. Placed the signal light within reach.	_____	_____	_____
24. Raised or lowered bed rails. Followed the care plan.	_____	_____	_____
25. Unscreened the person.	_____	_____	_____
26. Completed a safety check of the room as noted on the inside of the front textbook cover.	_____	_____	_____
27. Decontaminated your hands.	_____	_____	_____
28. Delivered the specimen and the requisition slip to the laboratory or storage area. Followed agency policy. Wore gloves.	_____	_____	_____
29. Reported and recorded your observations.	_____	_____	_____

Date of Satisfactory Completion _____   Instructor's Initials _____

Performing Range-of-Motion Exercises (NNAAP™)

Name: _____ Date: _____

	S	U	Comments

Quality of Life
- Knocked before entering the person's room.
- Addressed the person by name.
- Introduced yourself by name and title.
- Explained the procedure to the person before beginning and during the procedure.
- Protected the person's rights during the procedure.
- Handled the person gently during the procedure.

Pre-Procedure
1. Followed *Delegation Guidelines: Range-of-Motion Exercises*.
   Reviewed *Promoting Safety and Comfort: Range-of-Motion Exercises*.
2. Practiced hand hygiene.
3. Identified the person. Checked the ID bracelet against the assignment sheet. Called the person by name.
4. Obtained a bath blanket.
5. Provided for privacy.
6. Raised the bed for body mechanics. Bed rails were up if used.

Procedure
7. Lowered the bed rail near you if up.
8. Positioned the person supine.
9. Covered the person with a bath blanket. Fan-folded top linens to the foot of the bed.
10. Exercised the neck if allowed by your agency and if the RN instructed you to do so:
    a. Placed your hands over the person's ears to support the head. Supported the jaws with your fingers.
    b. Flexion—brought the head forward. The chin touched the chest.
    c. Extension—straightened the head.
    d. Hyperextension—brought the head backward until the chin pointed up.
    e. Rotation—turned the head from side to side.
    f. Lateral flexion—moved the head to the right and to the left.
    g. Repeated flexion, extension, hyperextension, rotation, and lateral flexion 5 times—or the number of times stated on the care plan.
11. Exercised the shoulder:
    a. Grasped the wrist with one hand. Grasped the elbow with the other hand.
    b. Flexion—raised the arm straight in front and over the head.
    c. Extension—brought the arm down to the side.
    d. Hyperextension—moved the arm behind the body. (Did this if the person was sitting in a straight-backed chair or was standing.)
    e. Abduction—moved the straight arm away from the side of the body.

Date of Satisfactory Completion _____ Instructor's Initials _____

Procedure—cont'd	S	U	Comments
f. Adduction—moved the straight arm to the side of the body.	___	___	_____
g. Internal rotation—bent the elbow. Placed it at the same level as the shoulder. Moved the forearm down toward the body.	___	___	_____
h. External rotation—moved the forearm toward the head.	___	___	_____
i. Repeated flexion, extension, hyperextension, abduction, adduction, and internal and external rotation 5 times—or the number of times stated on the care plan.	___	___	_____
12. Exercised the elbow:			
a. Grasped the person's wrist with one hand. Grasped the elbow with your other hand.	___	___	_____
b. Flexion—bent the arm so the same-side shoulder was touched.	___	___	_____
c. Extension—straightened the arm.	___	___	_____
d. Repeated flexion and extension 5 times—or the number of times stated on the care plan.	___	___	_____
13. Exercised the forearm:			
a. Continued to support the wrist and elbow.	___	___	_____
b. Pronation—turned the hand so the palm was down.	___	___	_____
c. Supination—turned the hand so the palm was up.	___	___	_____
d. Repeated pronation and supination 5 times—or the number of times stated on the care plan.	___	___	_____
14. Exercised the wrist:			
a. Held the wrist with both of your hands.	___	___	_____
b. Flexion—bent the hand down.	___	___	_____
c. Extension—straightened the hand.	___	___	_____
d. Hyperextension—bent the hand back.	___	___	_____
e. Radial flexion—turned the hand toward the thumb.	___	___	_____
f. Ulnar flexion—turned the hand toward the little finger.	___	___	_____
g. Repeated flexion, extension, hyperextension, and radial flexion and ulnar flexion 5 times—or the number of times stated on the care plan.	___	___	_____
15. Exercised the thumb:			
a. Held the person's hand with one hand. Held the thumb with your other hand.	___	___	_____
b. Abduction—moved the thumb out from the inner part of the index finger.	___	___	_____
c. Adduction—moved the thumb back next to the index finger.	___	___	_____
d. Opposition—touched each fingertip with the thumb.	___	___	_____
e. Flexion—bent the thumb into the hand.	___	___	_____
f. Extension—moved the thumb out to the side of the fingers.	___	___	_____
g. Repeated abduction, adduction, opposition, flexion, and extension 5 times—or the number of times stated on the care plan.	___	___	_____

Date of Satisfactory Completion _____   Instructor's Initials _____

Procedure—cont'd	S	U	Comments

16. Exercised the fingers:
   a. Abduction—spread the fingers and the thumb apart.
   b. Adduction—brought the fingers and thumb together.
   c. Flexion—made a fist.
   d. Extension—straightened the fingers so the fingers, hand, and arm were straight.
   e. Repeated abduction, adduction, flexion, and extension 5 times—or the number of times stated on the care plan.
17. Exercised the hip:
   a. Supported the leg. Placed one hand under the knee. Placed your other hand under the ankle.
   b. Flexion—raised the leg.
   c. Extension—straightened the leg.
   d. Abduction—moved the leg away from the body.
   e. Adduction—moved the leg toward the other leg.
   f. Internal rotation—turned the leg inward.
   g. External rotation—turned the leg outward.
   h. Repeated flexion, extension, abduction, adduction, and internal and external rotation 5 times—or the number of times stated on the care plan.
18. Exercised the knee:
   a. Supported the knee. Placed one hand under the knee. Placed your other hand under the ankle.
   b. Flexion—bent the leg.
   c. Extension—straightened the leg.
   d. Repeated flexion and extension of the knee 5 times—or the number of times stated on the care plan.
19. Exercised the ankle:
   a. Supported the foot and ankle. Placed one hand under the foot. Placed your other hand under the ankle.
   b. Dorsiflexion—pulled the foot forward. Pushed down on the heel at the same time.
   c. Plantar flexion—turned the foot down, or pointed the toes.
   d. Repeated dorsiflexion and plantar flexion 5 times—or the number of times stated on the care plan.
20. Exercised the foot:
   a. Continued to support the foot and ankle.
   b. Pronation—turned the outside of the foot up and the inside down.
   c. Supination—turned the inside of the foot up and the outside down.
   d. Repeated pronation and supination 5 times—or the number of times stated on the care plan.
21. Exercised the toes:
   a. Flexion—curled the toes.
   b. Extension—straightened the toes.
   c. Abduction—spread the toes apart.
   d. Adduction—pulled the toes together.
   e. Repeated flexion, extension, abduction, and adduction 5 times—or the number of times stated on the care plan.

Date of Satisfactory Completion _____   Instructor's Initials _____

Procedure—cont'd

	S	U	Comments
22. Covered the leg. Raised the bed rail if used.			
23. Went to the other side. Lowered the bed rail near you if up.			
24. Repeated steps 11 through 21.			
Post-Procedure			
25. Provided for comfort as noted on the inside of the front textbook cover.			
26. Removed the bath blanket.			
27. Placed the signal light within reach.			
28. Lowered the bed to its lowest level.			
29. Raised or lowered bed rails. Followed the care plan.			
30. Folded and returned the bath blanket to its proper place.			
31. Unscreened the person.			
32. Completed a safety check of the room as noted on the inside of the front textbook cover.			
33. Decontaminated your hands.			
34. Reported and recorded your observations.			

Date of Satisfactory Completion _____   Instructor's Initials _____

Helping the Person Walk (NNAAP™)

Name: _____   Date: _____

	S	U	Comments

Quality of Life
- Knocked before entering the person's room.
- Addressed the person by name.
- Introduced yourself by name and title.
- Explained the procedure to the person before beginning and during the procedure.
- Protected the person's rights during the procedure.
- Handled the person gently during the procedure.

Pre-Procedure
1. Followed *Delegation Guidelines: Ambulation.* Reviewed *Promoting Safety and Comfort: Ambulation.*
2. Practiced hand hygiene.
3. Collected the following:
   - Robe and non-skid shoes
   - Paper or sheet to protect bottom linens
   - Gait (transfer) belt
4. Identified the person. Checked the ID bracelet against the assignment sheet. Called the person by name.
5. Provided for privacy.

Procedure
6. Lowered the bed to its lowest position. Locked the bed wheels. Lowered the bed rail if up.
7. Fan-folded top linens to the foot of the bed.
8. Placed the paper or sheet under the person's feet. Put the shoes on the person. Fastened the shoes.
9. Helped the person to sit on the side of the bed. (See procedure *Sitting on the Side of the Bed [Dangling],* Chapter 13.)
10. Helped the person put on the robe.
11. Made sure the person's feet were flat on the floor.
12. Applied the gait belt. (See procedure *Applying a Transfer/Gait Belt,* Chapter 9.)
13. Helped the person stand. (See procedure *Transferring the Person to a Chair or Wheelchair,* Chapter 13.) Grasped the belt at each side. If not using a gait belt, placed your arms under the person's arms around to the shoulder blades.
14. Stood at the person's weak side while he or she gained balance. Held the belt at the side and back. If not using a gait belt, had one arm around the back and the other at the elbow to support the person.
15. Encouraged the person to stand erect with the head up and back straight.
16. Helped the person walk. Walked to the side and slightly behind the person on the person's weak side. Provided support with the gait belt. If not using a gait belt, had one arm around the back and the other at the elbow to support the person. Encouraged the person to use the hand rail on his or her strong side.
17. Encouraged the person to walk normally. (The heel should strike the floor first.) Discouraged shuffling, sliding, or walking on tip-toes.

Date of Satisfactory Completion _____   Instructor's Initials _____

Procedure—cont'd	S	U	Comments
18. Walked the required distance if the person tolerated the activity. Did not rush the person.	___	___	_____
19. Helped the person return to bed. Removed the gait belt. (See procedure *Transferring the Person From a Chair or Wheelchair to a Bed,* Chapter 13.)	___	___	_____
20. Lowered the head of the bed. Helped the person to the center of the bed.	___	___	_____
21. Removed the shoes. Removed and discarded the paper or sheet over the bottom sheet.	___	___	_____

Post-Procedure

	S	U	Comments
22. Provided for comfort as noted on the inside of the front textbook cover.	___	___	_____
23. Placed the signal light within reach.	___	___	_____
24. Raised or lowered bed rails. Followed the care plan.	___	___	_____
25. Returned the robe and shoes to their proper place.	___	___	_____
26. Unscreened the person.	___	___	_____
27. Completed a safety check of the room as noted on the inside of the front textbook cover.	___	___	_____
28. Decontaminated your hands.	___	___	_____
29. Reported and recorded your observations.	___	___	_____

Date of Satisfactory Completion _____   Instructor's Initials _____

Applying Elastic Stockings (NNAAP™)

View Video! **Video CLIP**

Name: _____   Date: _____

	S	U	Comments

Quality of Life

- Knocked before entering the person's room.
- Addressed the person by name.
- Introduced yourself by name and title.
- Explained the procedure to the person before beginning and during the procedure.
- Protected the person's rights during the procedure.
- Handled the person gently during the procedure.

Pre-Procedure

1. Followed *Delegation Guidelines: Elastic Stockings.* Reviewed *Promoting Safety and Comfort: Elastic Stockings.*
2. Practiced hand hygiene.
3. Obtained elastic stockings in the correct size and length.
4. Identified the person. Checked the ID bracelet against the assignment sheet. Called the person by name.
5. Provided for privacy.
6. Raised the bed for body mechanics. Bed rails were up if used.

Procedure

7. Lowered the bed rail near you if up.
8. Positioned the person supine.
9. Exposed the legs. Fan-folded top linens toward the thighs.
10. Turned the stocking inside out down to the heel.
11. Slipped the foot of the stocking over the toes, foot, and heel.
12. Grasped the stocking top. Pulled the stocking up the leg. The stocking turned right side out as it was pulled up. The stocking was even and snug.
13. Removed twists, creases, or wrinkles.
14. Repeated steps 10 through 13 for the other leg.

Post-Procedure

15. Covered the person.
16. Provided for comfort as noted on the inside of the front textbook cover.
17. Placed the signal light within reach.
18. Lowered the bed to its lowest position.
19. Raised or lowered bed rails. Followed the care plan.
20. Unscreened the person.
21. Completed a safety check of the room as noted on the inside of the front textbook cover.
22. Decontaminated your hands.
23. Reported and recorded your observations.

Date of Satisfactory Completion _____   Instructor's Initials _____

Applying Elastic Bandages

Name: _____　　Date: _____

	S	U	Comments

Quality of Life
- Knocked before entering the person's room.
- Addressed the person by name.
- Introduced yourself by name and title.
- Explained the procedure to the person before beginning and during the procedure.
- Protected the person's rights during the procedure.
- Handled the person gently during the procedure.

Pre-Procedure
1. Followed *Delegation Guidelines: Elastic Bandages*. Reviewed *Promoting Safety and Comfort: Elastic Bandages*.
2. Practiced hand hygiene.
3. Collected the following:
   - Elastic bandage as directed by the nurse
   - Tape or clips (unless the bandage had Velcro)
4. Identified the person. Checked the ID bracelet against the assignment sheet. Called the person by name.
5. Provided for privacy.
6. Raised the bed for body mechanics. Bed rails were up if used.

Procedure
7. Lowered the bed rail near you if up.
8. Helped the person to a comfortable position. Exposed the part to be bandaged.
9. Made sure the area was clean and dry.
10. Held the bandage so the roll was up. The loose end was on the bottom.
11. Applied the bandage to the smallest part of the wrist, foot, ankle, or knee.
12. Made two circular turns around the part.
13. Made overlapping spiral turns in an upward direction. Each turn overlapped about ½ to ⅔ of the previous turn. Made sure each overlap was equal.
14. Applied the bandage smoothly with firm, even pressure. It was not tight.
15. Ended the bandage with two circular turns.
16. Secured the bandage in place with Velcro, tape, or clips. The clips were not under the body part.
17. Checked the fingers or toes for coldness or cyanosis. Asked about pain, itching, numbness, or tingling. Removed the bandage if any were noted. Reported your observations to the nurse.

Post-Procedure
18. Provided for comfort as noted on the inside of the front textbook cover.
19. Placed the signal light within reach.
20. Lowered the bed to its lowest position.

Date of Satisfactory Completion _____　　Instructor's Initials _____

Post-Procedure—cont'd   S   U   Comments

21. Raised or lowered bed rails. Followed the care plan.   _____ _____ _____
22. Unscreened the person.   _____ _____ _____
23. Completed a safety check of the room as noted on the   _____ _____ _____
    inside of the front textbook cover.
24. Decontaminated your hands.   _____ _____ _____
25. Reported and recorded your observations.   _____ _____ _____

Date of Satisfactory Completion _____ Instructor's Initials _____

Applying a Dry, Non-Sterile Dressing

Name: _____   Date: _____

Quality of Life	S	U	Comments
• Knocked before entering the person's room.	___	___	_____
• Addressed the person by name.	___	___	_____
• Introduced yourself by name and title.	___	___	_____
• Explained the procedure to the person before beginning and during the procedure.	___	___	_____
• Protected the person's rights during the procedure.	___	___	_____
• Handled the person gently during the procedure.	___	___	_____

Pre-Procedure

	S	U	Comments
1. Followed *Delegation Guidelines: Applying Dressings.* Reviewed *Promoting Safety and Comfort: Applying Dressings.*	___	___	_____
2. Practiced hand hygiene.	___	___	_____
3. Collected the following:			
• Gloves	___	___	_____
• Personal protective equipment as needed	___	___	_____
• Tape or Montgomery ties	___	___	_____
• Dressings as directed by the nurse	___	___	_____
• Saline solution as directed by the nurse	___	___	_____
• Cleansing solution as directed by the nurse	___	___	_____
• Adhesive remover	___	___	_____
• Dressing set with scissors and forceps	___	___	_____
• Plastic bag	___	___	_____
• Bath blanket	___	___	_____
4. Decontaminated your hands.	___	___	_____
5. Identified the person. Checked the ID bracelet against the assignment sheet. Called the person by name.	___	___	_____
6. Provided for privacy.	___	___	_____
7. Arranged the work area so you would not have to reach over or turn your back on your work area.	___	___	_____
8. Raised the bed for body mechanics. Bed rails were up if used.	___	___	_____

Procedure

	S	U	Comments
9. Lowered the bed rail near you if up.	___	___	_____
10. Helped the person to a comfortable position.	___	___	_____
11. Covered the person with a bath blanket. Fan-folded top linens to the foot of the bed.	___	___	_____
12. Exposed the affected body part.	___	___	_____
13. Made a cuff on the plastic bag. Placed it within reach.	___	___	_____
14. Decontaminated your hands.	___	___	_____
15. Put on needed personal protective equipment. Put on gloves.	___	___	_____
16. Removed tape or undid Montgomery ties.			
a. Tape: held the skin down. Gently pulled the tape toward the wound.	___	___	_____
b. Montgomery ties: folded ties away from the wound.	___	___	_____
17. Removed any adhesive from the skin. Wet a 4 × 4 gauze dressing with the adhesive remover. Cleaned away from the wound.	___	___	_____

Date of Satisfactory Completion _____   Instructor's Initials _____

Procedure—cont'd	S	U	Comments

Procedure—cont'd

18. Removed gauze dressings. Started with the top dressing, and removed each layer. Kept the soiled side of each dressing away from the person's sight. Put dressings in the plastic bag. They did not touch the outside of the bag.
19. Removed the dressing over the wound very gently. Moistened the dressing with saline if it stuck to the wound.
20. Observed the wound, drain site, and wound drainage.
21. Removed the gloves and put them in the plastic bag. Decontaminated your hands.
22. Opened the new dressings.
23. Cut the length of tape needed.
24. Put on clean gloves.
25. Cleaned the wound with saline as directed by the nurse.
26. Applied dressings as directed by the nurse.
27. Secured the dressings in place. Used tape or Montgomery ties.
28. Removed the gloves. Put them in the bag.
29. Removed and discarded personal protective equipment.
30. Decontaminated your hands.
31. Covered the person. Removed the bath blanket.

Post-Procedure

32. Provided for comfort as noted on the inside of the front textbook cover.
33. Placed the signal light within reach.
34. Lowered the bed to its lowest position.
35. Raised or lowered bed rails. Followed the care plan.
36. Returned equipment and supplies to the proper place. Left extra dressings and tape in the room.
37. Discarded used supplies into the bag. Tied the bag closed. Discarded the bag following agency policy. Wore gloves.
38. Cleaned your work area. Followed the Bloodborne Pathogen Standard.
39. Unscreened the person.
40. Completed a safety check of the room as noted on the inside of the front textbook cover.
41. Decontaminated your hands.
42. Reported and recorded your observations.

Date of Satisfactory Completion _____ Instructor's Initials _____

Applying Heat and Cold Applications

Name: _____   Date: _____

	S	U	Comments
Quality of Life			
• Knocked before entering the person's room.	____	____	_____
• Addressed the person by name.	____	____	_____
• Introduced yourself by name and title.	____	____	_____
• Explained the procedure to the person before beginning and during the procedure.	____	____	_____
• Protected the person's rights during the procedure.	____	____	_____
• Handled the person gently during the procedure.	____	____	_____
Pre-Procedure			
1. Followed *Delegation Guidelines: Applying Heat and Cold.* Reviewed *Promoting Safety and Comfort: Applying Heat and Cold.*	____	____	_____
2. Practiced hand hygiene.	____	____	_____
3. Collected needed equipment.	____	____	_____
a. For a hot compress:			
• Basin	____	____	_____
• Bath thermometer	____	____	_____
• Small towel, washcloth, or gauze squares	____	____	_____
• Plastic wrap or aquathermia pad	____	____	_____
• Ties, tape, or rolled gauze	____	____	_____
• Bath towel	____	____	_____
• Waterproof pad	____	____	_____
b. For a hot soak:			
• Water basin or arm or foot bath	____	____	_____
• Bath thermometer	____	____	_____
• Waterproof pad	____	____	_____
• Bath blanket	____	____	_____
• Towel	____	____	_____
c. For a sitz bath:			
• Disposable sitz bath	____	____	_____
• Bath thermometer	____	____	_____
• Two bath blankets, bath towels, and a clean gown	____	____	_____
d. For a hot or cold pack:			
• Commercial pack	____	____	_____
• Pack cover	____	____	_____
• Ties, tape, or rolled gauze (if needed)	____	____	_____
• Waterproof pad	____	____	_____
e. For an aquathermia pad:			
• Aquathermia pad and heating unit	____	____	_____
• Distilled water	____	____	_____
• Flannel cover or other cover as directed by the nurse	____	____	_____
• Ties, tape, or rolled gauze	____	____	_____
f. For an ice bag, ice collar, ice glove, or dry cold pack:			
• Ice bag, collar, or glove or cold pack	____	____	_____
• Crushed ice (except for a cold pack)	____	____	_____
• Flannel cover or other cover as directed by the nurse	____	____	_____
• Paper towels	____	____	_____

Date of Satisfactory Completion _____   Instructor's Initials _____

Pre-Procedure—cont'd	S	U	Comments

g. For a cold compress:
   • Large basin with ice
   • Small basin with cold water
   • Gauze squares, washcloths, or small towels
   • Waterproof pad
4. Identified the person. Checked the ID bracelet against the assignment sheet. Called the person by name.
5. Provided for privacy.

Procedure
6. Positioned the person for the procedure.
7. Placed the waterproof pad (if needed) under the body part.
8. For a hot compress:
   a. Filled the basin ½ to ⅔ full with hot water as directed by the nurse. Measured water temperature.
   b. Placed the compress in the water.
   c. Wrung out the compress.
   d. Applied the compress over the area. Noted the time.
   e. Covered the compress quickly. Used one of the following as directed by the nurse:
      (1) Applied plastic wrap and then a bath towel. Secured the towel in place with ties, tape, or rolled gauze.
      (2) Applied an aquathermia pad.
9. For a hot soak:
   a. Filled the container ½ full with hot water as directed by the nurse. Measured water temperature.
   b. Placed the part into the water. Padded the edge of the container with a towel. Noted the time.
   c. Covered the person with a bath blanket for warmth.
10. For a sitz bath:
   a. Placed the disposable sitz bath on the toilet seat.
   b. Filled the sitz bath ⅔ full with water as directed by the nurse. Measured water temperature.
   c. Secured the gown above the waist.
   d. Helped the person sit on the sitz bath. Noted the time.
   e. Provided for warmth. Placed a bath blanket around the shoulders. Placed another over the legs.
   f. Stayed with the person if he or she was weak or unsteady.
11. For a hot or cold pack:
   a. Squeezed, kneaded, or struck the pack as directed by the manufacturer.
   b. Placed the pack in the cover.
   c. Applied the pack. Noted the time.
   d. Secured the pack in place with ties, tape, or rolled gauze. (Some secure with Velcro straps.)

Date of Satisfactory Completion _____   Instructor's Initials _____

Procedure—cont'd	S	U	Comments

12. For an aquathermia pad:
   a. Filled the heating unit to the fill line with distilled water.
   b. Removed the bubbles. Placed the pad and tubing below the heating unit. Tilted the heating unit from side to side.
   c. Set the temperature as the nurse directed (usually 105°F [40.5°C]). Removed the key. (Gave the key to the nurse after the procedure.)
   d. Placed the pad in the cover.
   e. Plugged in the unit. Let water warm to the desired temperature.
   f. Set the heating unit on the bedside stand. Kept the pad and connecting hoses level with the unit. Hoses did not have kinks.
   g. Applied the pad to the part. Noted the time.
   h. Secured the pad in place with ties, tape, or rolled gauze. Did not use pins.
13. For an ice bag, collar, or glove:
   a. Filled the device with water. Put in the stopper. Turned the device upside down to check for leaks.
   b. Emptied the device.
   c. Filled the device ½ to ⅔ full with crushed ice or ice chips.
   d. Removed excess air. Bent, twisted, or squeezed the device. Or pressed it against a firm surface.
   e. Placed the cap or stopper on securely.
   f. Dried the device with paper towels.
   g. Placed the device in the cover.
   h. Applied the device. Noted the time.
   i. Secured the device in place with ties, tape, or rolled gauze.
14. For a cold compress:
   a. Placed the small basin with cold water into the large basin with ice.
   b. Placed the compresses into the cold water.
   c. Wrung out a compress.
   d. Applied the compress to the part. Noted the time.
15. Placed the signal light within reach. Unscreened the person.
16. Raised or lowered bed rails. Followed the care plan.
17. Checked the person every 5 minutes. Checked for signs and symptoms of complications. Removed the application if any occurred. Told the nurse at once.
18. Checked the application every 5 minutes. Changed the application if cooling (hot applications) or warming (cold applications) occurred.
19. Removed the application at the specified time. (If bed rails were up, lowered the near one for this step.)

Post-Procedure

20. Provided for comfort as noted on the inside of the front textbook cover.
21. Placed the signal light within reach.
22. Raised or lowered bed rails. Followed the care plan.

Date of Satisfactory Completion _____   Instructor's Initials _____

Post-Procedure—cont'd	S	U	Comments
23. Unscreened the person.	_____	_____	_____
24. Cleaned and returned re-usable items to their proper place. Followed agency policy for soiled linen. Wore gloves for this step.	_____	_____	_____
25. Completed a safety check of the room as noted on the inside of the front textbook cover.	_____	_____	_____
26. Removed and discarded the gloves. Decontaminated your hands.	_____	_____	_____
27. Reported and recorded your observations.	_____	_____	_____

Date of Satisfactory Completion _____ Instructor's Initials _____

Assisting With Deep-Breathing and Coughing Exercises

View Video!

Name: _____   Date: _____

	S	U	Comments
Quality of Life			
• Knocked before entering the person's room.	___	___	_____
• Addressed the person by name.	___	___	_____
• Introduced yourself by name and title.	___	___	_____
• Explained the procedure to the person before beginning and during the procedure.	___	___	_____
• Protected the person's rights during the procedure.	___	___	_____
• Handled the person gently during the procedure.	___	___	_____

Pre-Procedure

1. Followed *Delegation Guidelines: Deep Breathing and Coughing.*
   Reviewed *Promoting Safety and Comfort: Deep Breathing and Coughing.*   ___ ___ _____
2. Practiced hand hygiene.   ___ ___ _____
3. Identified the person. Checked the ID bracelet against the assignment sheet. Called the person by name.   ___ ___ _____
4. Provided for privacy.   ___ ___ _____

Procedure

5. Lowered the bed rail if up.   ___ ___ _____
6. Helped the person to a comfortable sitting position: sitting on the side of the bed, semi-Fowler's, or Fowler's.   ___ ___ _____
7. Had the person deep breathe:
   a. Had the person place the hands over the rib cage.   ___ ___ _____
   b. Had the person take a deep breath. It was as deep as possible. Reminded the person to inhale through the nose.   ___ ___ _____
   c. Asked the person to hold the breath for 2 to 3 seconds.   ___ ___ _____
   d. Asked the person to exhale slowly through pursed lips. Asked the person to exhale until the ribs moved as far down as possible.   ___ ___ _____
   e. Repeated this step 4 more times.   ___ ___ _____
8. Asked the person to cough:
   a. Had the person place both hands over the incision. One hand was on top of the other. The person could hold a pillow or folded towel over the incision.   ___ ___ _____
   b. Had the person take in a deep breath as in step 7.   ___ ___ _____
   c. Asked the person to cough strongly twice with the mouth open.   ___ ___ _____

Post-Procedure

9. Provided for comfort as noted on the inside of the front textbook cover.   ___ ___ _____
10. Placed the signal light within reach.   ___ ___ _____
11. Raised or lowered bed rails. Followed the care plan.   ___ ___ _____
12. Unscreened the person.   ___ ___ _____
13. Completed a safety check of the room as noted on the inside of the front textbook cover.   ___ ___ _____
14. Decontaminated your hands.   ___ ___ _____
15. Reported and recorded your observations.   ___ ___ _____

Date of Satisfactory Completion _____   Instructor's Initials _____

Adult CPR—One Rescuer

Name: _____   Date: _____

Procedure	S	U	Comments
1. Made sure the scene was safe.	___	___	_____
2. Took 5 to 10 seconds to check for a response and breathing:			
a. Checked if the person is responding. Tapped or gently shook the person. Called the person by name, if known. Shouted, "Are you OK?"	___	___	_____
b. Checked for no breathing or no normal breathing (gasping).	___	___	_____
3. Called for help. Activated the EMS system or the agency's RRT if the person was not responding and not breathing or not breathing normally (gasping).	___	___	_____
4. Went to get an AED or asked someone to bring an AED if available.	___	___	_____
5. Positioned the person supine on a hard, flat surface. Logrolled the person so there was no twisting of the spine. Placed the arms alongside the body.	___	___	_____
6. Checked for a carotid pulse. This took 5 to 10 seconds. Started chest compressions if pulse was not felt.	___	___	_____
7. Exposed the person's chest.	___	___	_____
8. Gave chest compressions at a rate of at least 100 per minute. Pushed hard and fast. Established a regular rhythm. Counted out loud. Pressed down at least 2 inches. Allowed the chest to recoil between compressions. Gave 30 chest compressions.	___	___	_____
9. Opened the airway. Used the head tilt-chin lift method.	___	___	_____
10. Gave 2 breaths. Each breath took only 1 second. Each breath made the chest rise. (If the first breath did not make the chest rise, tried opening the airway again. Used the head tilt-chin lift method.)	___	___	_____
11. Continued the cycle of 30 chest compressions followed by 2 breaths. Limited interruptions in compressions to less than 10 seconds. Continued cycles until the AED arrived. Or continued until help arrived or the person began to move. If movement occurred, placed the person in the recovery position.	___	___	_____

Date of Satisfactory Completion _____   Instructor's Initials _____

Adult CPR—Two Rescuers

Name: ————————————————   Date: ————————————————————

Procedure	S	U	Comments

Procedure

1. Made sure the scene was safe.
2. *Rescuer 1*—took 5 to 10 seconds to check for a response and breathing:
   a. Checked if the person was responding. Tapped or gently shook the person. Called the person by name, if known. Shouted, "Are you OK?"
   b. Checked for no breathing or no normal breathing (gasping).
3. *Rescuer 2:*
   a. Activated the EMS system or the agency's RRT if the person was not responding and not breathing or not breathing normally (gasping).
   b. Got a defibrillator (AED) if one was available
4. *Rescuer 1:* Positioned the person supine on a hard, flat surface. Logrolled the person so there was no twisting of the spine. Placed the arms alongside the body. Began 1-rescuer CPR until the second rescuer returned.
5. When the second rescuer returned, performed 2-rescuer CPR.
   a. *Rescuer 1:* Gave chest compressions at a rate of at least 100 per minute. Pushed hard and fast. Established a regular rhythm. Counted out loud. Pressed down at least 2 inches. Allowed the chest to recoil between compressions. Gave 30 chest compressions. Paused to allow the other rescuer to give 2 breaths.
   b. *Rescuer 2:*
      (1) Opened the airway. Used the head tilt-chin lift method.
      (2) Gave 2 breaths after every 30 compressions. Each breath took only 1 second and made the chest rise. (If the first breath did not make the chest rise, tried opening the airway again. Used the head tilt-chin lift method.)
   c. Continued cycles of 30 compressions and 2 breaths.
   d. Changed positions every 2 minutes (after about 5 cycles of 30 compressions and 2 breaths). The switch took no more than 5 seconds.
   e. Continued until the AED arrived. Or continued until help took over or the person began to move. If movement occurred, placed the person in the recovery position.

Date of Satisfactory Completion ————————————   Instructor's Initials ————————————

Adult CPR With AED—Two Rescuers

Name: ————————————————————   Date: ————————————————————

Procedure	S	U	Comments
1. Made sure the scene was safe.	____	____	_____
2. *Rescuer 1*—Took 5 to 10 seconds to check for a response and breathing:			
a. Checked if the person was responding. Tapped or gently shook the person. Called the person by name, if known. Shouted, "Are you OK?"	____	____	_____
b. Checked for no breathing or no normal breathing (gasping).	____	____	_____
3. *Rescuer 2:*			
a. Activated the EMS system or the agency's RRT if the person was not responding and not breathing or not breathing normally (gasping).	____	____	_____
b. Got a defibrillator (AED) if one was available.	____	____	_____
4. *Rescuer 1:*			
a. Positioned the person supine on a hard, flat surface. Logrolled the person so there was no twisting of the spine. Placed the arms alongside the body.	____	____	_____
b. Checked for a carotid pulse. This took 5 to 10 seconds. Started chest compressions if pulse not felt.	____	____	_____
c. Exposed the person's chest.	____	____	_____
d. Gave chest compressions at a rate of at least 100 per minute. Pushed hard and fast. Established a regular rhythm. Counted out loud. Pressed down at least 2 inches. Allowed the chest to recoil between compressions. Gave 30 chest compressions.	____	____	_____
e. Opened the airway. Used the head tilt-chin lift method.	____	____	_____
f. Gave 2 breaths. Each breath took only 1 second. Each breath made the chest rise. (If the first breath did not make the chest rise, tried opening the airway again. Used the head tilt-chin lift method.)	____	____	_____
g. Continued the cycle of 30 chest compressions followed by 2 breaths. Limited interruptions in compressions to less than 10 seconds.	____	____	_____
5. *Rescuer 2:*			
a. Opened the case with the AED.	____	____	_____
b. Turned on the AED.	____	____	_____
c. Applied adult electrode pads to the person's chest. Followed the instructions and diagram provided with the AED.	____	____	_____
d. Attached the connecting cables to the AED.	____	____	_____
e. Cleared away from the person. Made sure no one was touching the person.	____	____	_____
f. Let the AED check the person's heart rhythm.	____	____	_____
g. Made sure everyone was clear of the person if the AED advised a "shock." Loudly instructed others not to touch the person. Said: "I am clear, you are clear, everyone is clear!" Looked to made sure no one was touching the person.	____	____	_____
h. Pressed the "SHOCK" button if the AED advised a "shock."	____	____	_____

Date of Satisfactory Completion ——————————————   Instructor's Initials ——————————————

Procedure—cont'd   S   U   Comments

6. *Rescuers 1 and 2:*
   a. Performed 2-person CPR: _____ _____ _____
      (1) Began with compressions. One rescuer gave _____ _____ _____
          chest compressions at a rate of at least 100 per
          minute. Pushed hard and fast. Established a
          regular rhythm. Counted out loud. Allowed the
          chest to recoil between compressions. Gave 30
          chest compressions. Paused to allow the other
          rescuer to give 2 breaths.
      (2) The other rescuer gave 2 breaths after every _____ _____ _____
          30 chest compressions.
7. After 2 minutes of CPR
   a. Cleared away from the person. Made sure no one _____ _____ _____
      was touching the person.
   b. Let the AED check the person's heart rhythm. _____ _____ _____
   c. Made sure everyone was clear of the person if _____ _____ _____
      the AED advised a "shock." Loudly instructed
      others not to touch the person. Said: "I am clear,
      you are clear, everyone is clear!" Looked to
      made sure no one was touching the person.
   d. Pressed the "SHOCK" button if the AED advised a _____ _____ _____
      "shock."
   e. Changed positions and continued CPR beginning _____ _____ _____
      with compressions.
8. Continued until help took over or the person began to _____ _____ _____
   move. If movement occurred, placed the person in the
   recovery position.

Date of Satisfactory Completion _____   Instructor's Initials _____

Assisting With Post-Mortem Care

Name: _____   Date: _____

	S	**U**	**Comments**

Pre-Procedure
1. Followed *Delegation Guidelines: Post-Mortem Care.* Reviewed *Promoting Safety and Comfort: Post-Mortem Care.*
2. Practiced hand hygiene.
3. Collected the following:
   - Post-mortem kit (shroud or body bag, gown, ID tags, gauze squares, safety pins)
   - Bed protectors
   - Wash basin
   - Bath towels and washcloths
   - Denture cup
   - Tape
   - Dressings
   - Gloves
   - Cotton balls
   - Valuables envelope
4. Provided for privacy.
5. Raised the bed for body mechanics.
6. Made sure the bed was flat.

Procedure
7. Put on the gloves.
8. Positioned the body supine. Arms and legs were straight. A pillow was under the head and shoulders. Or you raised the head of the bed 15 to 20 degrees per agency policy.
9. Closed the eyes. Gently pulled the eyelids over the eyes. Applied moist cotton balls gently over the eyelids if the eyes would not stay closed.
10. Inserted dentures if it was agency policy. If not, put them in a labeled denture cup.
11. Closed the mouth. If necessary, placed a rolled towel under the chin to keep the mouth closed.
12. Followed agency policy for jewelry. Removed all jewelry, except for wedding rings if this was agency policy. Listed the jewelry that you removed. Placed the jewelry and the list in a valuables envelope.
13. Placed a cotton ball over the rings. Taped them in place.
14. Removed drainage containers.
15. Removed tubes and catheters. Used the gauze squares as needed.
16. Bathed soiled areas with plain water. Dried thoroughly.
17. Placed a bed protector under the buttocks.
18. Removed soiled dressings. Replaced them with clean ones.
19. Put a clean gown on the body. Positioned the body as in step 8.
20. Brushed and combed the hair if necessary.
21. Covered the body to the shoulders with a sheet if the family would view the body.

Date of Satisfactory Completion _____   Instructor's Initials _____

Procedure—cont'd	S	U	Comments
22. Gathered the person's belongings. Put them in a bag labeled with the person's name. Made sure eyeglasses, hearing aids, and other valuables were included.	_____	_____	_____
23. Removed supplies, equipment, and linens. Straightened the room. Provided soft lighting.	_____	_____	_____
24. Removed the gloves. Decontaminated your hands.	_____	_____	_____
25. Let the family view the body. Provided for privacy. Returned to the room after they left.	_____	_____	_____
26. Decontaminated your hands. Put on gloves.	_____	_____	_____
27. Filled out the ID tags. Tied one to the ankle or to the right big toe.	_____	_____	_____
28. Placed the body in the body bag or covered it with a sheet. Or applied the shroud:			
a. Positioned the shroud under the body.	_____	_____	_____
b. Brought the top down over the head.	_____	_____	_____
c. Folded the bottom up over the feet.	_____	_____	_____
d. Folded the sides over the body.	_____	_____	_____
e. Pinned or taped the shroud in place.	_____	_____	_____
29. Attached the second ID tag to the shroud, sheet, or body bag.	_____	_____	_____
30. Left the denture cup with the body.	_____	_____	_____
31. Pulled the privacy curtain around the bed or closed the door.	_____	_____	_____

Post-Procedure

	S	U	Comments
32. Removed the gloves. Decontaminated your hands.	_____	_____	_____
33. Stripped the unit after the body was removed. Wore gloves for this step.	_____	_____	_____
34. Removed the gloves. Decontaminated your hands.	_____	_____	_____
35. Reported the following:			
• The time the body was taken by the funeral director	_____	_____	_____
• What was done with jewelry, other valuables, and personal items	_____	_____	_____
• What was done with dentures	_____	_____	_____

Date of Satisfactory Completion _____   Instructor's Initials _____

COMPETENCY EVALUATION REVIEW

PREPARING FOR THE COMPETENCY EVALUATION

After completing your state's training program, you need to pass the competency evaluation. The purpose of the competency evaluation is to make sure you can safely do your job. This section will help you prepare for the test.

COMPETENCY EVALUATION

The competency evaluation has a written test and a skills test. The number of questions varies with each state. Each question has four possible answers. Although some questions may appear to have more than one possible answer, there is only one best answer. You will have about 1 minute to read and answer each question. Some questions take less time to read and answer. Other questions take longer. You should have enough time to take the test without feeling rushed.

The content of the written test varies depending on your state. Content may include:
- Activities of Daily Living—hygiene, dressing and grooming, nutrition and hydration, elimination, rest/sleep/comfort
- Basic Nursing Skills—infection control, safety/emergency, therapeutic/technical procedures (e.g., vital signs, bedmaking), data collection and reporting
- Restorative Skills—prevention, self-care/independence
- Emotional and Mental Health Needs
- Spiritual and Cultural Needs
- The Person's Rights
- Legal and Ethical Behavior
- Being a member of the Health Care Team
- Communication

The written test is given as a paper and pencil test in most states. Some test sites may use computers. You do not need computer experience to take the test on the computer. If you have difficulty reading English, you may request to take an oral test. Talk with your instructor or employer about details for computer testing or oral testing.

The skills test involves performing five nursing skills that you learned in your training program. These skills are randomly chosen. You do not select the skills.

You are allowed about 30 minutes to do the skills. See p. 410 for more information about the skills test.

TAKING THE COMPETENCY EVALUATION

To register for the test, you need to complete an application. Your instructor or employer tells you when and where the tests are given. There is a fee for the evaluation. If you work in a nursing center, the employer may pay this fee. If you pay the fee, you may need to purchase a money order or certified check. Make sure your name is on the money order or certified check. Cash and personal checks may not be accepted.

Plan to arrive at the test site about 15 to 30 minutes before the evaluation begins. Most centers do not admit you if you are late. Know the exact location of the test site and room. Actually drive or take transportation to the test site a few days or a week before the test. Making a "dry run" lets you know how much time you need to travel, park, and get to the test site. It will also help decrease your anxiety level on the test day.

To be admitted to the test, you need two pieces of identification (ID). The first form of ID is a government-issued document such as a driver's license or passport. It must have a current photo and your signature. The name on the ID must be the same as the name on your application form. If your name has changed and you have not been able to have the name changed on your identification documents, ask your instructor or employer what to do. The second form of ID must include your name and signature. Examples include a library card, hunting license, or credit card.

Take several sharpened Number 2 pencils to the test. For the skills test you will need a watch with a second hand. You may need a person to play the role of the patient or resident. Ask your instructor or employer how this is done in your state.

Taking the written test and skills test may take several hours. You may want to bring snacks or lunch and a beverage to the testing site. Eating and drinking are not allowed during the test. However, you may be told where you can eat while waiting for the test.

You cannot bring textbooks, study notes, or other materials into the testing room. The only exception may be a language translation dictionary that you show to the proctor (a person who monitors the test) before the test begins. Cell phones, pagers, calculators, or other electronic devices are not permitted during testing. Children and pets are not allowed in the testing areas.

STUDYING FOR THE COMPETENCY EVALUATION

You began to prepare for the written and skills test during your training program. You learned the basic nursing content and skills needed to provide safe, quality care. The following suggestions can help you study for the competency evaluation:

- Begin to study at least 2 to 3 weeks before the test. Plan to study for 1 to 2 hours each day.
- Decide on a specific time to study. Choose a study time that is best for you. This may be early in the morning before others are awake. It may be in the evening after others go to sleep. Try to choose a time when you are mentally alert.
- Choose a specific area to study in. This area should be quiet, well lit and comfortable. You should have enough room to write and to spread out your books, notes, and other study aids—CD, DVD. The area does not need to be noise-free. The testing site is not absolutely quiet. You want to concentrate and not be distracted by the noise around you.
- Collect everything you need before settling down to study. This includes your textbook, notes, paper, highlighters, pens or pencils, CD, and DVD.
- Take short breaks when you need them. Take a break when your mind begins to wander or if you feel sleepy.
- Develop a study plan. Write your plan down so you can refer to it. Study one content area before going on to the next. For example, study personal hygiene before going on to vital signs. Do not jump from one subject to another.
- Use a variety of ways to study:
  - Use index cards to help you review abbreviations and terminology. Put the abbreviation or term on the front of the card and place the meaning on the back. Take the cards with you and review them whenever you have a break or are waiting.
  - Tape key points. You can listen to the tape while cooking or riding in the car.
  - Study groups are another way to prepare for a test. Group members can quiz each other.
- To remember what you are learning, try these ideas:
  - Relax when you study. When relaxed, you learn information quickly and recall it with greater ease.
  - Repeat what you are learning. Say it out loud. This helps you remember the idea.
  - Make the information you are learning meaningful. Think about how the information will help you be a good nursing assistant.
  - Write down what you are learning. Writing helps you remember information. Prepare study sheets.
  - Be positive about what you are learning. You remember what you find interesting.
- Suggestions for studying if you have children:
  - When you first come home from work or school, spend time with your children. Then plan study time.
  - Select educational programs on TV that your children can watch as you study. Or get a CD-ROM from the library.
  - When you take your study breaks, spend time with your children.
  - Ask other adults to take care of the children while you study.
- Take the two 75-question practice tests in this section. Each question has the correct answer and the reason why an answer is correct or incorrect. If you practice taking tests, you are more likely to pass them. Take the practice tests under conditions similar to the real test. Work within time limits.
- If your state has a practice test and a candidate handbook, study the content. Some states have practice tests on-line.

MANAGING ANXIETY

Almost everyone dreads taking tests. It is common and normal to experience anxiety before taking a test. If used wisely, anxiety can actually help you do well. When you are anxious, that means you are concerned. You may be concerned about how prepared you are to take the test. Or you may be concerned about how you will feel about yourself if you do not pass the test. Being concerned usually results in some action. To overcome anxiety before the test:

- Study and prepare for the test. That helps increase your confidence as you recall or clarify what you have learned. Anxiety decreases as confidence increases. When you think you know the information, keep studying. This reinforces your learning.
- Develop a positive mental attitude. You can pass this test. You took tests in your training program and passed them. Praise yourself. Talk to yourself in a positive way. If a negative thought enters your mind, stop it at once. Challenge the mental thought and tell yourself you will pass the test.
- Visualize success. Think about how wonderful you will feel when you are notified that you have passed the test.

- Perform breathing exercises. Breathe slowly and deeply.
- Perform regular exercise. Exercise helps you stay physically fit. It also helps keep you calm.
- Good nourishment helps you think clearly. Eat a nourishing meal before the test. Do not skip breakfast. Vitamin C helps fight short-term stress. Protein and calcium help overcome the effects of long-term stress. Complex carbohydrates (pasta, nuts, yogurt) can help settle your nerves. Eat familiar foods the day before and the day of the test. Do not eat foods that could cause stomach or intestinal upset.
- Maintain a normal routine the day before the test.
- Get a good night's sleep before the test. Go to bed early enough so you do not oversleep or are too tired to get up. Set your alarm clock properly. You may want to set two alarm clocks.
- Do not "cram" the evening before or the day of the test. Last minute cramming increases your anxiety. Do something relaxing with family and friends.
- Avoid drinking large amounts of coffee, colas, water, or other beverages. You do not want to be uncomfortable with a full bladder when you take the test.
- Wear comfortable clothes. Dress in layers so that you are prepared for a cold or warm room.
- If you are a woman, remember that worry and anxiety can affect your menstrual cycle. Wear a panty liner, sanitary napkin, or tampon if you think your period may start. This eliminates worry about soiling your clothing during the test.
- Allow plenty of time for travel, traffic, and parking.
- Arrive early enough to use the restroom before the test begins.
- Do not talk about the test with others. Their panic or anxiety may affect your self-confidence.

TAKING THE TEST

Follow these guidelines for taking the test:
- Listen carefully, and follow the instructions given by the proctor (person administering the test).
- When you receive the test, make certain you have all the test pages.
- Read and follow all directions carefully.
- You are not allowed to ask questions about the content of the test questions.
- Do deep-breathing and muscle-relaxation exercises as needed.
- Cheating of any kind is not allowed. If the proctor sees you giving or receiving any type of assistance, your test booklet is taken and you must leave the testing site.
- If using a computer answer sheet, completely fill in the bubble.

- If you make a mistake, erase the wrong answer completely. Do not make any stray marks on the paper. Not erasing completely or leaving stray marks could cause the computer to misread your answer.
- Do not worry or get anxious if people finish the test before you do. Persons who finish a test early do not necessarily have a better score than those who finish later.
- You cannot take any evaluation materials or notes out of the testing room.

ANSWERING MULTIPLE-CHOICE QUESTIONS

Pace yourself during the test. First, answer all the questions that you know. Then go back and answer skipped questions. Sometimes you will remember the answer later. Or another test question may give you a clue to the one you skipped. Spending too much time on a question can cost you valuable time later. To help you answer the questions or statements:
- Always read the questions or statements carefully. Do not scan or glance at questions. Scanning or glancing can cause you to miss important key words. Read each word of the question.
- Before reading the answers, decide what the answer is in your own words. Then read all four answers to the question. Select the one best answer.
- Do not read into a question. Take the question as it is asked. Do not add your own thoughts and ideas to the question. Do not assume or suppose "what if." Just respond to the information provided.
- Trust your common sense. If unsure of an answer, select your first choice. Do not change your answer unless you are absolutely sure of the correct answer. Your first reaction is usually correct.
- Look for key words in every question. Sometimes key words are in italics, highlighted, or underlined. Common key words are: *always, never, first, except, best, not, correct, incorrect, true,* or *false.*
- Know which words can make a statement correct (e.g., *may, can, usually, most, at least, sometimes*). The word "except" can make a question a false statement.
- Be careful of answers with these key words or phrases: *always, never, every, only, all, none, at all times,* or *at no time.* These words and phrases do not allow for exceptions. In nursing, exceptions are generally present. However, sometimes answers containing these words are correct. For example, which of the following is correct and which are incorrect?
  a. Always use a turning sheet.
  b. Never shake linens.
  c. Soap is used for all baths.
  d. The signal light must always be attached to the bed.

The correct answer is b. Incorrect answers are a, c, and d.

- Omit answers that are obviously wrong. Then choose the best of the remaining answers.
- Go back to the questions you skipped. Answer all questions by eliminating or narrowing your choices. Always mark an answer even if you are not sure.
- Review the test a second time for completeness and accuracy before turning it in.
- Make sure you have answered each question. Also check that you have given only one answer for each question.

- Remember, the test is not designed to trick or confuse you. The written competency evaluation tests what you know, not what you do not know. You know more than you are asked.

ON-LINE TESTING

The test may be given by computer at the test site. Ask your instructor what computer skills you will need. You usually do not need keyboard or typing skills. You will use a computer mouse to select answers. Also, you will usually receive instruction before the test begins. This will let you practice using the computer before starting the test.

TEXTBOOK CHAPTERS REVIEW

NOTE: This review covers selected chapters based on Competency Evaluation requirements.

CHAPTER 1 INTRODUCTION TO HOSPITALS AND NURSING CENTERS

HOSPITALS
- Provide emergency care, surgery, medical and nursing care, x-ray procedures and treatments, and laboratory testing.
- Hospitals also provide respiratory, physical, occupational, and speech therapies.

LONG-TERM CARE CENTERS
- Provide medical and nursing, dietary, recreational, rehabilitative, and social services. Housekeeping and laundry services are also provided.
- Most residents are older and may have chronic diseases, poor nutrition, or poor health.
- Some residents are disabled from birth defects, accidents, or diseases.
- Some residents have been discharged from hospitals and are recovering until they can return home.
- Long-term care centers include board and care homes, assisted-living residences, nursing centers, hospices, and Alzheimer's or dementia care units.

THE NURSING TEAM
- Provides quality care to people.
- Care is coordinated by an RN.

Nursing Assistants
- Report to the nurse supervising their work.
- Perform delegated nursing tasks under the supervision of a licensed nurse (RN or LPN/LVN).

THE OMNIBUS BUDGET RECONCILIATION ACT OF 1987 (OBRA)
- OBRA is a federal law.
- Nursing centers must provide care in a manner and in a setting that maintains or improves each person's quality of life, health, and safety.
- Resident rights are a major part of OBRA.

Resident Rights
- Centers must protect and promote residents' rights. Residents must be free to exercise their rights without interference. If residents are not able to exercise their rights, legal representatives do so for them.
- Residents are informed of their rights orally and in writing. This occurs before or during admission to the center. It is given in the language the person understands.

Information
- The right to information includes:
  - Access to medical records, incident reports, contracts, and financial records.
  - Information about his or her health condition.
  - Information about his or her doctor.
- Report any request for information to the nurse.

Refusing Treatment
- The person has the right to refuse treatment or to take part in research. If a person does not give consent or refuses treatment, it cannot be given. The center must find out what the person is refusing and why.
- Advance directives are part of the right to refuse treatment.
- Report any treatment refusal to the nurse.

Privacy and Confidentiality
- Residents have the right to:
  - Personal privacy. The person's body is not exposed unnecessarily. Only staff directly involved in care and treatments are present. The person must give consent for others to be present. A person has the right to use the bathroom in private. Privacy is maintained for all personal care measures.
  - Visit with others in private—in areas where others cannot see or hear them. This includes phone calls.
  - Send and receive mail without others interfering. No one can open mail the person sends or receives without his or her consent. Mail is given to the person within 24 hours of delivery to the center.
- Information about the person's care, treatment, and condition is kept confidential. So are medical

and financial records. Consent is needed to release information to other agencies or persons.

Personal Choice
- Residents have the right to:
  - Choose their own doctor.
  - Take part in planning and deciding their care and treatment.
  - Choose activities, schedules, and care based on their preferences.
  - Choose when to get up and go to bed, what to wear, what to eat, and how to spend their time.
  - Choose friends and visitors inside and outside the center.

Disputes and Grievances
- Residents have the right to voice concerns, ask questions, and complain about treatment or care. The center must promptly try to correct the matter. No one can punish the person in any way for voicing the grievance.

Work
- The person does not work for the center. However, the person can work or perform services if he or she wants to.

Taking Part in Resident and Family Groups
- The resident has the right to:
  - Form and take part in resident and family groups.
  - Take part in social, cultural, religious, and community events. The resident has the right to help in getting to and from events of his or her choice.

Care and Security of Personal Items
- The resident has the right to:
  - Keep and use personal items, such as clothing and some furnishings.
  - Have his or her property treated with care and respect. Items are labeled with the person's name.
- Protect yourself and the center from being accused of stealing a person's property. Do not go through a person's closet, drawers, purse, or other space without the person's knowledge and consent. If you have to inspect closets and drawers, follow center policy for reporting and recording the inspection.

Freedom From Abuse, Mistreatment, and Neglect
- Residents have the right to be free from:
  - Verbal, sexual, physical, or mental abuse.
  - Involuntary seclusion—separating a person from others against his or her will, confining

a person to a certain area, keeping the person away from his or her room without consent.
- No one can abuse, neglect, or mistreat a resident. This includes center staff, volunteers, staff from other agencies or groups, other residents, family members, visitors, and legal representatives.

Freedom From Restraint
- Residents have the right not to have body movements restricted by restraints or drugs. If a restraint is needed to protect the person or others from harm, a doctor's order is needed.

Quality of Life
- Residents must be cared for in a manner that promotes dignity and self-esteem. Physical, psychological, and mental well-being must be promoted. Review Box 1-3, OBRA-Required Actions to Promote Dignity and Privacy, in your textbook.
- Centers must provide activity programs that promote physical, intellectual, social, spiritual, and emotional well-being. Many centers provide religious services for spiritual health. You assist residents to and from activity programs. You may need to help them with activities.
- The center's environment must be clean, safe, comfortable, and as home-like as possible.

MEETING STANDARDS
- Surveys are done to see if agencies meet set standards. You have an important role in meeting standards and in the survey process. You must:
  - Provide quality care.
  - Protect the person's rights.
  - Provide for the person's and your own safety.
  - Help keep the agency clean and safe.
  - Conduct yourself in a professional manner.
  - Have good work ethics.
  - Follow agency policies and procedures.
  - Answer questions honestly and completely.

OMBUDSMAN
- The Older Americans Act requires an ombudsman program in every state. **Ombudsmen** protect the health, safety, welfare, and rights of residents. They also may investigate and resolve complaints, provide support to resident and family groups, and help the center manage difficult problems.
- Because a family or resident may share a concern with you, you must know the policies and procedures for contacting an ombudsman.

CHAPTER 1 REVIEW QUESTIONS
Circle the BEST answer.
1. Nursing assistants do all the following *except*
   a. Provide quality care
   b. Follow agency policies and procedures
   c. Conduct themselves in an unprofessional manner
   d. Help keep the agency clean and safe
2. Nursing assistants report to
   a. Other nursing assistants
   b. Licensed nurses
   c. The administrator
   d. The medical director
3. Nursing assistants perform nursing tasks delegated to them by an RN or LPN/LVN.
   a. True
   b. False
4. A resident asks you about his or her medical condition. You
   a. Tell the nurse about the resident's request
   b. Tell the resident what is in his or her medical record
   c. Ignore the question
   d. Tell another nursing assistant about the resident's request
5. Residents have all the following rights *except*
   a. Refusing a treatment
   b. Making a telephone call in private
   c. Choosing activities to attend
   d. Being punished for voicing a grievance
Answers to these questions are on p. 425.

CHAPTER 2 THE NURSING ASSISTANT
OBRA REQUIREMENTS
- OBRA requires that each state must have a nursing assistant training and competency evaluation program (NATCEP). Each state must also have a nursing assistant registry that lists persons who have successfully completed the NATCEP.
- Nursing assistants can have their certification, license, or registration denied, revoked, or suspended. The National Council of State Boards of Nursing (NCSBN) lists these reasons for doing so:
  - Substance abuse or dependency.
  - Abandoning a patient or resident.
  - Abusing a patient or resident.
  - Fraud or deceit. Examples include:
    - Filing false personal information
    - Providing false information when applying for initial certification
    - Providing false information when applying to have certification re-instated
    - Providing false information when applying for certification renewal
  - Neglecting a patient or resident.
  - Violating professional boundaries.
  - Giving unsafe care.
  - Performing acts beyond the nursing assistant role.
  - Misappropriation (stealing, theft) or misusing property.
  - Obtaining money or property from a patient or resident. Fraud, falsely representing oneself, and force are examples.
  - Having been convicted of a crime. Examples include murder, assault, kidnapping, rape or sexual assault, robbery, sexual crimes involving children, criminal mistreatment of children or a vulnerable adult, drug trafficking, embezzlement, theft, and arson.
  - Failing to conform to the standards of nursing assistants.
  - Putting patients and residents at risk for harm.
  - Violating the privacy of a patient or resident.
  - Failing to maintain the confidentiality of patient or resident information.

ROLES, RESPONSIBILITIES, AND STANDARDS
- OBRA, state laws, and legal and advisory opinions direct what you can do.
- Rules for you to follow:
  - You are an assistant to the nurse.
  - A nurse assigns and supervises your work.
  - You report observations about the person's physical and mental status to the nurse. Report changes in the person's condition or behavior at once.
  - The nurse decides what should be done for a person. You do not make these decisions.
  - Review directions and the care plan with the nurse before going to the person.
  - Perform no nursing task that you are not trained to do.
  - Perform no nursing task that you are not comfortable doing without a nurse's supervision.
  - Perform only the nursing tasks that your state and job description allow.
- Role limits for nursing assistants:
  - Never give drugs.
  - Never insert tubes or objects into body openings. Do not remove tubes from the body.
  - Never take oral or telephone orders from doctors.
  - Never perform procedures that require sterile technique.
  - Never tell the person or family the person's diagnosis or treatment plans.
  - Never diagnose or prescribe treatments or drugs for anyone.
  - Never supervise others, including other nursing assistants.

- Never ignore an order or request to do something.
- Review Box 2-4, Nursing Assistant Standards, in the textbook.
- Always obtain a written job description when you apply for a job. Do not take a job that requires you to:
  - Act beyond the legal limits of your role.
  - Function beyond your training limits.
  - Perform acts that are against your morals or religion.

DELEGATION

- RNs can delegate tasks to you. In some states, LPNs/LVNs can delegate tasks to you.
- You cannot delegate any task to other nursing assistants or to any other worker.
- Delegation decisions by the nurse must result in the best care for the person. If you perform a task that places the person at risk, you can face serious legal problems.
- The *Five Rights of Delegation* for Nursing Assistants:
  - *The right task*. Does your state allow you to perform the task? Were you trained to do the task? Do you have experience performing the task? Is the task in your job description?
  - *The right circumstances*. Do you have experience performing the task given the person's condition and needs? Do you understand the purposes of the task for the person? Can you perform the task safely under the current circumstances? Do you have the equipment and supplies to safely complete the task? Do you know how to use the equipment and supplies?
  - *The right person*. Are you comfortable performing the task? Do you have concerns about performing the task?
  - *The right directions and communication*. Did the nurse give clear directions and instructions? Did you review the task with the nurse? Do you understand what the nurse expects?
  - *The right supervision*. Is a nurse available to answer questions? Is a nurse available if the person's condition changes or if problems occur?
- When you agree to perform a task, you are responsible for your own actions. You must complete the task safely. Report to the nurse what you did and the observations you made.
- You should refuse to perform a task when:
  - The task is beyond the legal limits of your role.
  - The task is not in your job description.
  - You were not prepared to perform the task.
  - The task could harm the person.
  - The person's condition has changed.
  - You do not know how to use the supplies or equipment.

- Directions are not ethical or legal.
- Directions are against center policies.
- Directions are unclear or incomplete.
- A nurse is not available for supervision.
- Never ignore an order or request to do something. Tell the nurse about your concerns.

ETHICAL ASPECTS

- Ethics is the knowledge of what is right conduct and wrong conduct. It also deals with choices or judgments about what should or should not be done. An ethical person does not cause a person harm.
- Ethical behavior involves not being prejudiced or biased—to make judgments and have views before knowing the facts. You should not judge a person by your values and standards. Also, do not avoid persons whose standards and values differ from your own.

Boundaries

- **Professional boundaries** separate helpful behaviors from behaviors that are not helpful.
- A **boundary violation** is an act or behavior that meets your needs, not the person's. The act or behavior is unethical. Boundary violations include abuse, keeping secrets with a person, or giving a lot of personal information about yourself to another. Review Box 2-6, Code of Conduct for Nursing Assistants, in the textbook.
- **Professional sexual misconduct** is an act, behavior, or comment that is sexual in nature. It is sexual misconduct even if the person consents or makes the first move.
- To maintain professional boundaries, review Box 2-7, Rules for Maintaining Professional Boundaries. Be alert to **boundary signs** (acts, behaviors, or thoughts that warn of a boundary crossing or violation).

LEGAL ASPECTS

- **Negligence** is an unintentional wrong. The negligent person did not act in a reasonable and careful manner. As a result, harm was caused to the person or property of another. The person did not mean to cause harm.
- **Malpractice** is negligence by a professional person.
- You are legally responsible (liable) for your own actions. The nurse is liable as your supervisor.
- **Defamation** is injuring a person's name and reputation by making false statements to a third person. **Libel** is making false statements in print, writing, or through pictures or drawings. **Slander**

is making false statements orally. Never make false statements about a patient, resident, co-worker, or any other person.
- **False imprisonment** is the unlawful restraint or restriction of a person's freedom of movement. It involves threatening to restrain a person, restraining a person, and preventing a person from leaving the center.
- **Invasion of privacy** is violating a person's right not to have his or her name, photo, or private affairs exposed or made public without giving consent. Review Box 2-8, Protecting the Right to Privacy, in the textbook.
- The Health Insurance Portability and Accountability Act (HIPAA) protects the privacy and security of a person's health information. **Protected health information** refers to identifying information and information about the person's health care. Direct any questions about the person or the person's care to the nurse.
- **Fraud** is saying or doing something to trick, fool, or deceive a person. The act is fraud if it does or could cause harm to a person or the person's property.
- **Assault** is intentionally attempting or threatening to touch a person's body without the person's consent. The person fears bodily harm. **Battery** is touching a person's body without his or her consent. Protect yourself from being accused of assault and battery. Explain to the person what is to be done and get the person's consent.

Informed Consent
- A person has the right to decide what will be done to his or her body and who can touch his or her body. Consent is informed when the person clearly understands all aspects of treatment.
- Persons who cannot give consent are persons who are under the legal age or are mentally incompetent. Unconscious, sedated, or confused persons also do not give consent. Informed consent is given by a responsible party—wife, husband, daughter, son, legal representative.
- You are never responsible for obtaining written consent.

REPORTING ABUSE
- Abuse is the intentional mistreatment or harm of another person. Abuse has one or more of these elements:
  - Willful causing of injury
  - Unreasonable confinement
  - Intimidation (to make afraid with threats of force or violence)
  - Punishment

- Depriving the person of the goods or services needed for physical, mental, or psychosocial well-being
- Abuse causes physical harm, pain, or mental anguish.
- **Vulnerable adults** are persons 18 years old or older who have disabilities or conditions that make them at risk to be wounded, attacked, or damaged. They have problems caring for or protecting themselves due to:
  - A mental, emotional, physical, or developmental disability
  - Brain damage
  - Changes from aging
- Older persons and children are at risk for abuse.
- **Elder abuse** is any knowing, intentional, or negligent act by a person to an older adult. It may include physical abuse, neglect, verbal abuse, involuntary seclusion, financial exploitation, emotional abuse, sexual abuse, or abandonment. Review Box 2-9, Signs of Elder Abuse, in the textbook.
- If you suspect a person is being abused, report your observations to the nurse.

CHAPTER 2 REVIEW QUESTIONS
Circle the BEST answer.
1. You answer the telephone. The doctor starts to give you an order. You
   a. Take the order from the doctor
   b. Politely give your name and title, and ask the doctor to wait for the nurse. Promptly find the nurse
   c. Politely ask the doctor to call back later
   d. Ask the doctor if the nurse may call him back
2. You can have your certification revoked for all the following *except*
   a. Substance abuse or dependency
   b. Abandoning a patient or resident
   c. Performing acts beyond the nursing assistant role
   d. Giving safe care
3. When should you refuse a task?
   a. The task is not in your job description.
   b. The task is within the legal limits of your role.
   c. The directions for the task are clear.
   d. A nurse is available for questions and supervision.
4. A nurse delegates a task that you did not learn in your training. The task is in your job description. What is your appropriate response to the nurse?
   a. "I cannot do that task."
   b. "I did not learn that task in my training. Can you show me how to do it?"
   c. "I will ask the other nursing assistant to watch me do the task."

d. "I will ask the other nursing assistant to do the task for me."

5. You are busy with a new resident. It is time for another resident's bath. You may delegate the bath to another nursing assistant.
   a. True
   b. False

6. A resident offers you a gift certificate for being kind to her. You should
   a. Say "thank you" and accept the gift
   b. Accept the gift and give it to charity
   c. Thank the resident for thinking of you, then explain it is against policy for you to accept the gift
   d. Accept the gift and give it to your daughter

7. To protect a person's privacy, you should do the following *except*
   a. Keep all information about the person confidential
   b. Discuss the person's treatment or diagnosis with the nurse supervising your work
   c. Open the person's mail
   d. Allow the person to visit with others in private

8. What should you do if you suspect an older person is being abused?
   a. Report the situation to the health department.
   b. Notify the nurse and discuss the observations with him or her.
   c. Notify the doctor about the suspected abuse.
   d. Ask the family why they are abusing the person.

9. A resident needs help going to the bathroom. You do not answer her signal light promptly. She gets up without help, falls, and breaks a leg. This is an example of
   a. Negligence
   b. Defamation
   c. False imprisonment
   d. Slander

10. Examples of defamation include all the following *except*
    a. Implying or suggesting that a person uses drugs
    b. Saying that a person is insane or mentally ill
    c. Implying that a person steals money from staff
    d. Burning a resident with water that is too hot

11. Which statement about ethics is *false*?
    a. An ethical person does not judge others by his or her values and standards.
    b. An ethical person avoids persons whose standards and values differ from his or her own.
    c. An ethical person is not prejudiced or biased.

d. An ethical person does not cause harm to another person.

12. Examples of false imprisonment include all of the following *except*
    a. Threatening to restrain a resident
    b. Restraining a resident without a doctor's order
    c. Treating the resident with respect
    d. Preventing a resident from leaving the agency

13. To protect yourself from being accused of assault and battery, you should explain to the resident what you plan to do before touching him or her and get consent.
    a. True
    b. False

Answers to these questions are on p. 425.

CHAPTER 3 WORK ETHICS
HEALTH, HYGIENE, AND APPEARANCE

- To give safe and effective care, you must be physically and mentally healthy. You need a balanced diet, sleep and rest, and exercise on a regular basis.
- Personal hygiene needs careful attention. Bathe daily, use deodorant or antiperspirant, and brush your teeth often. Shampoo often. Keep fingernails clean, short, and neatly shaped.
- Review Box 3-1, Practices for a Professional Appearance, in your textbook.

TEAMWORK

- Practice good work ethics—work when scheduled, be cheerful and friendly, perform delegated tasks, be kind to others, be available to help others.
- Be ready to work when your shift starts. Arrive on your nursing unit a few minutes early.
  - Stay the entire shift. When it is time to leave, report off-duty to the nurse.
- A good attitude is needed. Review Box 3-2, Qualities and Traits for Good Work Ethics, in your textbook.
- Gossiping is unprofessional and hurtful. To avoid being a part of **gossip:**
  - Remove yourself from a group or situation where gossip is occurring.
  - Do not make or repeat any comment that can hurt another person.
  - Do not make or repeat any comment that you do not know to be true.
  - Do not talk about residents, family members, visitors, co-workers, or the center at home or in social settings.
- **Confidentiality** means trusting others with personal and private information. The person's

information is shared only among health team members involved in his or her care. Agency and co-worker information also is confidential.

- Your speech and language must be professional:
  - Do not swear or use foul, vulgar, or abusive language.
  - Do not use slang.
  - Speak softly, gently, and clearly.
  - Do not shout or yell.
  - Do not fight or argue with a resident, family member, visitor, or co-worker.
- A courtesy is a polite, considerate, or helpful comment or act.
  - Address others by Miss, Mrs., Ms., Mr., or Doctor. Use a first name only if the person asks you to do so.
  - Say "please" and "thank you." Say "I'm sorry" when you make a mistake or hurt someone.
  - Let residents, families, and visitors enter elevators first.
  - Be thoughtful—compliment others, give praise.
  - Wish the person and family well when they leave the center.
  - Hold doors open for others.
  - Help others willingly when asked.
  - Do not take credit for another person's deeds. Give the person credit for the action.
- Keep personal matters out of the workplace:
  - Make personal phone calls during meals and breaks.
  - Do not let family and friends visit you on the unit.
  - Do not use the agency's computers and other equipment for personal use.
  - Do not take agency supplies for personal use.
  - Do not discuss personal problems at work.
  - Control your emotions.
  - Do not borrow money from or lend money to co-workers.
  - Do not sell things or engage in fund-raising at work.
  - Do not have wireless phones or personal pagers on while at work.
- Leave for and return from breaks and meals on time. Tell the nurse when you leave and return to the unit.

MANAGING STRESS

- These guidelines can help you reduce or cope with stress:
  - Exercise regularly.
  - Get enough sleep or rest.
  - Eat healthy.

- Plan personal and quiet time for yourself.
- Use common sense about what you can do.
- Do one thing at a time.
- Do not judge yourself harshly.
- Give yourself praise.
- Have a sense of humor.
- Talk to the nurse if your work or a person is causing too much stress.

HARASSMENT

- **Harassment** means to trouble, torment, offend, or worry a person by one's behavior or comments. Harassment can be sexual. Or it can involve age, race, ethnic background, religion, or disability. You must respect others. Do not offend others by your gestures, remarks, or use of touch. Do not offend others with jokes, photos, or other pictures.

CHAPTER 3 REVIEW QUESTIONS
Circle the BEST answer.

1. You believe you have good work ethics. This means you do the following *except*
   a. Work when scheduled
   b. Act cheerful and friendly
   c. Refuse to help others
   d. Perform tasks assigned by the nurse
2. A nursing assistant is gossiping about a co-worker. You should
   a. Stay with the group and listen to what is being said
   b. Repeat the comment to your family
   c. Remove yourself from the group where gossip is occurring
   d. Repeat the comment to another co-worker
3. You want to maintain confidentiality about others. You do the following *except*
   a. Share information about a resident with a nurse who is on another unit
   b. Avoid talking about a resident in the elevator, hallway, or dining area
   c. Avoid talking about co-workers and residents when others are present
   d. Avoid eavesdropping
4. When you are at work, you should do which of the following?
   a. Swear and use foul language.
   b. Use slang.
   c. Argue with a visitor.
   d. Speak clearly and softly.
5. To give safe and effective care, you do all the following *except*
   a. Eat a balanced diet
   b. Get enough sleep and rest

c. Exercise on a regular basis

d. Drink too much alcohol

6. While at work, you should do all of the following *except*

a. Be courteous to others

b. Make personal phone calls

c. Admit when you are wrong or make mistakes

d. Respect others

Answers to these questions are on p. 425.

CHAPTER 4 COMMUNICATING WITH THE HEALTH TEAM

COMMUNICATION

- For good communication:
  - Use words that mean the same thing to you and the receiver of the message.
  - Use familiar words.
  - Be brief and concise.
  - Give information in a logical and orderly manner.
  - Give facts, and be specific.

THE MEDICAL RECORD

- The **medical record** is a way for the health team to share information about the person. It is a legal document.
- If you know a person in the agency, but you do not give care to that person, you have no right to review the person's chart. To do so is an invasion of privacy.
- A person or legal representative may ask you for the chart. Report the request to the nurse.
- Follow your agency's policies about recording in the medical record.

NURSING PROCESS

- The **nursing process** is the method nurses use to plan and deliver nursing care.
- You play a key role by making observations as you care and talk with the person.
- **Observation** is using the senses of sight, hearing, touch, and smell to collect information. Box 4-1, Basic Observations, in your textbook lists the basic observations you need to make and report to the nurse. Examples are:
  - Can the person give his or her name, the time, and location when asked?
  - Can the person move the arms and legs?
  - Is the skin pale or flushed?
  - Is there drainage from the eyes? What color is the drainage?
  - Does the person like the food served?
  - Can the person bathe without help?

- Observations you need to report to the nurse at once are:
  - A change in the person's ability to respond
  - A change in the person's mobility
  - Complaints of sudden, severe pain
  - A sore or reddened area on the person's skin
  - Complaints of a sudden change in vision
  - Complaints of pain or difficulty breathing
  - Abnormal respirations
  - Complaints of or signs of difficulty swallowing
  - Vomiting
  - Bleeding
  - Vital signs outside their normal ranges
- **Objective data (signs)** are seen, heard, felt, or smelled by an observer.
- **Subjective data (symptoms)** are things a person tells you about that you cannot observe through your senses.
- The RN may conduct a care conference to share information and ideas about the person's care. The RN, nursing assistants, and other health team members take part in the conference. The person has the right to take part in care planning conferences. Sometimes the family is involved. The person may refuse actions suggested by the health team.
- Use your assignment sheet to organize your work and set priorities:
  - What do you need to do first?
  - What can be done while the person is having breakfast, lunch, or dinner?
  - What can you do while the person is at a therapy or an activity?
  - Do you need to reserve the use of rooms or equipment?
  - What do you need help with?
  - How many co-workers are needed to complete nursing tasks?
  - Ask a co-worker to help you.
  - Check off tasks as you complete them.

REPORTING

- You report care and observations to the nurse. Follow these rules:
  - Be prompt, thorough, and accurate.
  - Give the person's name, and room and bed numbers.
  - Give the time your observations were made or the care was given.
  - Report only what you observed or did yourself.
  - Give reports as often as the person's condition requires or when the nurse asks you to.
  - Report any changes from normal or changes in the person's condition at once.

- Use your written notes to give a specific, concise, and clear report.

RECORDING

- Rules for recording are:
  - Always use ink. Use the color required by the center.
  - Include the date and time for every recording.
  - Make sure writing is readable and neat.
  - Use only center-approved abbreviations.
  - Use correct spelling, grammar, and punctuation.
  - Do not use ditto marks.
  - Never erase or use correction fluid. Follow the center's procedure for correcting errors.
  - Sign all entries with your name and title as required by center policy.
  - Do not skip lines.
  - Make sure each form is stamped with the person's name and other identifying information.
  - Record only what you observed and did yourself.
  - Never chart a procedure, treatment, or care measure until after it is completed.
  - Be accurate, concise, and factual. Do not record judgments or interpretations.
  - Record in a logical and sequential manner.
  - Be descriptive. Avoid terms with more than one meaning.
  - Use the person's exact words whenever possible. Use quotation marks to show that the statement is a direct quote.
  - Chart any changes from normal or changes in the person's condition. Also chart that you informed the nurse (include the nurse's name), what you told the nurse, and the time you made the report.
  - Do not omit information.
  - Record safety measures. Example: Reminding a person not to get out of bed.
- Review the 24-hour clock in Figure 4-6 in your textbook.

MEDICAL TERMINOLOGY AND ABBREVIATIONS

- Medical terminology and abbreviations are used in health care. Someone may use a word or phrase that you do not understand. If so, ask the nurse to explain its meaning.
- Review Box 4-5, Medical Terminology, in the textbook.
- Use only the abbreviations accepted by the center. If you are not sure that an abbreviation is acceptable, write the term out in full. See the inside of the back cover of the textbook for common abbreviations.

COMPUTERS AND OTHER ELECTRONIC DEVICES

- Computers contain vast amounts of information about a person. Therefore the right to privacy must be protected. If allowed access, you must follow the agency's policies. Review Box 4-6, Using the Agency's Computer and Other Electronic Devices, in your textbook.

PHONE COMMUNICATIONS

- Guidelines for answering phones:
  - Answer the call after the first ring if possible.
  - Do not answer the phone in a rushed or hasty manner.
  - Give a courteous greeting. Identify the nursing unit and your name and title.
  - When taking a message, write down the caller's name, phone number, date and time, and message.
  - Repeat the message and phone number back to the caller.
  - Ask the caller to "Please hold" if necessary.
  - Do not lay the phone down or cover the receiver with your hand when not speaking to the caller. The caller may hear confidential information.
  - Return to a caller on hold within 30 seconds.
  - Do not give confidential information to any caller.
  - Transfer a call if appropriate. Tell the caller you are going to transfer the call. Give the name and phone number in case the call gets disconnected.
  - End the conversation politely.
  - Give the message to the appropriate person.

DEALING WITH CONFLICT

- These guidelines can help you deal with conflict:
  - Ask your supervisor for some time to talk privately about the problem.
  - Approach the person with whom you have the conflict. Ask to talk privately. Be polite and professional.
  - Agree on a time and place to talk.
  - Talk in a private setting. No one should hear you or the other person.
  - Explain the problem and what is bothering you. Give facts and specific behaviors. Focus on the problem. Do not focus on the person.
  - Listen to the person. Do not interrupt.
  - Identify ways to solve the problem. Offer your thoughts. Ask for the co-worker's ideas.
  - Set a date and time to review the matter.
  - Thank the person for meeting with you.
  - Carry out the solution.
  - Review the matter as scheduled.

CHAPTER 4 REVIEW QUESTIONS
Circle the BEST answer.

1. For good communication, you should do the following *except*
   a. Use words with more than one meaning
   b. Use familiar words to the person or family
   c. Give facts in a brief and concise manner
   d. Give information in a logical and orderly manner
2. Which statement about observations is *false?*
   a. You make observations as you care and talk with people.
   b. Observation uses the senses of smell, sight, touch, and hearing.
   c. A reddened area on the person's skin is reported to the nurse at once.
   d. You report observations to the doctor.
3. Objective data include all the following *except*
   a. The person has pain in his abdomen
   b. The person's pulse is 76
   c. The person's urine is dark amber
   d. The person's breath has an odor
4. When reporting care and observations to the nurse, you do the following *except*
   a. Give the person's name and room and bed numbers
   b. Report only what you observed or did yourself
   c. Report any changes from normal or changes in the person's condition at once
   d. Report any changes from normal or changes in the person's condition at the end of the shift
5. When you record in a person's chart, you do the following *except*
   a. Record what you observed and did
   b. Record the person's response to the treatment or procedure
   c. Use abbreviations that are not on the accepted list for the center
   d. Record the time the observation was made or the treatment performed

Answers to these questions are on p. 425.

CHAPTER 5 UNDERSTANDING THE PERSON
CARING FOR THE PERSON
- The whole person needs to be considered when you provide care—physical, social, psychological, and spiritual parts. These parts are woven together and cannot be separated.
- Follow these rules to address persons with dignity and respect:
  - Call persons by their titles—Mrs. Dennison, Mr. Smith, Miss Turner, or Dr. Gonzalez.
  - Do not call persons by their first names unless they ask you to.
  - Do not call persons by any other name unless they ask you to.
  - Do not call persons Grandma, Papa, Sweetheart, Honey, or other name.

BASIC NEEDS
- A **need** is something necessary or desired for maintaining life and mental well-being.
- According to Maslow, basic needs must be met for a person to survive and function:
  - *Physiological or physical needs*—are required for life. They are oxygen, food, water, elimination, rest, and shelter.
  - *Safety and security needs*—relate to feeling safe from harm, danger, and fear.
  - *Love and belonging needs*—relate to love, closeness, affection, and meaningful relationships with others. Family, friends, and the health team can meet love and belonging needs.
  - *Self-esteem needs*—relate to thinking well of oneself and to seeing oneself as useful and having value. People often lack self-esteem when ill, injured, older, or disabled.
  - *The need for self-actualization*—involves learning, understanding, and creating to the limit of a person's capacity. Rarely, if ever, is it totally met.

CULTURE AND RELIGION
- **Culture** is the characteristics of a group of people. People come from many cultures, races, and nationalities. Family practices, food choices, hygiene habits, clothing styles, and language are part of their culture. The person's culture also influences health beliefs and practices.
- **Religion** relates to spiritual beliefs, needs, and practices. A person's religion influences health and illness practices. Many may want to pray and observe religious practices. Assist residents to attend religious services as needed. If a person wants to see a spiritual leader or advisor, tell the nurse. Provide privacy during the visit.
- A person may not follow all the beliefs and practices of his or her culture or religion. Some people do not practice a religion.
- Respect and accept the person's culture and religion. Learn about practices and beliefs different from your own. Do not judge a person by your standards.

BEHAVIOR ISSUES
- Many people do not adjust well to illness, injury, and disability. They have some of the following behaviors:

- *Anger.* Anger may be communicated verbally and nonverbally. Verbal outbursts, shouting, and rapid speech are common. Some people are silent. Others are uncooperative and may refuse to answer questions. Nonverbal signs include rapid movements, pacing, clenched fists, and a red face. Glaring and getting close to you when speaking are other signs. Violent behaviors can occur.
- *Demanding behavior.* Nothing seems to please the person. The person is critical of others.
- *Self-centered behavior.* The person cares only about his or her own needs. The needs of others are ignored. The person becomes impatient if needs are not met.
- *Aggressive behavior.* The person may swear, bite, hit, pinch, scratch, or kick. Protect the person, others, and yourself from harm.
- *Withdrawal.* The person has little or no contact with family, friends, and staff. Some people are generally not social and prefer to be alone.
- *Inappropriate sexual behavior.* Some people make inappropriate sexual remarks or touch others in the wrong way. These behaviors may be on purpose. Or they are caused by disease, confusion, dementia, or drug side effects.
- You cannot avoid persons with unpleasant behaviors or who lose control. Review Box 5-1, Dealing With Behavior Issues, in your textbook.

COMMUNICATING WITH THE PERSON
- For effective communication between you and the person, you must:
  - Follow the rules of communication in Chapter 4.
  - Understand and respect the patient or resident as a person.
  - View the person as a physical, psychological, social, and spiritual human being.
  - Appreciate the person's problems and frustrations.
  - Respect the person's rights.
  - Respect the person's religion and culture.
  - Give the person time to understand the information that you give.
  - Repeat information as often as needed.
  - Ask questions to see if the person understood you.
  - Be patient. People with memory problems may ask the same question many times.
  - Include the person in conversations when others are present.

Verbal Communication
- When talking with a person follow these rules:
  - Face the person.
  - Position yourself at the person's eye level.
  - Control the loudness and tone of your voice.
  - Speak clearly, slowly, and distinctly.
  - Do not use slang or vulgar words.
  - Repeat information as needed.
  - Ask one question at a time, and wait for an answer.
  - Do not shout, whisper, or mumble.
  - Be kind, courteous, and friendly.
- Use written words if the person cannot speak or hear but can read. Keep written messages brief and concise. Use a black felt pen on white paper, and print in large letters.
- Some persons cannot speak or read. Ask questions that have "yes" and "no" answers. A picture board may be helpful.

Nonverbal Communication
- Messages are sent with gestures, facial expressions, posture, body movements, touch, and smell. Nonverbal messages more accurately reflect a person's feelings than words do. A person may say one thing but act another way. Watch the person's eyes, hand movements, gestures, posture, and other actions.
- Touch conveys comfort, caring, love, affection, interest, trust, concern, and reassurance. Touch should be gentle. Touch means different things to different people. Some people do not like to be touched.
- People send messages through their **body language**—facial expressions, gestures, posture, hand and body movements, gait, eye contact, and appearance. Your body language should show interest, enthusiasm, caring, and respect for the person. Often you need to control your body language. Control reactions to odors from body fluids, secretions, or excretions.

Communication Methods
- *Listening* means to focus on verbal and nonverbal communication. You use sight, hearing, touch, and smell. To be a good listener:
  - Face the person.
  - Have good eye contact with the person.
  - Lean toward the person. Do not sit back with your arms crossed.
  - Respond to the person. Nod your head, and ask questions.
  - Avoid communication barriers.
- *Paraphrasing* is restating the person's message in your own words.
- *Direct questions* focus on certain information. You ask the person something you need to know.
- *Open-ended questions* lead or invite the person to share thoughts, feelings, or ideas. The person chooses what to talk about.

- *Clarifying* lets you make sure that you understand the message. You can ask the person to repeat the message, say you do not understand, or restate the message.
- *Focusing* deals with a certain topic. It is useful when a person wanders in thought.
- *Silence* is a very powerful way to communicate. Silence on your part shows caring and respect for the person's situation and feelings.

Communication Barriers

- *Language.* You and the person must use and understand the same language.
- *Cultural differences.* A person from another country may attach different meanings to verbal and nonverbal communication from what you intended.
- *Changing the subject.* Avoid changing the subject whenever possible.
- *Giving your opinions.* Opinions involve judging values, behavior, or feelings. Let others express feelings and concerns. Do not make judgments or jump to conclusions.
- *Talking a lot when others are silent.* Talking too much is usually because of nervousness and discomfort with silence.
- *Failure to listen.* Do not pretend to listen. It shows lack of caring and interest. You may miss complaints of pain, discomfort, or other symptoms that you must report to the nurse.
- *Pat answers.* "Don't worry." "Everything will be okay." These make the person feel that you do not care about his or her concerns, feelings, and fears.
- *Illness and disability.* Speech, hearing, vision, cognitive function, and body movements may be affected. Verbal and nonverbal communication is affected.
- *Age.* Values and communication styles vary among age-groups.

PERSONS WITH SPECIAL NEEDS

- Common courtesies and manners apply to any person with a disability. Review Box 5-2, Disability Etiquette, in the textbook.
- The person who is comatose is unconscious and cannot respond to others. Often the person can feel touch and pain. Assume that the person hears and understands you. Use touch, and give care gently. Practice these measures:
  - Knock before entering the person's room.
  - Tell the person your name, the time, and the place every time you enter the room.
  - Give care on the same schedule every day.
  - Explain what you are going to do.
  - Tell the person when you are finishing care.
  - Use touch to communicate care, concern, and comfort.
  - Tell the person what time you will be back to check on him or her.
  - Tell the person when you are leaving the room.

FAMILY AND FRIENDS

- If you need to give care when visitors are there, protect the person's right to privacy. Politely ask the visitors to leave the room when you give care. A partner or family member may help you if the patient or resident consents.
- Treat family and visitors with courtesy and respect.
- Do not discuss the person's condition with family and friends. Refer questions to the nurse. A visitor may upset or tire a person. Report your observations to the nurse.

CHAPTER 5 REVIEW QUESTIONS
Circle the BEST answer.

1. While caring for a person, you need to
   a. Consider only the person's physical and social needs
   b. Consider the person's physical, social, psychological, and spiritual needs
   c. Consider only the person's cultural needs
   d. Ignore the person's spiritual needs
2. When referring to residents, you should
   a. Refer to them by their room number
   b. Call them "Honey"
   c. Call them by their first name
   d. Call them by their name and title
3. Based on Maslow's theory of basic needs, which person's needs must be met first?
   a. The person who wants to talk about her granddaughter's wedding
   b. The person who is uncomfortable in the dining room
   c. The person who wants mail opened
   d. The person who asks for more water
4. Which statement about culture is *false?*
   a. A person's culture influences health beliefs and practices.
   b. You must respect a person's culture.
   c. You should ignore the person's culture while you give his or her care.
   d. You should learn about another person's culture that is different from yours.
5. Which statement about religion and spiritual beliefs is *false?*
   a. A person's religion influences health and illness practices.
   b. You should assist a person to attend services in the nursing center.
   c. Many people find comfort and strength from religion during illness.
   d. A person must follow all beliefs of his or her religion.

6. A person is angry and is shouting at you. You should do the following *except*
   a. Stay calm and professional
   b. Yell so the person will listen to you
   c. Listen to what the person is saying
   d. Report the person's behavior to the nurse

7. A person tries to scratch and kick you. You should
   a. Protect yourself from harm
   b. Argue with the person
   c. Become angry with the person
   d. Refuse to care for the person

8. When speaking with another person, you do the following *except*
   a. Position yourself at the person's eye level
   b. Speak slowly, clearly, and distinctly
   c. Shout, mumble, and whisper
   d. Ask one question at a time

9. Which statement about listening is *false?*
   a. You use sight, hearing, touch, and smell when you listen.
   b. You observe nonverbal cues.
   c. You have good eye contact with the person.
   d. You sit back with your arms crossed.

10. Which statement about silence is *false?*
    a. Silence is a powerful way to communicate.
    b. Silence gives people time to think.
    c. You should talk a lot when the other person is silent.
    d. Silence helps when the person is upset and needs to gain control.

11. A person speaks a foreign language. You should do the following *except*
    a. Keep messages short and simple
    b. Use gestures and pictures
    c. Shout or speak loudly
    d. Repeat the message in other words

12. When caring for a person who is comatose, you do the following *except*
    a. Tell the person your name when you enter the room
    b. Explain what you are doing
    c. Use touch to communicate care and comfort
    d. Make jokes about how sick the person is

13. A person is in a wheelchair. You should do all the following *except*
    a. Lean on a person's wheelchair
    b. Sit or squat to talk to a person in a wheelchair or chair
    c. Think about obstacles before giving directions to a person in a wheelchair
    d. Extend the same courtesies to the person as you would to anyone else

14. A person's daughter is visiting and you need to provide care to the person. You
    a. Expose the person's body in front of the visitor

b. Politely ask the visitor to leave the room
c. Decide to not provide the care at all
d. Discuss the person's condition with the visitor

Answers to these questions are on p. 425.

CHAPTER 7 CARE OF THE OLDER PERSON
GROWTH AND DEVELOPMENT

- Aging is normal. It is not a disease. Normal changes occur in body structure and function. Psychological and social changes also occur.
- **Growth** is the physical changes that are measured and that occur in a steady and orderly manner.
- **Development** relates to changes in mental, emotional, and social function.
- Growth and development occur in a sequence, order, and pattern. Review Box 7-1, Stages of Growth and Development, in your textbook.

SOCIAL CHANGES

- Physical reminders of growing old affect self-esteem and may threaten self-image, feelings of self-worth, and independence.
- People cope with aging in their own way. How they cope depends on their health status, life experiences, finances, education, and social support systems.
- *Retirement.* Many people enjoy retirement. Others are in poor health and have medical bills that can make retirement hard.
- *Reduced income.* Retirement usually means reduced income. The retired person still has expenses. Reduced income may force life-style changes. One example is the person avoids health care or needed drugs.
- *Social relationships.* Social relationships change throughout life. Family time helps prevent loneliness. So do hobbies, religious and community events, and new friends.
- *Children as caregivers.* Some older persons feel more secure when children care for them. Others feel unwanted and useless. Some lose dignity and self-respect. Tensions may occur among the child, parent, and other household members.
- *Death of a partner.* When death occurs, the person loses a lover, friend, companion, and confidant. Grief may be great. The person's life will likely change.

PHYSICAL CHANGES

- Body processes slow down. Energy level and body efficiency decline.

- *The integumentary system.* The skin loses its elasticity, strength, and fatty tissue layer. Wrinkles appear. Dry skin occurs and may cause itching. The skin is fragile and easily injured. The person is more sensitive to cold. Nails become thick and tough. Feet may have poor circulation. White or gray hair is common. Hair thins. Facial hair may occur in women. Hair is drier. The risk of skin cancer increases.
- *The musculoskeletal system.* Muscle and bone strength are lost. Bones become brittle and break easily. Vertebrae shorten. Joints become stiff and painful. Mobility decreases. There is a gradual loss of height.
- *The nervous system.* Confusion, dizziness, and fatigue may occur. Responses are slower. The risk for falls increases. Forgetfulness increases. Memory is shorter. Events from long ago are remembered better than recent ones. Older persons have a harder time falling asleep. Sleep periods are shorter. Older persons wake often during the night and have less deep sleep. Less sleep is needed. They may rest or nap during the day. They may go to bed early and get up early.
- *The senses.* Hearing and vision losses occur. Taste and smell dull. Touch and sensitivity to pain, pressure, hot, and cold are reduced.
- *The circulatory system.* The heart muscle weakens. Arteries narrow and are less elastic. Poor circulation occurs in many body parts.
- *The respiratory system.* Respiratory muscles weaken. Lung tissue becomes less elastic. Difficult, labored, or painful breathing may occur with activity. The person may lack strength to cough and clear the airway of secretions. Respiratory infections and diseases may develop.
- *The digestive system.* Less saliva is produced. The person may have difficulty swallowing (dysphagia). Indigestion may occur. Loss of teeth and ill-fitting dentures cause chewing problems and digestion problems. Flatulence and constipation can occur. Fewer calories are needed as energy and activity levels decline. More fluids are needed.
- *The urinary system.* Urine is more concentrated. Bladder muscles weaken. Bladder size decreases. Urinary frequency or urgency may occur. Many older persons have to urinate at night. Urinary incontinence may occur. In men, the prostate gland enlarges. This may cause difficulty urinating or frequent urination.
- *The reproductive system.* In men, testosterone decreases. An erection takes longer. Orgasm is less forceful. Women experience menopause. Female hormones of estrogen and progesterone decrease.

The uterus, vagina, and genitalia shrink (atrophy). Vaginal walls thin. There is vaginal dryness. Arousal takes longer. Orgasm is less intense.

NEEDING NURSING CENTER CARE
- The person needing nursing center care may suffer some or all of these losses:
  - Loss of identity as a productive member of a family and community
  - Loss of possessions—home, household items, car, and so on
  - Loss of independence
  - Loss of real-world experiences—shopping, traveling, cooking, driving, hobbies
  - Loss of health and mobility
- The person may feel useless, powerless, and hopeless. The health team helps the person cope with loss and improve quality of life. Treat the person with dignity and respect. Also practice good communication skills. Follow the care plan.

CHAPTER 7 REVIEW QUESTIONS
Circle the BEST answer.
1. Which is a developmental task of late adulthood?
   a. Accepting changes in appearance
   b. Adjusting to decreased strength
   c. Developing a satisfactory sex life
   d. Performing self-care
2. Which statement is *false?*
   a. Physical changes occur with aging.
   b. Energy level and body efficiency decline with age.
   c. Some people age faster than others.
   d. Normal aging means loss of health.
3. As a person ages, the integumentary system changes. Which statement is *false?*
   a. Dry skin and itching occur.
   b. Nails become thick and tough.
   c. The person is less sensitive to cold.
   d. Skin is injured more easily.
4. Which statement is *false* about the musculo-skeletal system and aging?
   a. Strength decreases.
   b. Vertebrae shorten.
   c. Mobility increases.
   d. Bone mass decreases.
5. Which statement about the nervous system and aging is *false?*
   a. Reflexes slow.
   b. Memory may be shorter.
   c. Sleep patterns change.
   d. Forgetfulness decreases.

6. Which statement about the digestive system and aging is *false?*
   a. Appetite decreases.
   b. Less saliva is produced.
   c. Flatulence and constipation may decrease.
   d. Teeth may be lost.
7. Which statement about the urinary system and aging is *false?*
   a. Urine becomes more concentrated.
   b. Urinary frequency may occur.
   c. Urinary urgency may occur.
   d. Bladder muscles become stronger.

Answers to these questions are on p. 425.

CHAPTER 8 PROMOTING SAFETY
ACCIDENT RISK FACTORS
- *Age.* Older persons are at risk for falls and other injuries.
- *Awareness of surroundings.* People need to know their surroundings to protect themselves from injury.
- *Agitated and aggressive behaviors.* Pain, confusion, fear, and decreased awareness of surroundings can cause these behaviors.
- *Impaired vision.* Persons can fall or trip over items. Some have problems reading labels on containers.
- *Impaired hearing.* Persons have problems hearing explanations and instructions. They may not hear warning signals or fire alarms. They do not know to move to safety.
- *Impaired smell and touch.* Illness and aging affect smell and touch.
- *Impaired mobility.* Some diseases and injuries affect mobility. A person may be aware of danger but is unable to move to safety.
- *Drugs.* Drugs have side effects. Report behavior changes and the person's complaints.

IDENTIFYING THE PERSON
- You must give the right care to the right person. To identify the person:
  - Compare identifying information on the assignment sheet or treatment card with that on the identification (ID) bracelet.
  - Call the person by name when checking the ID bracelet. Just calling the person by name is not enough to identify him or her. Confused, disoriented, drowsy, hard-of-hearing, or distracted persons may answer to any name.
  - Some nursing centers have photo ID systems. Use this system safely.
  - Alert and oriented persons may choose not to wear ID bracelets. Follow center policy and the care plan to identify the person.

PREVENTING BURNS
- Smoking, spilled hot liquids, very hot water, and electrical devices are common causes of burns. See p. 107 in your textbook for safety measures to prevent burns.

PREVENTING POISONING
- Drugs and household products are common poisons. Poisoning in adults may be from carelessness, confusion, or poor vision when reading labels. To prevent poisoning:
  - Make sure patients and residents cannot reach hazardous materials.
  - Follow agency policy for storing personal care items.

PREVENTING SUFFOCATION
- **Suffocation** is when breathing stops from the lack of oxygen. Death occurs if the person does not start breathing.
- To prevent suffocation, review Box 8-1, Safety Measures to Prevent Suffocation.

Choking
- Choking or foreign-body airway obstruction (FBAO) occurs when a foreign body obstructs the airway. Air cannot pass through the air passages to the lungs. The body does not get enough oxygen. This can lead to cardiac arrest.
- Choking often occurs during eating. A large, poorly chewed piece of meat is the most common cause. Other common causes include laughing and talking while eating.
- With *mild airway obstruction,* some air moves in and out of the lungs. The person is conscious. Usually the person can speak. Often forceful coughing can remove the object.
- With *severe airway obstruction,* the conscious person clutches at the throat—the "universal sign of choking." The person has difficulty breathing. Some persons cannot breathe, speak, or cough. The person appears pale and cyanotic. Air does not move in and out of the lungs. If the obstruction is not removed, the person will die. Severe airway obstruction is an emergency.
- Use abdominal thrusts to relieve FBAO. Chest thrusts are used for very obese persons and pregnant women.
- Call for help when a person has an obstructed airway. Report and record what happened, what you did, and the person's response.

PREVENTING EQUIPMENT ACCIDENTS
- All equipment is unsafe if broken, not used correctly, or not working properly. Inspect all

equipment before use. Review Box 8-2, Safety Measures to Prevent Equipment Accidents, in the textbook.

WHEELCHAIR AND STRETCHER SAFETY
- Review Box 8-3, Wheelchair and Stretcher Safety, in the textbook.

HANDLING HAZARDOUS SUBSTANCES
- A hazardous substance is any chemical in the workplace that can cause harm. Hazardous substances include oxygen, mercury, disinfectants, and cleaning agents.
- Hazardous substance containers must have a warning label. If a label is removed or damaged, do not use the substance. Take the container to the nurse. Do not leave the container unattended.
- Check the material safety data sheet (MSDS) before using a hazardous substance, cleaning up a leak or spill, or disposing of the substance. Tell the nurse about a leak or spill right away. Do not leave a leak or spill unattended.

FIRE SAFETY
- Faulty electrical equipment and wiring, overloaded electrical circuits, and smoking are major causes of fires.
- Safety measures are needed where oxygen is used and stored:
  - "NO SMOKING" signs are placed on the door and near the person's bed.
  - The person and visitors are reminded not to smoke in the room.
  - Smoking materials are removed from the room.
  - Electrical items are turned off before being unplugged.
  - Wool blankets and fabrics that cause static electricity are not used.
  - The person wears a cotton gown or pajamas.
  - Electrical items are in good working order.
  - Lit candles and other open flames are not allowed.
  - Materials that ignite easily are removed from the room.
- Review Box 8-4, Fire Prevention Measures, in the textbook.
- Know your center's policies and procedures for fire emergencies. Know where to find fire alarms, fire extinguishers, and emergency exits. Remember the word RACE:
  - R—*rescue*. Rescue persons in immediate danger. Move them to a safe place.
  - A—*alarm*. Sound the nearest fire alarm. Notify the telephone operator.
  - C—*confine*. Close doors and windows. Turn off oxygen or electrical items.
  - E—*extinguish*. Use a fire extinguisher on a small fire.
- Remember the word PASS for using a fire extinguisher:
  - P—*pull* the safety pin.
  - A—*aim* low. Aim at the base of the fire.
  - S—*squeeze* the lever. This starts the stream of water.
  - S—*sweep* back and forth. Sweep side to side at the base of the fire.
- Do not use elevators during a fire.

DISASTERS
- A **disaster** is a sudden catastrophic event. The agency has procedures for disasters that could occur in your area. Follow them to keep patients, residents, visitors, staff, and yourself safe.

WORKPLACE VIOLENCE
- **Workplace violence** is violent acts (including assault or threat of assault) directed toward persons at work or while on duty. Review Box 8-5, Measures to Deal With Agitated or Aggressive Persons, in the textbook.

CHAPTER 8 REVIEW QUESTIONS
Circle the BEST answer.
1. You see a water spill in the hallway. What will you do?
   a. Ask housekeeping to wipe up the spill right away.
   b. Wipe up the spill right away.
   c. Report the spill to the nurse.
   d. Ask the resident to walk around the spill.
2. An electrical outlet in a person's room does not work. What will you do?
   a. Tell the administrator about the problem.
   b. Tell another nursing assistant about the problem.
   c. Try to repair the electrical outlet.
   d. Follow the center's policy for reporting the problem.
3. Accident risk factors include all of the following *except*
   a. Walking without difficulty
   b. Hearing problems
   c. Dulled sense of smell
   d. Poor vision
4. To prevent a person from being burned, you should do the following *except*
   a. Supervise the smoking of persons who are confused
   b. Turn cold water on first; turn hot water off first
   c. Do not let the person sleep with a heating pad
   d. Allow smoking in bed

5. To prevent suffocation, you should do the following *except*
   a. Make sure dentures fit properly
   b. Check the care plan for swallowing problems before serving food or liquids
   c. Leave a person alone in a bathtub or shower
   d. Position the person in bed properly
6. Which statement about mild airway obstruction is *false*?
   a. Some air moves in and out of the lungs.
   b. The person is conscious.
   c. Usually the person cannot speak.
   d. Forceful coughing will often remove the object.
7. The "universal sign of choking" is
   a. Clutching at the chest
   b. Clutching at the throat
   c. Not being able to talk
   d. Not being able to breathe
8. Which statement about wheelchair safety is *false?*
   a. Lock the wheels before transferring a resident to or from a wheelchair.
   b. The person's feet should rest on the footplate when you are pushing the wheelchair.
   c. Let the footplates fall back onto a person's legs.
   d. Check for flat or loose tires.
9. Which of the following is *not* a safety measure with oxygen?
   a. "No Smoking" signs are placed on the resident's door and near the bed.
   b. Lit candles and other open flames are permitted in the room.
   c. Electrical items are turned off before being unplugged.
   d. The person wears a cotton gown or pajamas.
10. You have discovered a fire in the nursing center. You should do the following *except*
    a. Rescue persons in immediate danger
    b. Sound the nearest fire alarm
    c. Open doors and windows, and keep oxygen on
    d. Use a fire extinguisher on a small fire that has not spread to a larger area
11. When using a fire extinguisher, you do the following *except*
    a. Pull the safety pin on the fire extinguisher
    b. Aim at the top of the flames
    c. Squeeze the lever to start the stream
    d. Sweep the stream back and forth

Answers to these questions are on p. 425.

CHAPTER 9 PREVENTING FALLS

- Falls are a leading cause of injuries and deaths among older persons. A history of falls increases the risk of falling again.
- Most falls occur in resident rooms and bathrooms. Most occur between 1800 (6:00 PM) and 2100 (9:00 PM). Falls are more likely during shift changes.
- Causes for falls are poor lighting, cluttered floors, needing to use the bathroom, and out-of-place furniture. So are wet and slippery floors, bathtubs, and showers. Review Box 9-1, Factors Increasing the Risk of Falls, in the textbook.
- Agencies have fall prevention programs. Review Box 9-2, Safety Measures to Prevent Falls, in the textbook. The person's care plan also lists measures specific for the person.

BED RAILS

- A **bed rail** (*side rail*) is a device that serves as a guard or barrier along the side of the bed.
- The nurse and care plan tell you when to raise bed rails. They are needed by persons who are unconscious or sedated with drugs. Some confused and disoriented people need them. If a person needs bed rails, keep them up at all times except when giving bedside nursing care.
- Bed rails present hazards. The person can fall when trying to get out of bed. Or the person can get caught, trapped, entangled, or strangled.
- Bed rails are considered restraints if the person cannot get out of bed or lower them without help.
- Bed rails cannot be used unless they are needed to treat a person's medical symptoms. The person or legal representative must give consent for raised bed rails. The need for bed rails is carefully noted in the person's medical record and the care plan. If a person uses bed rails, check the person often. Record when you checked the person and your observations.
- To prevent falls:
  - Never leave the person alone when the bed is raised.
  - Always lower the bed to its lowest position when you are done giving care.
  - If a person does not use bed rails and you need to raise the bed, ask a co-worker to stand on the far side of the bed to protect the person from falling.
  - If you raise the bed to give care, always raise the far bed rail if you are working alone.
  - Be sure the person who uses raised bed rails has access to items on the bedside stand and overbed table. The signal light, water pitcher and cup, tissues, phone, and TV and light controls should be within the person's reach.

HAND RAILS AND GRAB BARS

- Hand rails give support to persons who are weak or unsteady when walking.
- Grab bars provide support for sitting down or getting up from a toilet. They also are used for getting in and out of the shower or tub.

WHEEL LOCKS

- Bed wheels are locked at all times except when moving the bed.
- Wheelchair and stretcher wheels are locked when transferring a person.

TRANSFER/GAIT BELTS

- Use a **transfer belt (gait belt)** to support a person who is unsteady or disabled. Always follow the manufacturer's instructions. Apply the belt over clothing and under the breasts. The belt buckle is never positioned over the person's spine. Tighten the belt so it is snug. You should be able to slide your open, flat hand under the belt. Tuck the excess strap under the belt. Remove the belt after the procedure.
- Check with the nurse and care plan before using a transfer/gait belt if the person has:
  - A colostomy, ileostomy, gastrostomy, urostomy
  - A gastric tube
  - Chronic obstructive pulmonary disease
  - An abdominal wound, incision, or drainage tube
  - A chest wound, incision, or drainage tube
  - Monitoring equipment
  - A hernia
  - Other conditions or care equipment involving the chest or abdomen

THE FALLING PERSON

- If a person starts to fall, do not try to prevent the fall. You could injure yourself and the person. Ease the person to the floor, and protect the person's head. Do not let the person get up before the nurse checks for injuries. An incident report is completed after all falls.

CHAPTER 9 REVIEW QUESTIONS
Circle the BEST answer.

1. Most falls occur in
   a. Resident rooms and bathrooms
   b. Dining rooms
   c. Hallways
   d. Activity rooms
2. Which statement about falls is *false*?
   a. Poor lighting, cluttered floors, and throw rugs may cause falls.
   b. Improper shoes and needing to use the bathroom may cause falls.
   c. Most falls occur between 6:00 PM and 9:00 PM.
   d. Falls are less likely to occur during shift changes.
3. You note the following after a person got dressed. Which is unsafe?
   a. Non-skid footwear is worn.
   b. Pant cuffs are dragging on the floor.
   c. Clothing fits properly.
   d. The belt is fastened.
4. Which statement about bed rails is *false*?
   a. The nurse and care plan tell you when to raise bed rails.

   b. Bed rails are considered restraints.
   c. You may leave a person alone when the bed is raised and the bed rails are down.
   d. Bed rails can present hazards because people try to climb over them.
5. Which statement about transfer/gait belts is *false*?
   a. To use the belt safely, follow the manufacturer's instructions.
   b. Always apply the belt over clothing.
   c. Tighten the belt so it is very snug and breathing is impaired.
   d. Place the belt buckle off center so it is not over the spine.
6. A person becomes faint in the hallway and begins to fall. You should do the following *except*
   a. Ease the person to the floor
   b. Protect the person's head
   c. Let the person get up before the nurse checks him or her
   d. Help the nurse complete the incident report

Answers to these questions are on p. 425.

CHAPTER 10 RESTRAINT ALTERNATIVES AND SAFE RESTRAINT USE

- The Centers for Medicare & Medicaid Services (CMS) has rules for using restraints. These rules protect the person's rights and safety.
- Restraints may only be used to treat a medical symptom or for the immediate physical safety of the person or others. Restraints may only be used when less restrictive measures fail to protect the person or others. They must be discontinued at the earliest possible time.
- A **physical restraint** is any manual method or physical or mechanical device, material, or equipment attached to or near the person's body that he or she cannot remove easily and that restricts freedom of movement or normal access to one's body.
- A **chemical restraint** is a drug that is used for discipline or convenience and not required to treat medical symptoms. The drug or dosage is not a standard treatment for the person's condition.
- Federal, state, and accrediting agencies have guidelines about restraint use. They do not forbid restraint use. They require considering or trying all other appropriate alternatives first.

RESTRAINT ALTERNATIVES

- Knowing and treating the cause for harmful behaviors can prevent restraint use. There are many alternatives to restraints, such as answering the signal light promptly. For other alternatives see Box 10-2, Alternatives to Restraint Use, in the textbook.

SAFE RESTRAINT USE
- Restraints are used only when necessary to treat a person's medical symptoms—physical, emotional, or behavioral problems. Sometimes restraints are needed to protect the person or others.

Physical and Chemical Restraints
- *Physical restraints* are applied to the chest, waist, elbows, wrists, hands, or ankles. They confine the person to a bed or chair. Or they prevent movement of a body part.
- Some furniture or barriers prevent free movement:
  - Geriatric chairs or chairs with attached trays
  - Any chair placed so close to the wall that the person cannot move
  - Bed rails
  - Sheets tucked in so tightly that they restrict movement
  - Wheelchair locks if the person cannot release them
- Drugs or drug dosages are *chemical restraints* if they:
  - Control behavior or restrict movement
  - Are not standard treatment for the person's condition

Complications of Restraint Use
- Restraints can cause many complications. Injuries occur as the person tries to get free of the restraint. Injuries also occur from using the wrong restraint, applying it wrong, or keeping it on too long. Cuts, bruises, and fractures are common. The most serious risk is death from strangulation. Review Box 10-1, Risks of Restraint Use, in the textbook.
- Restraints may also affect a person's dignity and self-esteem. Depression, anger, and agitation are common. So are embarrassment, humiliation, and mistrust.

Legal Aspects
- *Restraints must protect the person.* A restraint is used only when it is the best safety measure for the person.
- *A doctor's order is required.* The doctor gives the reason for the restraint, what body part to restrain, what to use, and how long to use it.
- *The least restrictive method is used.* It allows the greatest amount of movement or body access possible.
- *Restraints are used only after other measures fail to protect the person.* Box 10-2 lists alternatives to restraint use.
- *Unnecessary restraint is false imprisonment.* If you apply an unneeded restraint, you could face false imprisonment charges.

- *Consent is required.* The person must understand the reason for the restraint. If the person cannot give consent, his or her legal representative must give consent before a restraint can be used. The doctor or nurse provides the necessary information and obtains the consent. However, using restraints cannot be refused if used as a last resort because the person's behavior causes an immediate threat to self or others.

Safety Guidelines
- Review Box 10-3, Safety Measures for Using Restraints, in the textbook.
- *Observe for increased confusion and agitation.* Restraints can increase confusion and agitation. Restrained persons need repeated explanations and reassurance. Spending time with them has a calming effect.
- *Protect the person's quality of life.* Restraints are used for as short a time as possible. You must meet the person's physical, emotional, and social needs.
- *Follow the manufacturer's instructions.* The restraint must be snug and firm, but not tight. You could be negligent if you do not apply or secure a restraint properly.
- *Apply restraints with enough help to protect the person and staff from injury.*
- *Observe the person at least every 15 minutes or more often as noted in the care plan.* Injuries and deaths can result from improper restraint use and poor observation.
- *Remove or release the restraint, reposition the person, and meet basic needs at least every 2 hours or as often as noted in the care plan.* This includes food, fluid, comfort, safety, hygiene, and elimination needs and giving skin care. Perform range-of-motion exercises or help the person walk.

Reporting and Recording
- Report and record the following:
  - Type of restraint applied.
  - Body part or parts restrained.
  - Reason for the restraint.
  - Safety measures taken.
  - Time you applied the restraint.
  - Time you removed or released the restraint.
  - Care given when restraint was removed.
  - Person's vital signs.
  - Skin color and condition.
  - Condition of the limbs.
  - Pulse felt in the restrained part.
  - Changes in the person's behavior.
  - Complaints of discomfort; a tight restraint; difficulty breathing; or pain, numbness, or tingling in the restrained part. Report these complaints to the nurse at once.

CHAPTER 10 REVIEW QUESTIONS
Circle the BEST answer.

1. A geriatric chair or a bed rail may be considered a restraint if free movement is restricted.
   a. True
   b. False

2. Which statement about the use of restraints is *false?*
   a. A person may be embarrassed and humiliated when restraints are on.
   b. A person may experience depression and agitation when restraints are on.
   c. Restraints can be used for staff convenience.
   d. Restraints can cause serious injury and death.

3. Restraints can increase a person's confusion and agitation.
   a. True
   b. False

4. The person with a restraint should be observed at least every
   a. 15 minutes
   b. 30 minutes
   c. Hour
   d. 2 hours

5. Restraints need to be removed at least every
   a. Hour
   b. 2 hours
   c. 3 hours
   d. 4 hours

6. You should record all the following *except*
   a. The type of restraint used
   b. The consent for the restraint
   c. The time you removed the restraint
   d. The care you gave when the restraint was removed

Answers to these questions are on p. 425.

CHAPTER 11 PREVENTING INFECTION
MICROORGANISMS

- A **microorganism (microbe)** is a small *(micro)* living plant or animal *(organism)*.
- Some microbes are harmful and can cause infections **(pathogens).** Others do not usually cause infection **(non-pathogens).**

Multidrug-Resistant Organisms

- *Multidrug-resistant organisms (MDROs)* can resist the effects of antibiotics. Such organisms are able to change their structures to survive in the presence of antibiotics. The infections they cause are harder to treat.
- MDROs are caused by doctors prescribing antibiotics when they are not needed (over-prescribing). Not taking antibiotics for the prescribed length of time is also a cause.

- Two common types of MDROs are resistant to many antibiotics:
  - *Methicillin-resistant Staphylococcus aureus (MRSA)*
  - *Vancomycin-resistant Enterococcus (VRE)*

INFECTION

- An **infection** is a disease state resulting from the invasion and growth of microbes in the body.
- Review Box 11-1, Signs and Symptoms of Infection, in the textbook.

Healthcare-Associated Infection

- A **healthcare-associated infection (HAI)** is an infection that develops in a person cared for in any setting where health care is given. Hospitals, nursing centers, clinics, and home care settings are examples. HAIs also are called *nosocomial infections*.
- The health team must prevent the spread of HAIs by:
  - Medical asepsis. This includes hand hygiene.
  - Surgical asepsis.
  - Standard Precautions and Transmission-Based Precautions.
  - The Bloodborne Pathogen Standard.

Infection in Older Persons

- Older persons may not show the normal signs and symptoms of infection. The person may have only a slight fever or no fever at all. Redness and swelling may be very slight. The person may not complain of pain. Confusion and delirium may occur.
- Infections can become life-threatening before the older person has obvious signs and symptoms. Be alert to minor changes in the person's behavior or condition. Review Box 11-1, Signs and Symptoms of Infection, in the textbook. Report any concerns to the nurse at once.

MEDICAL ASEPSIS

- **Asepsis** is being free of disease-producing microbes.
- **Medical asepsis (clean technique)** refers to the practices used to:
  - Remove or destroy pathogens.
  - Prevent pathogens from spreading from one person or place to another person or place.

Common Aseptic Practices

- To prevent the spread of microbes, wash your hands:
  - After urinating or having a bowel movement.
  - After changing tampons or sanitary pads.
  - After contact with your own or another person's blood, body fluids, secretions, or excretions. This includes saliva, vomitus, urine, feces, vaginal discharge, mucus, semen, wound drainage, pus, and respiratory secretions.

- After coughing, sneezing, or blowing your nose.
- Before and after handling, preparing, or eating food.
- After smoking a cigarette, cigar, or pipe.
- Also do the following:
  - Provide all persons with their own linens and personal care items.
  - Cover your nose and mouth when coughing, sneezing, or blowing your nose.
  - Bathe, wash hair, and brush your teeth regularly.
  - Wash fruits and raw vegetables before eating or serving them.
  - Wash cooking and eating utensils with soap and water after use.

Hand Hygiene
- *Hand hygiene is the easiest and most important way to prevent the spread of infection.* Practice hand hygiene before and after giving care. Review Box 11-2, Rules of Hand Hygiene, in the textbook.

Supplies and Equipment
- Most health care equipment is disposable. Bedpans, urinals, wash basins, water pitchers, and drinking cups are multi-use items. Do not "borrow" them for another person.
- Non-disposable items are cleaned and then disinfected. Then they are sterilized.

Other Aseptic Measures
- Review Box 11-3, Aseptic Measures, in the textbook.

ISOLATION PRECAUTIONS
- Isolation Precautions prevent the spread of **communicable diseases (contagious diseases).** They are diseases caused by pathogens that spread easily.
- The CDC's isolation precautions guideline has two tiers of precautions:
  - Standard Precautions
  - Transmission-Based Precautions

Standard Precautions
- Standard Precautions reduce the risk of spreading pathogens and known and unknown infections. Standard Precautions are used for all persons whenever care is given. They prevent the spread of infection from:
  - Blood.
  - All body fluids, secretions, and excretions even if blood is not visible. Sweat is not known to spread infections.
  - Non-intact skin (skin with open breaks).
  - Mucous membranes.

- Review Box 11-4, Standard Precautions, in the textbook.

Transmission-Based Precautions
- Some infections require Transmission-Based Precautions. Review Box 11-5, Transmission-Based Precautions, in the textbook.
- Agency policies may differ from those in the book. The rules in Box 11-6, Rules for Isolation Precautions, in the textbook are a guide for giving safe care.

Protective Measures
- Isolation Precautions involve wearing PPE—gloves, a gown, a mask, and goggles or a face shield.
- Removing linens, trash, and equipment from the room may require double-bagging.
- Follow agency procedures when collecting specimens and transporting persons.
- Wear gloves whenever contact with blood, body fluids, secretions, excretions, mucous membranes, and non-intact skin is likely. Wearing gloves is the most common protective measure used with Standard Precautions and Transmission-Based Precautions. Remember the following when using gloves:
  - The outside of gloves is contaminated.
  - Gloves are easier to put on when your hands are dry.
  - Do not tear gloves when putting them on.
  - You need a new pair for every person.
  - Remove and discard torn, cut, or punctured gloves at once. Practice hand hygiene. Then put on a new pair.
  - Wear gloves once. Discard them after use.
  - Put on clean gloves just before touching mucous membranes or non-intact skin.
  - Put on new gloves whenever gloves become contaminated with blood, body fluids, secretions, or excretions. A task may require more than one pair of gloves.
  - Change gloves if interacting with the person involves touching portable computer keyboards or other mobile equipment that is transported from room to room.
  - Put on gloves last when worn with other PPE.
  - Change gloves whenever moving from a contaminated body site to a clean body site.
  - Make sure gloves cover your wrists. If you wear a gown, gloves cover the cuffs.
  - Remove gloves so the inside part is on the outside. The inside is clean.
  - Decontaminate your hands after removing gloves.
- Latex allergies are common and can cause skin rashes. Asthma and shock are more serious

problems. Report skin rashes and breathing problems at once. If you or a resident has a latex allergy, wear latex-free gloves.

- Gowns must completely cover your neck to your knees. The gown front and sleeves are considered contaminated. A wet gown is contaminated. Gowns are used once. When removing a gown, roll it away from you. Keep it inside out.
- Masks are disposable. A wet or moist mask is contaminated. When removing a mask, touch only the ties or elastic bands. The front of the mask is contaminated.
- The outside of goggles or a face shield is contaminated. Use the device's ties, headband, or ear pieces to remove the device.
- Contaminated items, linens, and trash are bagged to remove them from the person's room. Leak-proof plastic bags are used. They have the BIOHAZARD symbol. Double-bagging is not needed unless the outside of the bag is soiled.

Meeting Basic Needs

- Love, belonging, and self-esteem needs are often unmet when Transmission-Based Precautions are used. Visitors and staff often avoid the person. The person may feel lonely, unwanted, and rejected. He or she may feel dirty and undesirable. The person may feel ashamed and guilty for having a contagious disease. You can help meet the person's needs.

BLOODBORNE PATHOGEN STANDARD

- The health team is at risk for exposure to human immunodeficiency virus (HIV) and the hepatitis B virus (HBV). HIV and HBV are bloodborne pathogens found in the blood.
- The Bloodborne Pathogen Standard is intended to protect you from exposure.
- Staff at risk for exposure to HIV and HBV receive free training.
- *Hepatitis B vaccination.* You can receive the hepatitis B vaccination within 10 working days of being hired. The agency pays for it. If you refuse the vaccination, you must sign a statement. You can have the vaccination at a later date.

Engineering and Work Practice Controls

- *Engineering controls* reduce employee exposure in the workplace. There are special containers for contaminated sharps (needles, broken glass) and specimens. These containers are puncture-resistant, leak-proof, and color-coded in red. They have the BIOHAZARD symbol.
- *Work practice controls* reduce exposure risk. All tasks involving blood or other potentially infectious materials (OPIM) are done in ways

to limit splatters, splashes, and sprays. Other controls include:
- Do not eat, drink, smoke, apply cosmetics or lip balm, or handle contact lenses in areas of occupational exposure.
- Do not store food or drinks where blood or OPIM are kept.
- Practice hand hygiene after removing gloves.
- Wash hands as soon as possible after skin contact with blood or OPIM.
- Never recap, bend, or remove needles by hand.
- Never shear or break contaminated needles.
- Discard contaminated needles and sharp instruments (razors) in containers that are closable, puncture-resistant, and leak-proof.

Personal Protective Equipment (PPE)

- This includes gloves, goggles, face shields, masks, laboratory coats, gowns, shoe covers, and surgical caps. For safe handling and use of PPE:
  - Remove PPE before leaving the work area.
  - Remove PPE when a garment becomes contaminated.
  - Place used PPE in marked areas or containers when being stored, washed, decontaminated, or discarded.
  - Wear gloves when you expect contact with blood or OPIM.
  - Wear gloves when handling or touching contaminated items or surfaces.
  - Replace worn, punctured, or contaminated gloves.
  - Never wash or decontaminate disposable gloves for re-use.
  - Discard utility gloves that show signs of cracking, peeling, tearing, or puncturing. Utility gloves are decontaminated for re-use if the process will not ruin them.

Equipment

- Contaminated equipment is cleaned and decontaminated. Decontaminate work surfaces with a proper disinfectant:
  - Upon completing tasks
  - At once when there is obvious contamination
  - After any spill of blood or OPIM
  - At the end of the work shift when surfaces become contaminated

Laundry

- OSHA requires these measures for contaminated laundry:
  - Handle it as little as possible.
  - Wear gloves or other needed PPE.
  - Bag contaminated laundry where it is used.
  - Mark laundry bags or containers with the BIOHAZARD symbol for laundry sent off-site.

- Place wet, contaminated laundry in leak-proof containers before transport. The containers are color-coded in red or have the BIOHAZARD symbol.

Exposure Incidents

- Report exposure incidents at once. Medical evaluation, follow-up, and required tests are free. Your blood is tested for HIV and HBV. Confidentiality is important.

CHAPTER 11 REVIEW QUESTIONS

Circle the BEST answer.

1. A healthcare-associated infection (nosocomial infection) is
   a. An infection free of disease-producing microbes
   b. An infection that develops in a person cared for in any setting where health care is given
   c. An infection acquired by health care workers
   d. An infection acquired only by older persons
2. Which statement about hand hygiene is *false?*
   a. Hand hygiene is the easiest way to prevent the spread of infection.
   b. Hand hygiene is the most important way to prevent the spread of infection.
   c. Hand hygiene is practiced before and after giving care to a person.
   d. If hands are visibly soiled, hand hygiene can be done with an alcohol-based hand rub.
3. When washing your hands, you should do the following *except*
   a. Stand away from the sink so your clothes do not touch the sink
   b. Keep your hands lower than your elbows
   c. Wash your hands for at least 15 seconds
   d. Dry your arms from the forearms to the fingertips
4. Which statement about wearing gloves is *false?*
   a. The insides of gloves are contaminated.
   b. You need a new pair of gloves for each person you care for.
   c. Change gloves when moving from a contaminated body site to a clean body site.
   d. Gloves need to cover your wrists.
5. Which statement is *false?*
   a. Gowns must cover you from your neck to your waist.
   b. A moist mask is contaminated.
   c. The outside of goggles is contaminated.
   d. You should wash your hands after removing a gown, mask, or goggles.
6. Which statement about PPE is *false?*
   a. Remove PPE when a garment becomes contaminated.
   b. Wear gloves when handling or touching contaminated items or surfaces.
   c. Wash or decontaminate disposable gloves for re-use.
   d. Remove PPE before leaving the work area.

Answers to these questions are on p. 425.

CHAPTER 12 BODY MECHANICS

PRINCIPLES OF BODY MECHANICS

- Your strongest and largest muscles are in the shoulders, upper arms, hips, and thighs. Use these muscles to lift and move persons and heavy objects.
- For good body mechanics:
  - Bend your knees and squat to lift a heavy object. Do not bend from your waist.
  - Hold items close to your body and base of support.
- Review Box 12-1, Rules for Body Mechanics, in your textbook.

ERGONOMICS

- **Ergonomics** is the science of designing a job to fit the worker. The task, work station, equipment, and tools are changed to help reduce stress on the worker's body. The goal is to prevent injury and disorders of the muscles, tendons, ligaments, joints, cartilage, and nervous system.
- Early signs and symptoms of injury include pain, limited joint movement, or soft tissue swelling. Always report a work-related injury as soon as possible. Early attention can help prevent the problem from becoming worse.

POSITIONING THE PERSON

- The person must be properly positioned at all times. Regular position changes and good alignment promote comfort and well-being. Breathing is easier. Circulation is promoted. Pressure ulcers and contractures are prevented.
- Whether in bed or in a chair, the person is repositioned at least every 2 hours. To safely position a person:
  - Use good body mechanics.
  - Ask a co-worker to help you if needed.
  - Explain the procedure to the person.
  - Be gentle when moving the person.
  - Provide for privacy.
  - Use pillows as directed by the nurse for support and alignment.
  - Provide for comfort after positioning.
  - Place the signal light within reach after positioning.
  - Complete a safety check before leaving the room.

- Use pillows and positioning devices to support body parts and keep the person in good alignment.
- **Fowler's position** is a semi-sitting position. The head of the bed is raised between 45 and 60 degrees. The knees may be slightly elevated.
- The **supine position (dorsal recumbent position)** is the back-lying position.
- A person in the **prone position** lies on the abdomen with the head turned to one side.
- A person in the **lateral position (side-lying position)** lies on one side or the other.
- The **Sims' position (semi-prone side position)** is a left side-lying position.
- Persons who sit in chairs must hold their upper bodies and heads erect. For good alignment:
  - The person's back and buttocks are against the back of the chair.
  - Feet are flat on the floor or wheelchair footplates. Never leave feet unsupported.
  - Backs of the knees and calves are slightly away from the edge of the seat.

CHAPTER 12 REVIEW QUESTIONS
Circle the BEST answer.

1. To lift and move residents and heavy objects you should
   a. Use the muscles in your lower arms
   b. Use the muscles in your legs
   c. Use the muscles in your shoulders, upper arms, hips, and thighs
   d. Use the muscles in your abdomen
2. For good body mechanics, you should do all of the following *except*
   a. Bend your knees and squat to lift a heavy object
   b. Bend from your waist to lift a heavy object
   c. Hold items close to your body and base of support
   d. Bend your legs; do not bend your back
3. Which statement is *false?*
   a. A person must be properly positioned at all times.
   b. Regular position changes and good alignment promote comfort and well-being.
   c. Regular position changes and good alignment promote pressure ulcers and contractures.
   d. When a person is in good alignment, breathing is easier and circulation is promoted.
4. In Fowler's position
   a. The head of the bed is flat
   b. The head of the bed is raised to 90 degrees
   c. The head of the bed is raised between 45 and 60 degrees
   d. The head of the bed is raised between 30 and 35 degrees

Answers to these questions are on p. 425.

CHAPTER 13 SAFELY HANDLING, MOVING, AND TRANSFERRING THE PERSON
PREVENTING WORK-RELATED INJURIES
- To prevent work-related injuries:
  - Wear shoes that provide good traction.
  - Use assistive equipment and devices whenever possible.
  - Get help from other staff.
  - Plan and prepare for the task. Know what equipment you will need and on what side of the bed to place the chair or wheelchair.
  - Schedule harder tasks early in your shift.
  - Tell the resident what he or she can do to help. Give clear, simple instructions.
  - Do not hold or grab the person under the arms.
- For additional guidelines, review Box 13-1, Preventing Work-Related Injuries, in the textbook.

PROTECTING THE SKIN
- Protect the person's skin from fiction and shearing. Both cause infection and pressure ulcers. To reduce friction and shearing:
  - Roll the person.
  - Use a lift sheet (turning sheet).
  - Use a turning pad, slide board, slide sheet, or a large incontinence product.

MOVING PERSONS IN BED
- Before moving a person in bed, you need to know from the nurse and care plan:
  - What procedure to use
  - How many workers are needed to safely move the person
  - Position limits and restrictions
  - How far you can lower the head of the bed
  - Any limits in the person's ability to move or be repositioned
  - What equipment is needed—trapeze, lift sheet, slide sheet, mechanical lift
  - How to position the person
  - If the person uses bed rails
  - What observations to report and record:
    - Who helped you with the procedure
    - How much help the person needed
    - How the person tolerated the procedure
    - How you positioned the person
    - Complaints of pain or discomfort
  - When to report observations
  - What specific concerns to report at once

Moving the Person Up in Bed
- You can sometimes move lightweight adults up in bed alone if they can assist and use a trapeze. Two or more staff members are needed to move heavy, weak, and very old persons up in bed. Always protect the person and yourself from injury.

- Assist devices are used to reduce shearing and friction. Such assist devices include a drawsheet (lift sheet), flat sheet folded in half, turning pad, slide sheet, and large incontinence product.

TURNING PERSONS

- Turning persons onto their sides helps prevent complications from bedrest. Certain procedures and care measures also require the side-lying position. After the person is turned, position him or her in good alignment. Use pillows as directed to support the person in the side-lying position.
- **Logrolling** is turning the person as a unit, in alignment, with one motion. The spine is kept straight.

SITTING ON THE SIDE OF THE BED (DANGLING)

- Many older persons become dizzy or faint when getting out of bed too fast. They need to sit on the side of the bed before walking or transferring. Some persons increase activity in stages—bedrest, to sitting on the side of the bed, to sitting in a chair, to walking.
- While dangling, the person coughs and deep breathes. He or she moves the legs back and forth in circles to stimulate circulation. Provide for warmth during dangling.
- Observations to report and record:
  - Pulse and respiratory rates
  - Pale or bluish skin color (cyanosis)
  - Complaints of light-headedness, dizziness, or difficulty breathing
  - How well the activity was tolerated
  - The length of time the person dangled
  - The amount of help needed
  - Other observations and complaints

TRANSFERRING PERSONS

- The rules of body mechanics apply during transfers.
- Arrange the room so there is enough space for a safe transfer. Correct placement of the chair, wheelchair, or other device also is needed for a safe transfer.
- Have the person wear non-skid footwear for transfers.
- Lock the wheels of the bed, wheelchair, stretcher, or other assist device.
- After the transfer, position the person in good alignment.
- Transfer belts (gait belts) are used to support persons during transfers and reposition persons in chairs and wheelchairs.

Bed to Chair or Wheelchair Transfers

- Safety is important for transfers. In transferring, the strong side moves first. Help the person out of bed on his or her strong side. Help the person from the wheelchair to the bed on his or her strong side.
- The person must not put his or her arms around your neck.

Mechanical Lifts

- Persons who cannot help themselves are transferred with mechanical lifts. So are persons who are too heavy for the staff to transfer.
- Before using a mechanical lift, you must be trained in its use. The sling, straps, hooks, and chains must be in good repair. The person's weight must not exceed the lift's capacity. At least two staff members are needed. Always follow the manufacturer's instructions for using the lift.
- Falling from the lift is a common fear. To promote the person's mental comfort, always explain the procedure before you begin. Also show the person how the lift works.

CHAPTER 13 REVIEW QUESTIONS
Circle the BEST answer.

1. Friction and shearing are reduced by doing the following *except*
   a. Rolling the person
   b. Using a lift sheet or turning pad
   c. Using a pillow
   d. Using a slide board or slide sheet
2. After a person is turned, you must position him or her in good alignment.
   a. True
   b. False
3. Which statement about dangling is *false?*
   a. Many older persons become dizzy or faint when they first dangle.
   b. The person should cough and deep breathe while dangling.
   c. The person moves his or her legs before dangling.
   d. You should cover the person's shoulders with a robe or blanket while dangling.
4. You are transferring a person from the bed to a wheelchair. Which statement is *false?*
   a. The person should wear non-skid footwear.
   b. The person may put his or her arm around your neck.
   c. You should use a gait/transfer belt.
   d. You should lock the wheelchair wheels.
5. A person has a weak left side and a strong right side. In transferring the person from the bed to the wheelchair, his or her strong (right) side moves first.
   a. True
   b. False

6. Before using a mechanical lift, you do all the following *except*
   a. Check the sling, straps, and chains to ensure good repair
   b. Check the person's weight to be sure it does not exceed the lift's capacity
   c. Follow the manufacturer's instructions for using the lift
   d. Operate the lift without a co-worker

Answers to these questions are on p. 425.

CHAPTER 14 ASSISTING WITH COMFORT
- Comfort is a state of well-being. Many factors affect comfort.

THE PERSON'S UNIT
- Patient and resident rooms are designed to provide comfort, safety, and privacy. In nursing centers, resident rooms are as personal and home-like as possible. You need to help keep the person's unit clean, neat, safe, and comfortable.
- Review Box 14-1, Maintaining the Person's Unit, in your textbook.

Temperature and Ventilation
- Older persons, and those who are ill, may need higher temperatures for comfort.
- To protect older and ill persons from cool areas and drafts:
  - Keep room temperatures warm.
  - Make sure they wear the correct clothing.
  - Offer lap robes to cover the legs.
  - Provide enough blankets for warmth.
  - Cover them with bath blankets when giving care.
  - Move them from drafty areas.

Odors
- To reduce odors in nursing centers:
  - Empty, clean, and disinfect bedpans, urinals, commodes, and kidney basins promptly.
  - Check to make sure toilets are flushed.
  - Check incontinent people often.
  - Clean persons who are wet or soiled from urine, feces, or wound drainage.
  - Change wet or soiled linens and clothing promptly.
  - Keep laundry containers closed.
  - Follow agency policy for wet or soiled linens and clothing.
  - Dispose of incontinence and ostomy products promptly.
  - Provide good hygiene to prevent body and breath odors.
  - Use room deodorizers as needed.

- If you smoke, practice hand washing after handling smoking materials and before giving care. Give careful attention to your uniform, hair, and breath because of smoke odors.

Noise
- To decrease noise:
  - Control your voice.
  - Handle equipment carefully.
  - Keep equipment in good working order.
  - Answer phones, signal lights, and intercoms promptly.

Lighting
- Adjust lighting to meet the person's needs. Glares, shadows, and dull lighting can cause falls, headaches, and eyestrain. A bright room is cheerful. Dim light is better for relaxing and rest. Persons with poor vision need bright light. Always keep light controls within the person's reach.

ROOM FURNITURE AND EQUIPMENT
- Rooms are furnished and equipped to meet basic needs.

The Bed
- Beds are raised to give care. They are positioned at the lowest level when not giving care.
- Bed wheels are locked at all times except when moving the bed.
- Use bed rails as the nurse and care plan direct.
- Basic bed positions:
  - *Flat*—the usual sleeping position.
  - *Fowler's position*—a semi-sitting position. The head of the bed is raised between 45 and 60 degrees.
  - *High-Fowler's position*—a semi-sitting position. The head of the bed is raised 60 to 90 degrees.
  - *Semi-Fowler's position*—the head of the bed is raised 30 degrees. Some agencies define semi-Fowler's position as when the head of the bed is raised 30 degrees and the knee portion is raised 15 degrees. Know the definition used by your agency.
  - *Trendelenburg's position*—the head of the bed is lowered and the foot of the bed is raised. A doctor orders the position.
  - *Reverse Trendelenburg's position*—the head of the bed is raised and the foot of the bed is lowered. A doctor orders the position.

Bed Safety
- *Entrapment* means the person can get caught, trapped, or entangled in spaces created by bed rails, the mattress, the bed frame, or the

headboard and footboard. Serious injuries and deaths have occurred from entrapment. If a person is at risk for entrapment, report your concerns to the nurse at once. If a person is caught, trapped, or entangled, try to release the person. Call for the nurse at once.

The Overbed Table

- Only clean and sterile items are placed on the table. Never place bedpans, urinals, or soiled linen on the overbed table or on top of the bedside stand.
- Clean the table and bedside stand after using them for a work surface.

Privacy Curtains

- Always pull the curtain completely around the bed before giving care. Privacy curtains do not block sound or conversations.

The Call System

- The signal light must always be kept within the person's reach—in the room, bathroom, and shower or tub room. You must:
  - Place the signal light on the person's strong side.
  - Remind the person to signal when help is needed.
  - Answer signal lights promptly.
  - Answer bathroom and shower or tub room signal lights at once.
- Persons with limited hand mobility may need special communication measures.
- Be careful when using the intercom. Remember confidentiality. Persons nearby can hear what you and the person say.

Closet and Drawer Space

- The person must have free access to the closet and its contents. You must have the person's permission to open or search closets or drawers.
- Agency staff can inspect a person's closet or drawers if hoarding is suspected. The person is informed of the inspection and is present when it takes place. Have a co-worker present when you inspect a person's closet.

BEDMAKING

- Clean, dry, and wrinkle-free linens promote comfort. Skin breakdown and pressure ulcers are prevented. Do the following to keep beds neat and clean:
  - Straighten linens whenever loose or wrinkled and at bedtime.
  - Check for and remove food and crumbs after meals.
  - Check linens for dentures, eyeglasses, hearing aids, sharp objects, and other items.

- Change linens whenever they become wet, soiled, or damp.
- Follow Standard Precautions and the Bloodborne Pathogen Standard.
- When handling linens and making beds:
  - Practice medical asepsis.
  - Always hold linen away from your body and uniform. Your uniform is considered dirty.
  - Never shake linen.
  - Place clean linens on a clean surface.
  - Never put clean or dirty linen on the floor.
- Do not bring unneeded linens into the person's room. Once in the room, extra linen is considered contaminated. It cannot be used for another person.
- Roll each piece of dirty linen away from you. The side that touched the person is inside the roll and away from you.

Making Beds

- When making beds, safety and medical asepsis are important. Use good body mechanics. Follow the rules for safe resident handling, moving, and transfers. Practice hand hygiene before handling clean linen and after handling dirty linen. To save time and energy, make beds with a co-worker.
- Review Box 14-2, Rules for Bedmaking, in the textbook.

The Occupied Bed

- You make an occupied bed when the person stays in bed. Keep the person in good alignment. Follow restrictions or limits in the person's movement or position. Explain each procedure step to the person before it is done. This is important even if the person cannot respond to you.

ASSISTING WITH PAIN RELIEF

- **Pain** means to ache, hurt, or be sore. Pain is subjective. You cannot see, hear, touch, or smell pain or discomfort. You must rely on what the person says.
- Report the person's complaints of pain and your observations to the nurse.
- Review Box 14-3, Nursing Measures to Promote Comfort and Relieve Pain, in the textbook.

Factors Affecting Pain

- *Past experience.* The severity of pain, its cause, how long it lasted, and if relief occurred all affect the person's current response to pain.
- *Anxiety.* Pain and anxiety are related. Pain can cause anxiety. Anxiety increases how much pain the person feels. Reducing anxiety helps lessen pain.
- *Rest and sleep.* Pain seems worse when a person is tired or restless.

- *Attention*. The more a person thinks about pain, the worse it seems.
- *Personal and family duties*. Often pain is ignored when there are children to care for. Some deny pain if a serious illness is feared.
- *The value or meaning of pain*. To some people, pain is a weakness. For some persons, pain means avoiding daily routines and people. Some people like doting and pampering by others. The person values pain and wants such attention.
- *Support from others*. Dealing with pain is often easier when family and friends offer comfort and support. Just being nearby helps. Facing pain alone is hard for persons.
- *Culture*. Culture affects pain responses. Non–English-speaking persons may have problems describing pain.
- *Illness*. Some diseases cause decreased pain sensations.
- *Age*. Older persons may have decreased pain sensations. They may not feel pain or it may not feel severe. The person is at risk for undetected disease or injury. Chronic pain may mask new pain.
- *Persons with dementia*. Persons with dementia may not be able to complain of pain. Changes in usual behavior may signal pain. Loss of appetite also signals pain. Report any changes in a person's usual behavior to the nurse.

PROMOTING SLEEP
- Sleep is a basic need. Tissue healing and repair occur during sleep. Sleep lowers stress, tension, and anxiety. It refreshes and renews the person. The person regains energy and mental alertness. The person thinks and functions better after sleep.

Factors Affecting Sleep
- *Illness*. Illness increases the need for sleep.
- *Nutrition*. Sleep needs increase with weight gain. Foods with caffeine prevent sleep.
- *Exercise*. People tire after exercise. Being tired helps people sleep well. Exercise before bedtime interferes with sleep. Exercise is avoided 2 hours before bedtime.
- *Environment*. People adjust to their usual sleep settings.
- *Drugs and other substances*. Sleeping pills promote sleep. Drugs for anxiety, depression, and pain may cause the person to sleep.
- *Emotional problems*. Fear, worry, depression, and anxiety affect sleep.

Sleep Disorders
- **Insomnia** is a chronic condition in which the person cannot sleep or stay asleep all night.

- **Sleep deprivation** means that the amount and quality of sleep are decreased. Sleep is interrupted.
- **Sleep-walking** is when the person leaves the bed and walks about. If a person is sleep-walking, protect the person from injury. Guide sleep-walkers back to bed. They startle easily. Awaken them gently.

Promoting Sleep
- To promote sleep, allow a flexible bedtime, provide a comfortable room temperature, and have the person void before going to bed. Review Box 14-4, Nursing Measures to Promote Sleep, in the textbook for other measures.

CHAPTER 14 REVIEW QUESTIONS
Circle T if the statement is true. Circle F if the statement is false.
1. T F Serious injuries and death have occurred from entrapment.
2. T F You should never place bedpans, urinals, or soiled linen on the overbed table.
3. T F You should clean the bedside stand if you use it for a work surface.
4. T F Once in the person's room, extra linen is considered contaminated. It can be used for another person.
5. T F Roll each piece of dirty linen away from you. The side that touched the person is inside the roll.
6. T F Wear gloves when removing linen from the person's bed.

Circle the BEST answer.
7. The following protect a person from drafts *except*
   a. Wearing enough clothing
   b. Lap robes
   c. Using a sheet when giving care
   d. Providing blankets
8. To reduce odors, you do the following *except*
   a. Empty bedpans and commodes promptly
   b. Keep laundry containers open
   c. Check to make sure toilets are flushed
   d. Clean persons who are wet or soiled from urine or feces
9. Which statement about the signal light is *false?*
   a. The signal light must always be within the person's reach.
   b. Place the signal light on the person's strong side.
   c. You have to answer the signal lights only for residents assigned to you.
   d. Answer signal lights promptly.

10. You suspect a person is hoarding food in her closet. Before you inspect the closet, what do you do?
    a. Tell another nursing assistant what you suspect
    b. Inspect the closet without telling the resident
    c. Tell the family
    d. Tell the resident you are going to inspect the closet
11. To keep beds neat and clean, do the following *except*
    a. Straighten linens whenever loose or wrinkled
    b. Check for and remove food and crumbs after meals
    c. Check linens for dentures, eyeglasses, and hearing aids
    d. Change linen monthly
12. Which statement is *false?*
    a. Practice medical asepsis when handling linen.
    b. Always hold linens away from your body and uniform.
    c. Shake linens to remove crumbs.
    d. Put dirty linens in the dirty laundry bin.
13. You can promote rest for a person by doing the following *except*
    a. Ask the person if he or she would like coffee or tea
    b. Place the signal light within reach
    c. Provide a quiet setting
    d. Follow the person's routines and rituals before rest
14. To promote sleep for a person, you should do the following *except*
    a. Follow the person's wishes
    b. Follow the care plan
    c. Follow the person's rituals and routines before bedtime
    d. Tell the person when to go to bed

Answers to these questions are on p. 425.

CHAPTER 15 ASSISTING WITH HYGIENE

• Besides cleansing, good hygiene prevents body and breath odors. It is relaxing and increases circulation.
• Culture and personal choice affect hygiene.

DAILY CARE

• Most people have hygiene routines and habits. Hygiene measures are often done before and after meals and at bedtime. You assist with hygiene whenever it is needed. Protect the person's right to privacy and to personal choice.

ORAL HYGIENE

• Oral hygiene keeps the mouth and teeth clean. It prevents mouth odors and infections, increases

comfort, and makes food taste better. Mouth care also reduces the risk for cavities and periodontal disease.
• Assist with oral hygiene after sleep, after meals, and at bedtime. Follow the care plan.
• Follow Standard Precautions and the Bloodborne Pathogen Standard.
• Report and record:
  • Dry, cracked, swollen, or blistered lips
  • Mouth or breath odor
  • Redness, swelling, irritation, sores, or white patches in the mouth or on the tongue
  • Bleeding, swelling, or redness of the gums
  • Loose teeth
  • Rough, sharp, or chipped areas on dentures

Brushing and Flossing Teeth

• Flossing removes plaque and tartar from the teeth as well as food from between the teeth. Flossing is usually done after brushing. If done once a day, bedtime is the best time to floss.
• Some persons need help gathering and setting up equipment for oral hygiene. You may have to perform oral care for persons who are weak, cannot move their arms, or are too confused to brush their teeth.

Mouth Care for the Unconscious Person

• Unconscious persons have dry mouths and crusting on the tongue and mucous membranes. Oral hygiene keeps the mouth clean and moist. It also helps prevent infection.
• Use sponge swabs to apply the cleaning agent. To prevent cracking of the lips, apply a lubricant to the lips. Check the care plan.
• To prevent aspiration on the unconscious person:
  • Position the person on one side with the head turned well to the side.
  • Use only a small amount of fluid to clean the mouth.
  • Do not insert dentures. Dentures are not worn when the person is unconscious.
• When giving oral hygiene, keep the person's mouth open with a padded tongue blade.
• Mouth care is given at least every 2 hours. Follow the nurse's direction and the care plan.

Denture Care

• Mouth care is given and dentures are cleaned as often as natural teeth. Dentures are usually removed at bedtime. Remind people not to wrap dentures in tissues or napkins.
• Dentures are slippery when wet. Hold them firmly. During cleaning, hold them over a basin of water lined with a towel. Use a cleaning agent, and follow the manufacturer's instructions.

- Hot water causes dentures to lose their shape. If dentures are not worn after cleaning, store them in a container with cool water or a denture soaking solution.
- Label the denture cup with the person's name, room number, and bed number. Report lost or damaged dentures to the nurse at once. Losing or damaging dentures is negligent conduct.
- Many people do not like being seen without their dentures. Privacy is important. If you clean dentures, return them to the person as quickly as possible.
- Persons with partial dentures have some natural teeth. They need to brush and floss the natural teeth.

BATHING

- Bathing cleans the skin. The mucous membranes of the genital and anal areas are cleaned as well. A bath is refreshing and relaxing. Circulation is stimulated and body parts exercised. You have time to talk to the person. You also can make observations.
- Review Box 15-1, Rules for Bathing, in the textbook.
- Soap dries the skin. Therefore older persons usually need a complete bath or shower twice a week. Partial baths are taken the other days. Some bathe daily but not with soap. Thorough rinsing is needed when using soap. Lotions and oils keep the skin soft.
- Water temperature for complete bed baths and partial bed baths is between 110° F and 115° F. Older persons have fragile skin and need lower water temperatures. Measure water temperature according to agency policy.
- Report and record:
  - The color of the skin, lips, nail beds, and sclera
  - The location and description of rashes
  - Dry skin
  - Bruises or open areas
  - Pale or reddened areas, particularly over bony parts
  - Drainage or bleeding from wounds or body openings
  - Swelling of the feet and legs
  - Corns or calluses on the feet
  - Skin temperature
  - Complaints of pain or discomfort
- Before bathing, assist the person with elimination needs.
- Provide for warmth. Cover the person with a bath blanket.
- Follow Standard Precautions and the Bloodborne Pathogen Standard.
- Use caution when applying powders. Do not use powders near persons with respiratory disorders. Do not sprinkle or shake powder onto the person. To safely apply powder:

- Turn away from the person.
- Sprinkle a small amount onto your hands or a cloth.
- Apply the powder in a thin layer.
- Make sure powder does not get on the floor. Powder is slippery and can cause falls.

The Complete Bed Bath

- The complete bed bath involves washing the person's entire body in bed. Wash around the person's eyes with water. Do not use soap. Gently wipe from the inner to the outer aspect of the eye. Use a clean part of the washcloth for each stroke. Ask the person if you should use soap to wash the face. Let the person wash the genital area if he or she is able.
- Give a back massage after the bath. Apply deodorant or antiperspirant, lotion, and powder as requested. Comb and brush the hair. Empty and clean the wash basin.

The Partial Bath

- The partial bath involves bathing the face, hands, axillae (underarms), back, buttocks, and perineal area. You assist the person as needed. Most need help washing the back.

Tub Baths and Showers

- Falls, burns, and chilling from water are risks. Review Box 15-2, Safety Measures for Tub Baths and Showers, in the textbook.
- A tub bath can cause a person to feel faint, weak, or tired. The person may need a transfer bench, a tub with a side entry door, a wheelchair or stretcher lift, or a mechanical lift to get in and out of the tub.
- Some people can use a regular shower. Have the person use the grab bars for support during the shower. Use a bath mat if the shower does not have non-skid surfaces. Never let weak or unsteady persons stand in the shower. They may need to use shower chairs, shower stalls or cabinets, or shower trolleys. Some shower rooms have two or more stations. Protect the person's privacy. Properly screen and cover the person.
- Water temperature for tub baths and showers is usually 105° F. Report and record dizziness and light-headedness.

THE BACK MASSAGE

- The back massage relaxes muscles and stimulates circulation.
- Massages are given after the bath and with evening care. You also can give back massages at other times, such as after repositioning a person.
- Observe the skin for breaks, bruises, reddened areas, and other signs of skin breakdown.

- Lotion reduces friction during the massage. It is warmed before applying.
- Use firm strokes. Keep your hands in contact with the person's skin.
- After the massage, apply some lotion to the elbows, knees, and heels.
- Back massages are dangerous for persons with certain heart diseases, back injuries, back surgeries, skin diseases, and some lung disorders. Check with the nurse and the care plan before giving back massages to persons with these conditions.
- Do not massage reddened bony areas. Reddened areas signal skin breakdown and pressure ulcers. Massage can lead to more tissue damage.
- Wear gloves if the person's skin is not intact. Always follow Standard Precautions and the Bloodborne Pathogen Standard.
- Report and record skin breakdown, redness, and bruising.

PERINEAL CARE

- Perineal care involves cleaning the genital and anal areas. It is done daily during the bath and whenever the area is soiled with urine or feces. The person does perineal care if able.
- Perineal and perineum are not common terms. Most people understand privates, private parts, crotch, genitals, or the area between the legs. Use terms the person understands.
- Standard Precautions, medical asepsis, and the Bloodborne Pathogen Standard are followed.
- Work from the cleanest area to the dirtiest—commonly called cleaning from "front to back." On a woman, clean from the urethra (cleanest) to the anal (dirtiest) area. On a male, start at the meatus of the urethra and work outward.
- Use warm water. Use washcloths, towelettes, cotton balls, or swabs according to center policy. Rinse thoroughly. Pat dry. Water temperature is usually 105° F to 109° F.
- Report and record:
  - Bleeding, redness, swelling, irritation
  - Complaints of pain or burning
  - Signs of urinary or fecal incontinence
  - Signs of skin breakdown
  - Discharge from the vagina or urinary tract
  - Odors

CHAPTER 15 REVIEW QUESTIONS
Circle the BEST answer.

1. Oral hygiene does the following *except*
   a. Keeps the mouth and teeth clean
   b. Prevents mouth odors and infections
   c. Decreases comfort
   d. Makes food taste better

2. When giving oral hygiene, you should report and record the following *except*
   a. Dry, cracked, swollen, or blistered lips
   b. Redness, sores, or white patches in the mouth
   c. Bleeding, swelling, or redness of the gums
   d. The number of fillings a person has

3. A person is unconscious. When you do mouth care, you do the following *except*
   a. Use only a small amount of fluid to clean the mouth
   b. Use your fingers to keep the mouth open
   c. Explain what you are doing
   d. Give mouth care at least every 2 hours

4. Which statement about dentures is *false?*
   a. Dentures are slippery when wet.
   b. During cleaning, hold dentures over a basin of water lined with a towel.
   c. Store dentures in cool water.
   d. Remind people to wrap their dentures in tissues or napkins.

5. Bathing does the following *except*
   a. Cleanses the skin
   b. Stimulates circulation
   c. Makes a person tense
   d. Permits you to observe the person's skin

6. The water temperature for a complete bed bath is
   a. 102° F to 108° F
   b. 110° F to 115° F
   c. 115° F to 120° F
   d. 120° F to 125° F

7. Which statement is *false?*
   a. Use powder near persons with respiratory disorders.
   b. Before applying powder, check with the nurse and the care plan.
   c. Before applying powder, sprinkle a small amount of powder onto your hands.
   d. Apply powder in a thin layer.

8. When washing a person's eyes, you should do the following *except*
   a. Use only water
   b. Gently wipe from the inner to the outer aspect of the eye
   c. Gently wipe from the outer to the inner aspect of the eye
   d. Use a clean part of the washcloth for each stroke

9. Which statement is *false?*
   a. A back massage relaxes and stimulates circulation.
   b. Massages are given after the bath and with evening care.
   c. You can observe the person's skin before beginning the massage.
   d. You should use cold lotion for the massage.

10. When giving female perineal care, you should work from the urethra to the anal area.
    a. True
    b. False
11. When giving male perineal care, start at the meatus and work outward.
    a. True
    b. False

Answers to these questions are on p. 425.

CHAPTER 16 ASSISTING WITH GROOMING
- Hair care, shaving, and nail and foot care prevent infection and promote comfort. They also affect love, belonging, and self-esteem needs.

HAIR CARE
- You assist patients and residents with brushing and combing hair and with shampooing according to the care plan. The nursing process reflects the person's culture, personal choice, skin and scalp condition, health history, and self-care ability.

Brushing and Combing Hair
- Brushing and combing prevent tangled and matted hair.
- When brushing and combing hair, start at the scalp and brush or comb to the hair ends.
- Never cut hair for any reason. Tell the nurse if you think the person's hair needs to be cut.
- Special measures are needed for curly, coarse, and dry hair. Check the care plan.
- When giving hair care, place a towel across the person's back and shoulders to protect garments from falling hair. If the person is in bed, give hair care before changing the linens and pillowcase.

Shampooing
- Shampooing frequency depends on the person's needs and preferences. Usually shampooing is done weekly on the person's bath or shower day.
- Hair is dried and styled as quickly as possible after the shampoo.
- During shampooing, report and record:
  - Scalp sores
  - Flaking
  - Itching
  - Presence of nits or lice
  - Patches of hair loss
  - Very dry or very oily hair
  - Matted or tangled hair
  - How the person tolerated the procedure
- Keep shampoo away from and out of eyes. Have the person hold a washcloth over the eyes.
- Wear gloves if the person has scalp sores.
- Follow Standard Precautions and the Bloodborne Pathogen Standard.

SHAVING
- Review Box 16-1, Rules for Shaving, in your textbook.

Caring for Mustaches and Beards
- Wash and comb mustaches and beards daily and as needed. Ask the person how to groom his mustache or beard.
- Never trim a mustache or beard without the person's consent.

Shaving Legs and Underarms
- Many women shave their legs and underarms. This practice varies among cultures. Legs and underarms are shaved after bathing when the skin is soft.

NAIL AND FOOT CARE
- Nail and foot care prevent infection, injury, and odors.
- Nails are easier to trim and clean right after soaking or bathing.
- Use nail clippers to cut fingernails. Never use scissors. Use extreme caution to prevent damage to nearby tissues.
- Follow Standard Precautions and the Bloodborne Pathogen Standard.
- Report and record:
  - Reddened, irritated, or calloused areas
  - Breaks in the skin
  - Corns on top of and between the toes
  - Very thick nails
  - Loose nails
- You do not cut or trim toenails if a person has diabetes or poor circulation to the legs and feet or takes drugs that affect blood clotting. Also, do not cut or trim toenails if the person has very thick nails or ingrown toenails. The nurse or podiatrist cuts toenails and provides foot care for these persons.
- When doing foot care, check between the toes for cracks and sores. If left untreated, a serious infection could occur.
- The feet of persons with decreased sensation or circulatory problems may easily burn because they do not feel hot temperatures.
- After soaking, apply lotion to the feet. Because the lotion can cause slippery feet, help the person put on non-skid footwear before you transfer the person or let the person walk.

CHANGING CLOTHING AND HOSPITAL GOWNS
- Garments are changed after the bath and whenever wet or soiled.
- When changing clothing:
  - Provide for privacy.
  - Encourage the person to do as much as possible.

- Let the person choose what to wear. Make sure the right undergarments are chosen.
- Remove clothing from the strong or "good" (unaffected) side first.
- Put clothing on the weak (affected) side first.
- Support the arm or leg when removing or putting on a garment.

CHAPTER 16 REVIEW QUESTIONS

Circle T if the statement is true. Circle F if the statement is false.

1. T F Hair care, shaving, and nail and foot care prevent infection and promote comfort.
2. T F If a person's hair is matted, you may cut the hair.
3. T F When giving hair care, place a towel across the person's back and shoulders to protect garments from falling hair.
4. T F You should wear gloves when shampooing a person who has scalp sores.
5. T F A person takes an anticoagulant. Therefore he shaves with a blade razor.
6. T F You should wear gloves when shaving a person.
7. T F Never trim a mustache or beard without the person's consent.
8. T F Mustaches and beards need daily care.
9. T F A person has diabetes. You can cut his or her toenails.

Circle the BEST answer.

10. Fingernails are cut with
    a. Scissors
    b. Nail clippers
    c. An emery board
    d. A nail file
11. Which statement is *false?*
    a. Provide privacy when a person is changing clothes.
    b. Most residents wear street clothes during the day.
    c. Let the person choose what to wear.
    d. You may tear a person's clothing.

Answers to these questions are on p. 425.

CHAPTER 17 ASSISTING WITH URINARY ELIMINATION
NORMAL URINATION

- The healthy adult produces about 1500 mL of urine a day.
- The frequency of urination is affected by amount of fluid intake, habits, availability of toilet facilities, activity, work, and illness. People usually void at bedtime, after sleep, and before meals.

Some people void every 2 to 3 hours. The need to void at night disturbs sleep. Review Box 17-1, Rules for Normal Urination, in the textbook.

Observations

- Observe urine for color, clarity, odor, amount, and particles. Normal urine is pale yellow, straw-colored, or amber. It is clear with no particles. A faint odor is normal.
- Some foods and drugs affect urine color. Ask the nurse to observe urine that looks or smells abnormal.
- Report the following urinary problems:
  - **Dysuria**—painful or difficult urination
  - **Hematuria**—blood in the urine
  - **Nocturia**—frequent urination at night
  - **Oliguria**—scant amount of urine; less than 500 mL in 24 hours
  - **Polyuria**—abnormally large amounts of urine
  - **Urinary frequency**—voiding at frequent intervals
  - **Urinary incontinence**—the loss of bladder control
  - **Urinary urgency**—the need to void at once

Bedpans

- Follow Standard Precautions and the Bloodborne Pathogen Standard when handling bedpans, urinals, commodes, and their contents.
- Thoroughly clean and disinfect bedpans, urinals, and commodes after use.

Urinals

- Some men need support when standing to use the urinal.
- You may have to place and hold the urinal for some men. This may embarrass both the person and you. Act in a professional manner at all times.
- Remind men to hang urinals on bed rails and to signal after using them.

URINARY INCONTINENCE

- **Urinary incontinence** is the loss of bladder control.
- If urinary incontinence is a new problem, tell the nurse at once.
- Incontinence is embarrassing. Garments are wet, and odors develop. Skin irritation, infection, and pressure ulcers are risks. The person's pride, dignity, and self-esteem are affected. Social isolation, loss of independence, and depression are common.
- Good skin care and dry garments and linens are essential. Promoting normal urinary elimination prevents incontinence in some people. Other people may need bladder training.

- Review Box 17-2, Nursing Measures for Persons With Urinary Incontinence, in the textbook.
- Caring for persons with incontinence is stressful. Remember, the person does not choose to be incontinent. If you find yourself becoming short-tempered and impatient, talk to the nurse at once. Kindness, empathy, understanding, and patience are needed.

CATHETERS

- An *indwelling catheter (retention or Foley catheter)* drains urine constantly into a drainage bag.
- The catheter must not pull at the insertion site. Hold the catheter securely during catheter care. Then properly secure the catheter. Also make sure the tubing is not under the person. Besides obstructing urine flow, lying on the tubing is uncomfortable. It can also cause skin breakdown.
- Follow Standard Precautions and the Bloodborne Pathogen Standard. Review Box 17-3, Caring for Persons With Indwelling Catheters, in the textbook.
- Report and record:
  - Complaints of pain, burning, irritation, or the need to void
  - Crusting, abnormal drainage, or secretions
  - The color, clarity, and odor of urine
  - Particles in the urine
  - Urine leaking at the insertion site
  - Drainage system leaks

Drainage Systems

- A closed drainage system is used for indwelling catheters. The drainage bag hangs from the bed frame, chair, or wheelchair. It must not touch the floor. The bag is always kept lower than the person's bladder. Do not hang the drainage bag on a bed rail.
- If the drainage system is disconnected accidentally, tell the nurse at once. Do not touch the ends of the catheter or tubing. Do the following:
  - Practice hand hygiene. Put on gloves.
  - Wipe the end of the tube with an antiseptic wipe.
  - Wipe the end of the catheter with another antiseptic wipe.
  - Do not put the ends down. Do not touch the ends after you clean them.
  - Connect the tubing to the catheter.
  - Discard the wipes into a BIOHAZARD bag.
  - Remove the gloves. Practice hand hygiene.
- Check with the nurse and care plan about when to empty and measure the urine in the drainage bag. Follow Standard Precautions and the Bloodborne Pathogen Standard.

- A leg bag is a drainage system that attaches to the thigh or calf. Empty and measure a leg bag when it is half full.
- Report and record:
  - The amount of urine measured
  - The color, clarity, and odor of urine
  - Particles in the urine
  - Complaints of pain, burning, irritation, or the need to urinate
  - Drainage system leaks

Condom Catheters

- Condom catheters are often used for incontinent men. They are also called external catheters, Texas catheters, and urinary sheaths.
- These catheters are changed daily after perineal care.
- To apply a condom catheter, follow the manufacturer's instructions. Thoroughly wash and dry the penis before applying the catheter.
- Some condom catheters are self-adhering. Other catheters are secured in place with elastic tape in a spiral manner. Never use adhesive tape to secure catheters. It does not expand. Blood flow to the penis is cut off, injuring the penis.
- When removing or applying a condom catheter, report and record the following observations:
  - Reddened or open areas on the penis
  - Swelling of the penis
  - Color, clarity, and odor of urine
  - Particles in the urine
- Do not apply a condom catheter if the penis is red, is irritated, or shows signs of skin breakdown. Report your observations to the nurse at once.

BLADDER TRAINING

- Bladder training helps some persons with urinary incontinence. Control of urination is the goal. Bladder control promotes comfort and quality of life. It also increases self-esteem. You assist with bladder training as directed by the nurse and the care plan.

CHAPTER 17 REVIEW QUESTIONS
Circle the BEST answer.

1. Which statement is *false?*
   a. Normal urine is yellow, straw-colored, or amber.
   b. Urine with a strong odor is normal.
   c. A person normally voids 1500 mL a day.
   d. Observe urine for color, clarity, odor, amount, and particles.
2. Which observation does *not* need to be reported to the nurse promptly?
   a. Complaints of urgency
   b. Burning on urination
   c. Painful or difficult urination
   d. Clear amber urine

3. Which statement is *false*?
   a. Incontinence is embarrassing.
   b. Caring for persons with incontinence may be stressful.
   c. Incontinence is a personal choice.
   d. Be kind and patient to persons who are incontinent.
4. A person with a catheter complains of pain. You should notify the nurse at once.
   a. True
   b. False
5. Which statement is *false*?
   a. The urine drainage system should hang from the bed frame or chair.
   b. The urine drainage system should hang on a bed rail.
   c. The urine drainage system must be off the floor.
   d. The urine drainage system must be kept lower than the person's bladder.
6. Which statement is *false*?
   a. Condom catheters are changed daily.
   b. Follow the manufacturer's instructions when applying a condom catheter.
   c. Use adhesive tape to secure a condom catheter in place.
   d. Report and record open or reddened areas on the penis at once.
7. The goal of bladder training is to
   a. Allow the person to use the toilet
   b. Keep the catheter
   c. Gain control of urination
   d. Decrease self-esteem

Answers to these questions are on p. 425.

CHAPTER 18 ASSISTING WITH BOWEL ELIMINATION
NORMAL BOWEL ELIMINATION
Observations

- Stools are normally brown, soft, formed, moist, and shaped like the rectum. They have a normal odor caused by bacterial action in the intestines. Certain foods and drugs cause odors.
- Carefully observe stools before disposing of them. Observe and report the color, amount, consistency, odor, and shape of stools. Also, observe and report the presence of blood or mucus, frequency of defecation, and any complaints of pain or discomfort.

Factors Affecting Bowel Elimination

- *Privacy*. Bowel elimination is a private act.
- *Habits*. Many people have a bowel movement after breakfast. Some read. Defecation is easier when a person is relaxed.
- *Diet—high-fiber foods*. Fiber helps prevent constipation.
- *Diet—other foods*. Some foods cause constipation. Other foods cause frequent stools or diarrhea.
- *Fluids*. Drinking 6 to 8 glasses of water daily promotes normal bowel elimination. Warm fluids—coffee, tea, hot cider, warm water—increase peristalsis.
- *Activity*. Exercise and activity maintain muscle tone and stimulate peristalsis.
- *Drugs*. Drugs can prevent constipation or control diarrhea. Some have diarrhea or constipation as side effects.
- *Disability*. Some people cannot control bowel movements. A bowel training program is needed.
- *Aging*. Older persons are at risk for constipation. Some older persons lose bowel control and have fecal incontinence.
- To provide comfort and safety during bowel elimination, review Box 18-1, Safety and Comfort During Bowel Elimination, in the textbook. Follow Standard Precautions and the Bloodborne Pathogen Standard.

COMMON PROBLEMS

- Common problems include constipation, fecal impaction, diarrhea, fecal incontinence, and flatulence.

Constipation

- **Constipation** is the passage of a hard, dry stool.
- Common causes of constipation are a low-fiber diet and ignoring the urge to defecate. Other causes include decreased fluid intake, inactivity, drugs, aging, and certain diseases.
- Dietary changes, fluids, and activity prevent or relieve constipation. So do drugs and enemas.

Fecal Impaction

- A **fecal impaction** is the prolonged retention and buildup of feces in the rectum.
- Fecal impaction results if constipation is not relieved. The person cannot defecate. Liquid feces pass around the hardened fecal mass in the rectum. The liquid feces seep from the anus.
- Abdominal discomfort, abdominal distention, nausea, cramping, and rectal pain are common. Older persons have poor appetite or confusion. Some persons have a fever. Report these signs and symptoms to the nurse.

Diarrhea

- **Diarrhea** is the frequent passage of liquid stools.
- The need to have a bowel movement is urgent. Some people cannot get to a bathroom in time. Abdominal cramping, nausea, and vomiting may occur.
- Assist with elimination needs promptly, dispose of stools promptly, and give good skin care. Liquid stools irritate the skin. So does frequent wiping with toilet paper. Skin breakdown and pressure ulcers are risks.
- Follow Standard Precautions and the Bloodborne Pathogen Standard when in contact with stools.
- Report signs of diarrhea at once. Ask the nurse to observe the stool.

Fecal Incontinence

- **Fecal incontinence** is the inability to control the passage of feces and gas through the anus.
- Fecal incontinence affects the person emotionally. Frustration, embarrassment, anger, and humiliation are common. The person may need:
  - Bowel training
  - Help with elimination after meals and every 2 to 3 hours
  - Incontinence products to keep garments and linens clean
  - Good skin care

Flatulence

- **Flatulence** is the excessive formation of gas or air in the stomach and intestines.
- Causes include swallowing air while eating and drinking and bacterial action in the intestines. Other causes may be gas-forming foods, constipation, bowel and abdominal surgeries, and drugs that decrease peristalsis.
- If flatus is not expelled, the intestines distend (swell or enlarge from the pressure of gases). Abdominal cramping or pain, shortness of breath, and a swollen abdomen occur. "Bloating" is a common complaint. Exercise, walking, moving in bed, and the left side-lying position often produce flatus. Enemas and drugs may be ordered.

BOWEL TRAINING

- Bowel training has two goals:
  - To gain control of bowel movements.
  - To develop a regular pattern of elimination. Fecal impactions, constipation, and fecal incontinence are prevented.
- Factors that promote elimination are part of the care plan and bowel training program.

ENEMAS

- An **enema** is the introduction of fluid into the rectum and lower colon.
- Doctors order enemas:
  - To remove feces
  - To relieve constipation, fecal impaction, or flatulence
  - To clean the bowel of feces before certain surgeries and diagnostic procedures
- Review Box 18-2, Safety and Comfort Measures for Giving Enemas, in the textbook.

THE PERSON WITH AN OSTOMY

- Sometimes part of the intestines is removed surgically. An ostomy is sometimes necessary. An **ostomy** is a surgically created opening. The opening is called a **stoma.** The person wears a pouch over the stoma to collect stools and flatus.
- Stools irritate the skin. Skin care prevents skin breakdown around the stoma. The skin is washed and dried. Then a skin barrier is applied around the stoma. It prevents stools from having contact with the skin. The skin barrier is part of the pouch or a separate device.
- The pouch has an adhesive backing that is applied to the skin. Sometimes pouches are secured to ostomy belts.
- The pouch is changed every 3 to 7 days and when it leaks. Frequent pouch changes can damage the skin.
- Many pouches have a drain at the bottom that closes with a clip, clamp, or wire closure. The drain is opened to empty the pouch. The drain is wiped with toilet tissue before it is closed.

CHAPTER 18 REVIEW QUESTIONS
Circle the BEST answer.

1. Which statement is *false*?
   a. Lack of privacy can prevent defecation.
   b. Low-fiber foods promote defecation.
   c. Drinking 6 to 8 glasses of water daily promotes normal bowel elimination.
   d. Exercise stimulates peristalsis.
2. Which of the following does *not* prevent constipation?
   a. A high-fiber diet
   b. Increased fluid intake
   c. Exercise
   d. Ignoring the urge to defecate
3. A person has fecal incontinence. You should do the following *except*
   a. Be patient
   b. Help with elimination after meals
   c. Provide good skin care
   d. Scold the person for being incontinent

4. The preferred position for an enema is the
   a. Sims' position or the left side-lying position
   b. Prone position
   c. Supine position
   d. Trendelenburg's position
Answers to these questions are on p. 425.

CHAPTER 19 ASSISTING WITH NUTRITION AND FLUIDS

- Food and water are necessary for life. A poor diet and poor eating habits:
  - Increase the risk for infection
  - Cause healing problems
  - Affect physical and mental function, increasing the risk for accidents and injuries

BASIC NUTRITION

- **Nutrition** is the process involved in the ingestion, digestion, absorption, and use of foods and fluids by the body. Good nutrition is needed for growth, healing, and body functions.
- A *nutrient* is a substance that is ingested, digested, absorbed, and used by the body.

Nutrients

- A well-balanced diet ensures an adequate intake of essential nutrients.
- *Protein*—is needed for tissue growth and repair. Sources include meat, fish, poultry, eggs, milk and milk products, cereals, beans, peas, and nuts.
- *Carbohydrates*—provide energy and fiber for bowel elimination. They are found in fruits, vegetables, breads, cereals, and sugar.
- *Fats*—provide energy, add flavor to food, and help the body use certain vitamins. Sources include meats, lard, butter, shortening, oils, milk, cheese, egg yolks, and nuts.
- *Vitamins*—are needed for certain body functions. The body stores vitamins A, D, E, and K. Vitamin C and the B complex vitamins must be ingested daily.
- *Minerals*—are needed for bone and tooth formation, nerve and muscle function, fluid balance, and other body processes.
- *Water*—is needed for all body processes.

FACTORS AFFECTING EATING AND NUTRITION

- *Age.* Many changes occur in the digestive system with aging.
- *Culture.* Culture influences dietary practices, food choices, and food preparation.
- *Religion.* Selecting, preparing, and eating food often involve religious practices. A person may follow all, some, or none of the dietary practices of his or her faith.

- *Appetite.* Illness, drugs, anxiety, pain, and depression can cause loss of appetite. Unpleasant sights, thoughts, and smells are other causes.
- *Personal choice.* Food likes and dislikes are influenced by foods served in the home. Usually food likes expand with age and social experiences.
- *Body reactions.* People usually avoid foods that cause allergic reactions. They also avoid foods that cause nausea, vomiting, diarrhea, indigestion, gas, or headaches.
- *Illness.* Appetite usually decreases during illness and recovery from injuries. However, nutritional needs are increased.
- *Disability.* Disease or injury can affect the hands, wrists, and arms. Adaptive equipment lets the person eat independently.

OBRA DIETARY REQUIREMENTS

- OBRA has requirements for food served in nursing centers:
  - Each person's nutritional and dietary needs are met.
  - The person's diet is well-balanced. It is nourishing and tastes good. Food is well-seasoned.
  - Food is appetizing. It has an appealing aroma and is attractive.
  - Hot food is served hot. Cold food is served cold.
  - Food is served promptly.
  - Food is prepared to meet each person's needs. Some people need food cut, ground, or chopped. Others have special diets ordered by the doctor.
  - Other foods are offered if the person refused the food served. Substituted food must have a similar nutritional value to the first foods served.
  - Each person receives at least 3 meals a day. A bedtime snack is offered.
  - The center provides needed adaptive equipment and utensils.

SPECIAL DIETS
The Sodium-Controlled Diet

- A sodium-controlled diet decreases the amount of sodium in the body. The diet involves:
  - Omitting high-sodium foods. Review Box 19-2, High-Sodium Foods, in the textbook.
  - Not adding salt when eating.
  - Limiting the amount of salt used in cooking.

Diabetes Meal Planning

- Diabetes meal planning is for people with diabetes. It involves the person's food preferences and calories needed. It also involves eating meals and snacks at regular times.

- Serve the person's meals and snacks on time to maintain a certain blood sugar level.
- Always check the tray to see what was eaten. Tell the nurse what the person did and did not eat. If not all the food was eaten, a between-meal nourishment is needed. The nurse tells you what to give. Tell the nurse about changes in the person's eating habits.

The Dysphagia Diet

- **Dysphagia** means difficulty swallowing. Food thickness is changed to meet the person's needs. Review Box 19-3, Dysphagia Diet, in the textbook.
- You may need to feed a person with dysphagia. To promote the person's comfort:
  - Know the signs and symptoms of dysphagia. Review Box 19-4 in the textbook.
  - Feed the person according to the care plan and swallow guide.
  - Follow aspiration precautions. Review Box 19-5 in the textbook.
  - Report changes in how the person eats.
  - Report choking, coughing, or difficulty breathing during or after meals. Also report abnormal breathing or respiratory sounds. Report these observations at once.

FLUID BALANCE

- Fluid balance is needed for health. The amount of fluid taken in **(input)** and the amount of fluid lost **(output)** must be equal. If fluid intake exceeds fluid output, body tissues swell with water **(edema).**
- **Dehydration** is a decrease in the amount of water in body tissues. Fluid output exceeds intake. Common causes are poor fluid intake, vomiting, diarrhea, bleeding, excess sweating, and increased urine production.

Normal Fluid Requirements

- An adult needs 1500 mL of water daily to survive. About 2000 to 2500 mL of fluid per day is needed for normal fluid balance. Water requirements increase with hot weather, exercise, fever, illness, and excess fluid loss.
- Older persons may have a decreased sense of thirst. Their bodies need water, but they may not feel thirsty. Offer fluids according to the care plan.

Special Fluid Orders

- The doctor may order the amount of fluid a person can have in 24 hours. Intake and output (I&O) records are kept.
- *Encourage fluids.* The person drinks an increased amount of fluid.
- *Restrict fluids.* Fluids are limited to a certain amount.

- *Nothing by mouth (NPO).* The person cannot eat or drink.
- *Thickened liquids.* All liquids are thickened, including water.

MEETING FOOD AND FLUID NEEDS
Preparing for Meals

- Preparing residents for meals promotes their comfort:
  - Assist with elimination needs.
  - Provide oral hygiene. Make sure dentures are in place.
  - Make sure eyeglasses and hearing aids are in place.
  - Make sure incontinent persons are clean and dry.
  - Position the person in a comfortable position.
  - Assist with hand washing.

Serving Meal Trays

- Food is served in containers that keep foods at the correct temperature. Hot food is kept hot. Cold food is kept cold.
- Prompt serving keeps food at the correct temperature.

Feeding the Person

- Serve food and fluid in the order the person prefers. Offer fluids during the meal.
- Use teaspoons to feed the person.
- Persons who need to be fed are often angry, humiliated, and embarrassed. Some are depressed or refuse to eat. Let them do as much as possible. If strong enough, let them hold milk or juice glasses. Never let them hold hot drinks.
- Tell the visually impaired person what is on the tray. Describe what you are offering. For persons who feed themselves, use the numbers on the clock for the location of foods.
- Many people pray before eating. Allow time and privacy for prayer.
- Meals provide social contact with others. Engage the person in pleasant conversations. Also, sit facing the person.
- Report and record:
  - The amount and kind of food eaten
  - Complaints of nausea or dysphagia
  - Signs and symptoms of dysphagia
  - Signs and symptoms of aspiration
- The person will eat better if not rushed.
- Wipe the person's hands, face, and mouth as needed during the meal.

Between-Meal Snacks

- Many special diets involve between-meal snacks. These snacks are served upon arrival on the nursing unit. Follow the same considerations and procedures for serving meal trays and feeding persons.

Calorie Counts
- Calorie records are kept for some people. On a flow sheet, note what the person ate and how much. A nurse or dietitian converts these portions into calories.

Providing Drinking Water
- Patients and residents need fresh drinking water. Follow the agency's procedure for providing fresh water.
- Water glasses and pitchers can spread microbes. To prevent the spread of microbes:
  - Label the water pitcher with the person's name and room and bed numbers.
  - Do not touch the rim or inside of the water glass, cup, or pitcher.
  - Do not let the ice scoop touch the rim or inside of the water glass, cup, or pitcher.
  - Place the ice scoop in the holder or on a towel, not in the ice container or dispenser.
  - Make sure the person's water pitcher and cup are clean and free of cracks and chips.

CHAPTER 19 REVIEW QUESTIONS
Circle the BEST answer.
1. A person is on a sodium-controlled diet. Which statement is *true*?
   a. High-sodium foods are allowed.
   b. Salt is added at the table.
   c. Pretzels and potato chips are a good snack.
   d. The amount of salt used in cooking is limited.
2. A person is a diabetic. You should do the following *except*
   a. Serve his meals and snacks late
   b. Always check his tray to see what he ate
   c. Tell the nurse what he ate and did not eat
   d. Provide a between-meal snack as the nurse directs
3. A person has dysphagia. You should do the following *except*
   a. Report choking and coughing during a meal at once
   b. Report difficulty in breathing during a meal at the end of the shift
   c. Report changes in how the person eats
   d. Follow aspiration precautions
4. Older persons have a decreased sense of thirst.
   a. True
   b. False
5. When feeding a person, you do the following *except*

a. Use a teaspoon to feed the person
b. Offer fluids during the meal
c. Let the person do as much as possible
d. Stand so you can feed 2 people at once

6. A person is visually impaired. You do the following *except*
   a. Tell the person what is on the tray
   b. Use the numbers on a clock to tell the person the location of food
   c. If feeding the person, describe what you are offering
   d. Let the person guess what is served

Answers to these questions are on p. 425.

CHAPTER 20 ASSISTING WITH ASSESSMENT
VITAL SIGNS
- Accuracy is essential when you measure, record, and report vital signs. If unsure of your measurements, promptly ask the nurse to take them again.
- Report the following at once:
  - Any vital sign that is changed from a prior measurement
  - Vital signs above or below the normal range

BODY TEMPERATURE
- Thermometers are used to measure temperature. It is measured using the Fahrenheit (F) and centigrade or Celsius (C) scales.
- Temperature sites are the mouth, rectum, axilla (underarm), tympanic membrane (ear), and temporal artery (forehead).
- Review Box 20-1, Temperature Sites, in the textbook.
- Normal range for body temperatures depends on the site:
  - Oral: 97.6° F to 99.6° F
  - Rectal: 98.6° F to 100.6° F
  - Axillary: 96.6° F to 98.6° F
  - Tympanic membrane: 98.6° F
  - Temporal artery: 99.6° F
- Older persons have lower body temperatures than younger persons.

Glass Thermometers
- If a mercury-glass thermometer breaks, tell the nurse at once. Do not touch the mercury. The agency must follow special procedures for handling all hazardous materials.
- When using a glass thermometer:
  - Use the person's thermometer.
  - Use a rectal thermometer only for rectal temperatures.
  - Rinse the thermometer under cold, running water if it was soaking in a disinfectant. Dry it from the stem to the bulb end with tissues.

- Discard the thermometer if broken, cracked, or chipped.
- Shake down the thermometer to below 94° F or 34° C before using it.
- Clean and store the thermometer following center policy.
- Use plastic covers following center policy.
- Practice medical asepsis.
- Follow Standard Precautions and the Bloodborne Pathogen Standard.

Taking Temperatures

- *The oral site.* The glass thermometer remains in place 2 to 3 minutes or as required by center policy.
- *The rectal site.* Lubricate the bulb end of the rectal thermometer. Insert the glass thermometer 1 inch into the rectum. Hold the thermometer in place for 2 minutes or as required by center policy. Privacy is important.
- *The axillary site.* The axilla must be dry. The glass thermometer stays in place for 5 to 10 minutes or as required by center policy.

Electronic Thermometers

- Tympanic membrane thermometers are gently inserted into the ear. The temperature is measured in 1 to 3 seconds. These thermometers are not used if there is ear drainage.
- Temporal artery thermometers measure body temperature at the temporal artery in the forehead. These thermometers measure body temperature in 3 to 4 seconds. Follow the manufacturer's instructions for using, cleaning, and storing the device.

PULSE
Pulse Rate

- The adult pulse rate is between 60 and 100 beats per minute. Report these abnormal rates to the nurse at once:
  - *Tachycardia*—the heart rate is more than 100 beats per minute.
  - *Bradycardia*—the heart rate is less than 60 beats per minute.

Rhythm and Force of the Pulse

- The rhythm of the pulse should be regular. Report and record an irregular pulse rhythm.
- Report and record if the pulse force is strong, full, bounding, weak, thready, or feeble.

Taking Pulses

- The radial pulse is used for routine vital signs. Do not use your thumb to take a pulse. Count the pulse for 30 seconds and multiply by 2 if the agency policy permits. If the pulse is irregular,

count it for 1 minute. Report and record if the pulse is regular or irregular.
- The apical pulse is on the left side of the chest slightly below the nipple. Count the apical pulse for 1 minute.

RESPIRATIONS

- The healthy adult has 12 to 20 respirations per minute. Respirations are normally quiet, effortless, and regular. Both sides of the chest rise and fall equally.
- Count respirations when the person is at rest. Count respirations right after taking a pulse.
- Count respirations for 30 seconds and multiply the number by 2 if the agency policy permits. If an abnormal pattern is noted, count the respirations for 1 minute.
- Report and record:
  - The respiratory rate
  - Equality and depth of respirations
  - If the respirations were regular or irregular
  - If the person has pain or difficulty breathing
  - Any respiratory noises
  - An abnormal respiratory pattern

BLOOD PRESSURE
Normal and Abnormal Blood Pressures

- Blood pressure has normal ranges:
  - *Systolic pressure* (upper number)—less than 120 mm Hg
  - *Diastolic pressure* (lower number)—less than 80 mm Hg
- **Hypertension**—blood pressure measurements that remain above a systolic pressure of 140 mm Hg or a diastolic pressure of 90 mm Hg. Report any systolic measurement above 120 mm Hg. Also report a diastolic pressure above 80 mm Hg.
- **Hypotension**—when the systolic blood pressure is below 90 mm Hg and the diastolic pressure is below 60 mm Hg. Report a systolic pressure below 90 mm Hg. Also report a diastolic pressure below 60 mm Hg.
- Review Box 20-2, Guidelines for Measuring Blood Pressure, in your textbook.

PAIN

- Pain is personal. It differs for each person. If a person complains of pain or discomfort, the person has pain or discomfort. You must believe the person.

Signs and Symptoms

- You cannot see, hear, touch, or smell the person's pain. Rely on what the person tells you. Promptly report any information you collect about pain. Use the person's exact words when reporting and recording pain. The nurse needs the following information:

- *Location*. Where is the pain?
- *Onset and duration*. When did the pain start? How long has it lasted?
- *Intensity*. Ask the person to rate the pain. Use a pain scale.
- *Description*. Ask the person to describe the pain.
- *Factors causing pain*. Ask when the pain started and what the person was doing.
- *Factors affecting pain*. Ask what makes the pain better and what makes it worse.
- *Vital signs*. Increases often occur with acute pain. They may be normal with chronic pain.
- *Other signs and symptoms*. Dizziness, nausea, vomiting, weakness, numbness, and tingling. Review Box 20-3, Signs and Symptoms of Pain, in the textbook.

INTAKE AND OUTPUT

- All fluids taken by mouth are measured and recorded—water, milk, and so forth. So are foods that melt at room temperature—ice cream, sherbet, pudding, gelatin, and Popsicles.
- Output includes urine, vomitus, diarrhea, and wound drainage.

Measuring Intake and Output

- To measure intake and output, you need to know:
  - 1 ounce (oz) equals 30 mL
  - A pint is about 500 mL
  - A quart is about 1000 mL
  - The serving sizes of bowls, dishes, cups, pitchers, glasses, and other containers
- An I&O record is kept at the bedside. Record I&O measurements in the correct column. Amounts are totaled at the end of the shift. The totals are recorded in the person's chart.
- The urinal, commode, bedpan, or specimen pan is used for voiding. Remind the person not to void in the toilet. Also remind the person not to put toilet tissue into the receptacle.

WEIGHT AND HEIGHT

- When weighing a person, follow the manufacturer's instructions and center procedures for using the scales. Follow these guidelines when measuring weight and height:
  - The person wears only a gown or pajamas. No footwear is worn.
  - The person voids before being weighed.
  - Weigh the person at the same time of day. Before breakfast is the best time.
- Use the same scale for daily, weekly, and monthly weights.
- Balance the scale at zero before weighing the person.

CHAPTER 20 REVIEW QUESTIONS
Circle the BEST answer.

1. Which statement about taking a rectal temperature is *false*?
   a. The bulb end of the thermometer needs to be lubricated.
   b. The thermometer is held in place for 5 minutes.
   c. Privacy is important.
   d. The normal range is 98.6° F to 100.6° F.
2. Which pulse rate should you report at once?
   a. A pulse rate of 52 beats per minute
   b. A pulse rate of 60 beats per minute
   c. A pulse rate of 76 beats per minute
   d. A pulse rate of 100 beats per minute
3. Which statement is *false*?
   a. An irregular pulse is counted for 1 minute.
   b. You may use your thumb to take a radial pulse rate.
   c. The radial pulse is usually used to count a pulse rate.
   d. Tachycardia is a fast pulse rate.
4. Which blood pressure should you report?
   a. 120/80 mm Hg
   b. 88/62 mm Hg
   c. 110/70 mm Hg
   d. 92/68 mm Hg
5. A person is on intake and output. He just ate ice cream. This is recorded as intake.
   a. True
   b. False
6. A person drank a pint of milk at lunch. You know he drank
   a. 250 mL of milk
   b. 350 mL of milk
   c. 500 mL of milk
   d. 750 mL of milk
7. The soup bowl holds 6 ounces. A person ate all of the soup. You record his intake as
   a. 50 mL
   b. 120 mL
   c. 180 mL
   d. 200 mL
8. A person complains of pain. You will do the following *except*
   a. Ask where the pain is
   b. Ask when the pain started
   c. Ask what the intensity of the pain is on a scale of 1 to 10
   d. Ask why he or she is complaining about pain

Answers to these questions are on p. 425.

CHAPTER 22 ASSISTING WITH EXERCISE AND ACTIVITY
BEDREST
- The doctor may order bedrest to treat a health problem.

Complications of Bedrest
- Pressure ulcers, constipation, and fecal impactions can result. Urinary tract infections and renal calculi (kidney stones) can occur. So can blood clots and pneumonia.
- The musculoskeletal system is affected by lack of exercise and activity. These complications must be prevented to maintain normal movement:
  - A **contracture** is the lack of joint mobility caused by abnormal shortening of a muscle. Common sites are the fingers, wrists, elbows, toes, ankles, knees, and hips. The person is permanently deformed and disabled.
  - **Atrophy** is the decrease in size or the wasting away of tissue. Tissues shrink in size.
- **Orthostatic hypotension (postural hypotension)** is abnormally low blood pressure when the person suddenly stands up. The person is dizzy and weak and has spots before the eyes. Fainting can occur. To prevent orthostatic hypotension, have the person change slowly from a lying or sitting position to a standing position.

Positioning
- Supportive devices are often used to support and maintain the person in a certain position:
  - *Bedboards*—are placed under the mattress to prevent the mattress from sagging.
  - *Footboards*—are placed at the foot of mattresses to prevent plantar flexion that can lead to footdrop.
  - *Trochanter rolls*—prevent the hips and legs from turning outward (external rotation).
  - *Hip abduction wedges*—keep the hips abducted.
  - *Handrolls or handgrips*—prevent contractures of the thumb, fingers, and wrist.
  - *Splints*—keep the elbows, wrists, thumbs, fingers, ankles, and knees in normal position.
  - *Bed cradles*—keep the weight of top linens off the feet and toes.

RANGE-OF-MOTION EXERCISES
- **Range-of-motion (ROM)** exercises involve moving the joints through their complete range of motion. They are usually done at least 2 times a day.
- *Active ROM*—exercises are done by the person.
- *Passive ROM*—someone moves the joints through their range of motion.
- *Active-assistive ROM*—the person does the exercises with some help.
- Review Box 22-1, Joint Movements, in the textbook.

- Range-of-motion exercises can cause injury if not done properly. Practice these rules:
  - Exercise only the joints the nurse tells you to exercise.
  - Expose only the body part being exercised.
  - Use good body mechanics.
  - Support the part being exercised.
  - Move the joint slowly, smoothly, and gently.
  - Do not force a joint beyond its present range of motion.
  - Do not force a joint to the point of pain.
  - Ask the person if he or she has pain or discomfort.
  - Perform ROM exercises to the neck only if allowed by center policy.

AMBULATION
- **Ambulation** is the act of walking.
- Follow the care plan when helping a person walk. Use a gait (transfer) belt if the person is weak or unsteady. The person uses hand rails along the wall. Always check the person for orthostatic hypotension.
- When you help the person walk, walk to the side and slightly behind the person on the person's weak side. Encourage the person to use the hand rail on his or her strong side.

Walking Aids
- A cane is held on the strong side of the body. The cane tip is about 6 to 10 inches to the side of the foot. It is about 6 to 10 inches in front of the foot on the strong side. The grip is level with the hip. To walk:
  - Step A: The cane is moved forward 6 to 10 inches.
  - Step B: The weak leg (opposite the cane) is moved forward even with the cane.
  - Step C: The strong leg is moved forward and ahead of the cane and the weak leg.
- A walker gives more support than a cane. Wheeled walkers are common. They have wheels on the front legs and rubber tips on the back legs. The person pushes the walker about 6 to 8 inches in front of his or her feet.
- Braces support weak body parts, prevent or correct deformities, or prevent joint movement. A brace is applied over the ankle, knee, or back. Skin and bony points under braces are kept clean and dry. Report redness or signs of skin breakdown at once. Also report complaints of pain or discomfort.

CHAPTER 22 REVIEW QUESTIONS
Circle the BEST answer.
1. To prevent orthostatic hypotension, you should
   a. Move a person from the lying position to the sitting position quickly
   b. Move a person from the sitting position to the standing position quickly
   c. Move a person from the lying or sitting position to a standing position slowly
   d. Keep the person in bed

2. Exercise helps prevent contractures and muscle atrophy.
   a. True
   b. False
3. When performing ROM exercises, you should force a joint to the point of pain.
   a. True
   b. False
4. A person's left leg is weaker than his right. The person holds the cane on his right side.
   a. True
   b. False

Answers to these questions are on p. 425.

CHAPTER 23 ASSISTING WITH WOUND CARE

- A **wound** is a break in the skin or mucous membrane.
- The wound is a portal of entry for microbes. Infection is a major threat. Wound care involves preventing infection and further injury to the wound and nearby tissues.

PRESSURE ULCERS

- A **pressure ulcer** is a localized injury to the skin and/or underlying tissue. Pressure ulcers usually occur over a bony prominence—the back of the head, shoulder blades, elbows, hips, spine, sacrum, knees, ankles, heels, and toes.
- *Decubitus ulcer, bed sore,* and *pressure sore* are other terms for pressure ulcer.
- Pressure, shearing, and friction are common causes of skin breakdown and pressure ulcers. Risk factors include breaks in the skin, poor circulation to an area, moisture, dry skin, and irritation by urine and feces.

Persons at Risk

- Persons at risk for pressure ulcers are those who:
  - Are confined to a bed or chair
  - Need some or total help in moving
  - Are agitated or have involuntary muscle movements
  - Have loss of bowel or bladder control
  - Are exposed to moisture
  - Have poor nutrition
  - Have poor fluid balance
  - Have lowered mental awareness
  - Have problems sensing pain or pressure
  - Have circulatory problems
  - Are older
  - Are obese or very thin

Pressure Ulcer Stages

- In persons with light skin, a reddened bony area is the first sign of a pressure ulcer. In persons with dark skin, a bony area may appear red, blue, or purple. The area may feel warm or cool. The person may complain of pain, burning, tingling, or itching in the area.
- Figure 23-4 in the textbook shows the stages of pressure ulcers.

Prevention and Treatment

- Preventing pressure ulcers is much easier than trying to heal them. Review Box 23-1, Measures to Prevent Pressure Ulcers, in the textbook.
- The person at risk for pressure ulcers may be placed on a foam, air, alternating air, gel, or water mattress.
- Protective devices are often used to prevent and treat pressure ulcers and skin breakdown. Protective devices include:
  - Bed cradle
  - Heel and elbow protectors
  - Heel and foot elevators
  - Gel or fluid-filled pads and cushions
  - Eggcrate-type pads
  - Special beds
  - Other equipment—pillows, trochanter rolls, and footboards

SKIN TEARS

- A **skin tear** is a break or rip in the skin.
- Skin tears are caused by friction, shearing, pulling, or pressure on the skin. Bumping a hand, arm, or leg on any hard surface can cause a skin tear. Beds, bed rails, chairs, wheelchair footplates, and tables are dangers. So is holding the person's arm or leg too tight.
- Skin tears are painful. They are portals of entry for microbes. Wound complications can develop. Tell the nurse at once if you cause or find a skin tear.
- Review Box 23-2, Measures to Prevent Skin Tears, in the textbook.

CIRCULATORY ULCERS

- *Circulatory ulcers (vascular ulcers)* are open sores on the lower legs or feet. They are caused by decreased blood flow through the arteries or veins.
- Review Box 23-3, Measures to Prevent Circulatory Ulcers, in the textbook.
- *Venous ulcers (stasis ulcers)* are open sores on the lower legs or feet. They are caused by poor blood flow through the veins. The heels and inner aspect of the ankles are common sites for venous ulcers.

- *Arterial ulcers* are open wounds on the lower legs or feet caused by poor arterial blood flow. They are found between the toes, on top of the toes, and on the outer side of the ankle.
- A *diabetic foot ulcer* is an open wound on the foot caused by complications from diabetes. When nerves are affected, the person can lose sensation in a foot or leg. The person may not feel pain, heat, or cold. Therefore the person may not feel a cut, blister, burn, or other trauma to the foot. Infection and a large sore can develop. When blood flow to the foot decreases, tissues and cells do not get needed oxygen and nutrients. A sore does not heal properly. Tissue death (gangrene) can occur.

Prevention and Treatment
- Check the person's feet and legs every day. Report any sign of a problem to the nurse at once. Follow the care plan to prevent and treat circulatory ulcers.

Elastic Stockings
- Elastic stockings also are called anti-embolism or anti-embolic (AE) stockings. They also are called TED hose.
- The person usually has two pairs of stockings. One pair is washed; the other pair is worn.
- Stockings should not have twists, creases, or wrinkles after you apply them.
- Stockings are applied before the person gets out of bed.

HEAT AND COLD APPLICATIONS
Heat Applications
- Heat relieves pain, relaxes muscles, promotes healing, reduces tissue swelling, and decreases joint stiffness.

Complications
- High temperatures can cause burns. Report pain, excessive redness, and blisters at once. Also observe for pale skin.
- Metal implants pose risks. Pacemakers and joint replacements are made of metal. Do not apply heat to an implant area.

Cold Applications
- Cold applications reduce pain, prevent swelling, and decrease circulation and bleeding.

Complications
- Complications include pain, burns, blisters, and poor circulation. Burns and blisters occur from intense cold. They also occur when dry cold is in direct contact with the skin.

Applying Heat and Cold
- Protect the person from injury during heat and cold applications. Review Box 23-6, Rules for Applying Heat and Cold, in the textbook.

CHAPTER 23 REVIEW QUESTIONS
Circle the BEST answer.
1. The following can cause a skin tear *except*
   a. Friction and shearing
   b. Holding a person's arm or leg too tight
   c. Rings, watches, bracelets
   d. Trimmed, short nails
2. You may expect to find a pressure ulcer at all of the following sites *except*
   a. Back of the head
   b. Ears
   c. Top of the thigh
   d. Toes
3. In obese people, pressure ulcers can occur between abdominal folds.
   a. True
   b. False
4. A person is diabetic. Which statement is *false?*
   a. The person may not feel pain in her feet.
   b. The person may not feel heat or cold in her feet.
   c. You need to check her feet weekly for foot problems.
   d. The person is at risk for diabetic foot ulcers.
5. Which statement about elastic stockings is *false?*
   a. Elastic stockings are also called anti-embolic stockings.
   b. Elastic stockings should be wrinkle-free after being applied.
   c. A person usually has two pairs of elastic stockings.
   d. Elastic stockings are applied after a person gets out of bed.
6. Complications from a heat application include the following *except*
   a. Excessive redness
   b. Blisters
   c. Pale skin
   d. Cyanotic (bluish) nail beds
7. When applying heat or cold, you should do the following *except*
   a. Ask the nurse what the temperature of the application should be
   b. Cover dry heat or cold applications before applying them
   c. Observe the skin every 2 hours
   d. Know how long to leave the application in place

Answers to these questions are on p. 425.

CHAPTER 24 ASSISTING WITH OXYGEN NEEDS
ALTERED RESPIRATORY FUNCTION
- Hypoxia means that cells do not have enough oxygen.
- Restlessness, dizziness, and disorientation are signs of hypoxia.
- Review Box 24-1, Signs and Symptoms of Hypoxia, in the textbook. Report signs and symptoms of hypoxia to the nurse at once. Hypoxia is life-threatening.

Abnormal Respirations
- Adults normally have 12 to 20 respirations per minute. They are quiet, effortless, and regular. Both sides of the chest rise and fall equally. Report these observations at once:
  - **Tachypnea**—rapid breathing. Respirations are 20 or more per minute.
  - **Bradypnea**—slow breathing. Respirations are fewer than 12 per minute.
  - **Apnea**—lack or absence of breathing.
  - **Hypoventilation**—respirations are slow, shallow, and sometimes irregular.
  - **Hyperventilation**—respirations are rapid and deeper than normal.
  - **Dyspnea**—difficult, labored, painful breathing.
  - **Cheyne-Stokes respirations**—respirations gradually increase in rate and depth. Then they become shallow and slow. Breathing may stop for 10 to 20 seconds.
  - **Orthopnea**—breathing deeply and comfortably only when sitting.
  - **Kussmaul respirations**—very deep and rapid respirations.

PROMOTING OXYGENATION
Positioning
- Breathing is usually easier in semi-Fowler's and Fowler's positions. Persons with difficulty breathing often prefer the **orthopneic position** (sitting up and leaning over a table to breathe).

Deep Breathing and Coughing
- Deep breathing moves air into most parts of the lungs. Coughing removes mucus. Deep breathing and coughing are usually done every 2 hours while the person is awake.

ASSISTING WITH OXYGEN THERAPY
Oxygen Devices
- A nasal cannula allows eating and drinking. Tight prongs can irritate the nose. Pressure on the ears and cheekbones is possible.

- A simple face mask covers the nose and mouth. Talking and eating are hard to do with a mask. Listen carefully. Moisture can build up under the mask. Keep the face clean and dry. Masks are removed for eating. Usually oxygen is given by cannula during meals.

Oxygen Flow Rates
- When giving care and checking the person, always check the flow rate. Tell the nurse at once if it is too high or too low. A nurse or respiratory therapist will adjust the flow rate.

Oxygen Safety
- You do not give oxygen. You assist the nurse in providing safe care.
- Always check the oxygen level when you are with or near persons using oxygen systems that contain a limited amount of oxygen. Oxygen tanks and liquid oxygen systems are examples. Report a low oxygen level to the nurse at once.
- Follow the rules for fire and the use of oxygen in Chapter 8.
- Never remove the oxygen device.
- Make sure the oxygen device is secure but not tight.
- Check for signs of irritation from the oxygen device—behind the ears, under the nose, around the face, and cheekbones.
- Keep the face clean and dry when a mask is used.
- Never shut off the oxygen flow.
- Do not adjust the flow rate unless allowed by your state and agency.
- Tell the nurse at once if the flow rate is too high or too low.
- Tell the nurse at once if the humidifier is not bubbling.
- Secure tubing to the person's garment. Follow agency policy.
- Make sure there are no kinks in the tubing.
- Make sure the person does not lie on any part of the tubing.
- Report signs of hypoxia, respiratory distress, or abnormal breathing to the nurse at once.
- Give oral hygiene as directed. Follow the care plan.
- Make sure the oxygen device is clean and free of mucus.

CHAPTER 24 REVIEW QUESTIONS
Circle the BEST answer.
1. Which statement is *false?*
   a. Restlessness, dizziness, and disorientation are signs of hypoxia.
   b. Hypoxia is life-threatening.
   c. Report signs and symptoms of hypoxia at the end of the shift.

d. Anything that affects respiratory function can cause hypoxia.
2. Adults normally have
  a. 8 to 10 respirations per minute
  b. 12 to 20 respirations per minute
  c. 10 to 12 respirations per minute
  d. 20 to 24 respirations per minute
3. Dyspnea is
  a. Difficult, labored, or painful breathing
  b. Slow breathing with fewer than 12 respirations per minute
  c. Rapid breathing with 24 or more respirations per minute
  d. Lack or absence of breathing
4. Which statement about positioning is *false*?
  a. Breathing is usually easier in semi-Fowler's or Fowler's position.
  b. Persons with difficulty breathing often prefer the orthopneic position.
  c. Position changes are needed at least every 4 hours.
  d. Follow the person's care plan for positioning preferences.
5. A person has a nasal cannula. Which statement is *false*?
  a. You will leave the nasal cannula on while the person is eating.
  b. You will watch the nose area for irritation.
  c. You will watch the ears and cheekbones for skin breakdown.
  d. You will take the nasal cannula off while the person is eating.

Answers to these questions are on p. 425.

CHAPTER 25 ASSISTING WITH REHABILITATION AND RESTORATIVE NURSING CARE

- A **disability** is any lost, absent, or impaired physical or mental function.
- **Rehabilitation** is the process of restoring the person to his or her highest possible level of physical, psychological, social, and economic function. The focus is on improving abilities. This promotes function at the highest level of independence.

REHABILITATION AND THE WHOLE PERSON

- Rehabilitation takes longer in older persons. Changes from aging affect healing, mobility, vision, hearing, and other functions. Chronic health problems can slow recovery.

Physical Aspects

- Rehabilitation starts when the person first seeks health care. Complications, such as contractures and pressure ulcers, are prevented.

- *Self-care.* Self-care for activities of daily living (ADL) is a major goal. Self-help devices are often needed.
- *Elimination.* Bowel or bladder training may be needed. Fecal impaction, constipation, and fecal incontinence are prevented.
- *Mobility.* The person may need crutches, a walker, a cane, a brace, or a wheelchair.
- *Nutrition.* The person may need a dysphagia diet or enteral nutrition.
- *Communication.* Speech therapy and communication devices may be helpful.

Psychological and Social Aspects

- A disability can affect function and appearance. Self-esteem and relationships may suffer. The person may feel unwhole, useless, unattractive, unclean, or undesirable. The person may deny the disability. The person may expect therapy to correct the problem. He or she may be depressed, angry, and hostile.
- Successful rehabilitation depends on the person's attitude. The person must accept his or her limits and be motivated. The focus is on abilities and strengths. Despair and frustration are common. Progress may be slow. Old fears and emotions may recur.
- Remind persons of their progress. They need help accepting disabilities and limits. Give support, reassurance, and encouragement. Spiritual support helps some people. Psychological and social needs are part of the care plan.

THE REHABILITATION TEAM

- Rehabilitation is a team effort. The person is the key member. The health team and family help the person set goals and plan care. All help the person regain function and independence.

Your Role

- Every part of your job focuses on promoting the person's independence. Preventing decline in function also is a goal. Review Box 25-1, Assisting With Rehabilitation and Restorative Care, in the textbook.

Quality of Life

- To promote quality of life:
  - *Protect the right to privacy.* The person relearns old or practices new skills in private. Others do not need to see mistakes, falls, spills, clumsiness, anger, or tears.
  - *Encourage personal choice.* This gives the person control.

- *Protect the right to be free from abuse and mistreatment*. Sometimes improvement is not seen for weeks. Repeated explanations and demonstrations may have little or no results. You and other staff and family may become upset and short-tempered. However, no one can shout, scream, or yell at the person. Nor can they call the person names or hit or strike the person. Unkind remarks are not allowed. Report signs of abuse or mistreatment.
- *Learn to deal with your anger and frustration*. The person does not choose loss of function. If the process upsets you, discuss your feelings with the nurse.
- *Encourage activities*. Provide support and reassurance to the person with the disability. Remind the person that others with disabilities can give support and understanding.
- *Provide a safe setting*. The setting must meet the person's needs. The overbed table, bedside stand, and signal light are moved to the person's strong side.
- *Show patience, understanding, and sensitivity*. The person may be upset and discouraged. Give support, encouragement, and praise when needed. Stress the person's abilities and strengths. Do not give pity or sympathy.

CHAPTER 25 REVIEW QUESTIONS
Circle the BEST answer.

1. Successful rehabilitation depends on the person's attitude.
   a. True
   b. False
2. A person with a disability may be depressed, angry, and hostile.
   a. True
   b. False
3. A person needs rehabilitation. You should do the following *except*
   a. Let the person relearn old skills in private
   b. Let the person practice new skills in private
   c. Encourage the person to make choices
   d. Shout at the person
4. You saw a family member hit and scream at a person. You need to report your observations to the nurse.
   a. True
   b. False
5. A person has a weak left arm. You will
   a. Place the signal light on his left side
   b. Place the signal light on his right side
   c. Give him sympathy
   d. Give him pity

Answers to these questions are on p. 425.

CHAPTER 26 CARING FOR PERSONS WITH COMMON HEALTH PROBLEMS
CANCER
- Cancer is the second leading cause of death in the United States.
- Review Box 26-1, Some Signs and Symptoms of Cancer, in the textbook.
- Surgery, radiation therapy, and chemotherapy are the most common treatments.
- Persons with cancer have many needs. They include:
  - Pain relief or control
  - Rest and exercise
  - Fluids and nutrition
  - Preventing skin breakdown
  - Preventing bowel problems (constipation, diarrhea)
  - Dealing with treatment side effects
  - Psychological and social needs
  - Spiritual needs
  - Sexual needs
- Anger, fear, and depression are common. Some surgeries are disfiguring. The person may feel unwhole, unattractive, or unclean. The person and family need support.
- Talk to the person. Do not avoid the person because you are uncomfortable. Use touch and listening to show that you care.
- Spiritual needs are important. A spiritual leader may provide comfort.

MUSCULOSKELETAL DISORDERS
Arthritis
- Arthritis means joint inflammation.
- *Osteoarthritis (Degenerative Joint Disease)*. The fingers, spine (neck and lower back), and weight-bearing joints (hips, knees, and feet) are often affected. Treatment involves pain relief, heat applications, exercise, rest and joint care, weight control, and a healthy life-style. Falls are prevented. Help is given with ADL as needed. Toilet seat risers are helpful when hips and knees are affected. So are chairs with higher seats and armrests. Some people need joint replacement surgery.
- *Rheumatoid Arthritis*. Rheumatoid arthritis (RA) causes joint pain, swelling, stiffness, and loss of function. Joints are tender, warm, and swollen. Fatigue and fever are common. The person does not feel well. The person's care plan may include rest balanced with exercise, proper positioning, joint care, weight control, measures to reduce stress, and measures to prevent falls. Drugs are ordered for pain relief and to reduce inflammation. Heat and cold applications may be ordered. Some persons need joint replacement

surgery. Emotional support is needed. Persons with RA need to stay as active as possible. Give encouragement and praise. Listen when the person needs to talk.

NERVOUS SYSTEM DISORDERS
Stroke
- Stroke is also called a brain attack or cerebrovascular accident (CVA). It is the third leading cause of death in the United States. Review Box 26-6, Warning Signs of Stroke, in the textbook.
- The effects of stroke include:
  - Loss of face, hand, arm, leg, or body control
  - **Hemiplegia**—paralysis on one side of the body
  - Changing emotions (crying easily or mood swings, sometimes for no reason)
  - Difficulty swallowing (dysphagia)
  - Aphasia or slowed or slurred speech
  - Changes in sight, touch, movement, and thought
  - Impaired memory
  - Urinary frequency, urgency, or incontinence
  - Loss of bowel control or constipation
  - Depression and frustration
- The health team helps the person regain the highest possible level of function. Review Box 26-7, Care of the Person With a Stroke, in the textbook.

Aphasia
- **Aphasia** is the total or partial loss of the ability to use or understand language.
- *Expressive aphasia* relates to difficulty expressing or sending out thoughts. Thinking is clear. The person knows what to say but has difficulty or cannot speak the words.
- *Receptive aphasia* relates to difficulty understanding language. The person has trouble understanding what is said or read. People and common objects are not recognized.

Parkinson's Disease
- Parkinson's disease is a slow, progressive disorder with no cure. Persons over the age of 50 are at risk. Signs and symptoms become worse over time. They include:
  - *Tremors*—often start in one finger and spread to the whole arm. Pill-rolling movements—rubbing the thumb and index finger—may occur. The person may have trembling in the hands, arms, legs, jaw, and face.
  - *Rigid, stiff muscles*—in the arms, legs, neck, and trunk.
  - *Slow movements*—the person has a slow, shuffling gait.
  - *Stooped posture and impaired balance*—it is hard to walk. Falls are a risk.
  - *Mask-like expression*—the person cannot blink and smile. A fixed stare is common.
- Other signs and symptoms that develop over time include swallowing and chewing problems, constipation, and bladder problems. Sleep problems, depression, and emotional changes (fear, insecurity) can occur. So can memory loss and slow thinking. The person may have slurred, monotone, and soft speech. Some people talk too fast or repeat what they say.
- Drugs are ordered to treat and control the disease. Exercise and physical therapy improve strength, posture, balance, and mobility. Therapy is needed for speech and swallowing problems. The person may need help with eating and self-care. Safety measures are needed to prevent falls and injury.

Multiple Sclerosis
- Multiple sclerosis (MS) is a chronic disease. The myelin (which covers nerve fibers) in the brain and spinal cord is destroyed. Nerve impulses are not sent to and from the brain in a normal manner. Functions are impaired or lost. There is no cure.
- Symptoms usually start between the ages of 20 and 40. Signs and symptoms depend on the damaged area. They may include vision problems, muscle weakness in the arms and legs, balance problems that affect standing and walking. Tingling, prickling, or numb sensations may occur. Also, partial or complete paralysis and pain may occur.
- Persons with MS are kept active as long as possible and as independent as possible. Skin care, hygiene, and range-of-motion exercises are important. So are turning, positioning, and deep breathing and coughing. Bowel and bladder elimination is promoted. Injuries and complications from bedrest are prevented.

Spinal Cord Injury
- Spinal cord injuries can permanently damage the nervous system. Common causes are stab or gunshot wounds, motor vehicle crashes, falls, and sports injuries.
- The higher the level of injury, the more functions lost:
  - Lumbar injuries—sensory and muscle function in the legs is lost. The person has **paraplegia**—paralysis in legs and lower trunk.
  - Thoracic injuries—sensory and muscle function below the chest is lost. The person has paraplegia.
  - Cervical injuries—sensory and muscle function of the arms, legs, and trunk is lost. Paralysis in

the arms, legs, and trunk is called **quadriplegia** or **tetraplegia.**
- Review Box 26-8, Care of Persons With Paralysis, in the textbook.

HEARING LOSS
- Obvious signs and symptoms of hearing loss include:
  - Speaking too loudly
  - Leaning forward to hear
  - Turning and cupping the better ear toward the speaker
  - Answering questions or responding inappropriately
  - Asking for words to be repeated
  - Asking others to speak louder or to speak more slowly and clearly
  - Having trouble hearing over the phone
  - Finding it hard to follow conversations when two or more people are talking
  - Turning up the TV, radio, or music volume so loud that others complain
- Persons with hearing loss may wear hearing aids or lip-read (speech-read). They watch facial expressions, gestures, and body language. Some people learn American Sign Language (ASL). Others may have hearing assistance dogs.
- Review Box 26-9, Measures to Promote Hearing, in the textbook.
- Hearing aids are battery-operated. If they do not seem to work properly:
  - Check if the hearing aid is on. It has an on and off switch.
  - Check the battery position.
  - Insert a new battery if needed.
  - Clean the hearing aid. Follow the nurse's direction and the manufacturer's instructions.
- Hearing aids are turned off when not in use. The battery is removed.
- Handle and care for hearing aids properly. If lost or damaged, report it to the nurse at once.

EYE DISORDERS
- *Glaucoma.* Glaucoma results when fluid builds up in the eye and causes pressure on the optic nerve. The optic nerve is damaged. Vision loss with eventual blindness occurs. Drugs and surgery can control glaucoma and prevent further damage to the optic nerve. Prior damage cannot be reversed.
- *Cataract.* Cataract is a clouding of the lens in the eye. Signs and symptoms include cloudy, blurry, or dimmed vision. Persons may also be sensitive to light and glares or see halos around lights. Poor vision at night and double vision in one eye are other symptoms. Surgery is the only treatment.

Review Box 26-10, Nursing Measures After Cataract Surgery, in the textbook.

Impaired Vision and Blindness
- Birth defects, accidents, and eye diseases are among the many causes of impaired vision and blindness. They also are complications of some diseases.
- Review Box 26-11, Caring for Blind and Visually Impaired Persons, in the textbook.

Corrective Lenses
- Clean eyeglasses daily and as needed.
- Protect eyeglasses from loss or damage. When not worn, put them in their case.
- Contact lenses are cleaned, removed, and stored according to the manufacturer's instructions.

CARDIOVASCULAR DISORDERS
Angina
- Angina is chest pain. It is from reduced blood flow to part of the heart muscle. Chest pain is described as tightness, pressure, squeezing, or burning in the chest. Pain can occur in the shoulders, arms, neck, jaw, or back. The person may be pale, feel faint, and perspire. Dyspnea is common. Nausea, fatigue, and weakness may occur. Some persons complain of "gas" or indigestion.
- Rest often relieves symptoms in 3 to 15 minutes. Chest pain lasting longer than a few minutes and not relieved by rest and nitroglycerin may signal heart attack. The person needs emergency care.

Myocardial Infarction
- Myocardial infarction (MI) also is called *heart attack, acute myocardial infarction (AMI),* and *acute coronary syndrome (ACS).*
- Blood flow to the heart muscle is suddenly blocked. Part of the heart muscle dies. MI is an emergency. Sudden cardiac death *(sudden cardiac arrest)* can occur.
- Review Box 26-13, Signs and Symptoms of Myocardial Infarction, in the textbook.

Heart Failure
- Heart failure or congestive heart failure (CHF) occurs when the heart is weakened and cannot pump normally. Blood backs up. Tissue congestion occurs.
- Drugs are given to strengthen the heart. They also reduce the amount of fluid in the body. A sodium-controlled diet is ordered. Oxygen is given. Semi-Fowler's position is preferred for breathing. I&O, daily weight, elastic stockings, and range-of-motion exercises are part of the care plan.

RESPIRATORY DISORDERS
Chronic Obstructive Pulmonary Disease
- Two disorders are grouped under chronic obstructive pulmonary disease (COPD). They are chronic bronchitis and emphysema. These disorders obstruct airflow. Lung function is gradually lost.
- *Chronic Bronchitis.* Bronchitis means inflammation of the bronchi. Chronic bronchitis occurs after repeated episodes of bronchitis. Smoking is the major cause. Smoker's cough in the morning is often the first symptom of chronic bronchitis. Over time, the cough becomes more frequent. The person has difficulty breathing and tires easily. The person must stop smoking. Oxygen therapy and breathing exercises are often ordered. If a respiratory tract infection occurs, the person needs prompt treatment.
- *Emphysema.* In emphysema, the alveoli enlarge and become less elastic. They do not expand and shrink normally when breathing in and out. Air becomes trapped when exhaling. Smoking is the most common cause. The person has shortness of breath and a cough. Sputum may contain pus. Fatigue is common. The person works hard to breathe in and out. Breathing is easier when the person sits upright and slightly forward. The person must stop smoking. Respiratory therapy, breathing exercises, oxygen, and drug therapy are ordered.

Asthma
- In asthma, the airway becomes inflamed and narrow. Extra mucus is produced. Dyspnea results. Wheezing and coughing are common. So are pain and tightening in the chest. Asthma usually is triggered by allergies. Other triggers include air pollutants and irritants, smoking and second-hand smoke, respiratory tract infections, exertion, and cold air. Asthma is treated with drugs. Severe attacks may require emergency care.

Pneumonia
- Pneumonia is an inflammation and infection of lung tissue. Bacteria, viruses, and other microbes are causes.
- High fever, chills, painful cough, chest pain on breathing, and rapid pulse occur. Shortness of breath and rapid breathing also occur. Cyanosis may be present. Sputum is thick and white, green, yellow, or rust-colored. Other signs and symptoms are nausea, vomiting, headache, tiredness, and muscle aches.
- Drugs are ordered for infection and pain. Fluid intake is increased. Intravenous therapy and oxygen may be needed. Semi-Fowler's position eases breathing. Rest is important. Standard

Precautions are followed. Isolation Precautions are used depending on the cause.

Tuberculosis
- Tuberculosis (TB) is a bacterial infection in the lungs. TB is spread by airborne droplets with coughing, sneezing, speaking, singing, or laughing. Those who have close, frequent contact with an infected person are at risk. TB is more likely to occur in close, crowded areas. Age, poor nutrition, and HIV infection are other risk factors.
- Signs and symptoms are tiredness, loss of appetite, weight loss, fever, and night sweats. Cough and sputum production increase over time. Sputum may contain blood. Chest pain occurs.
- Drugs for TB are given. Standard Precautions and Isolation Precautions are needed. The person must cover the mouth and nose with tissues when sneezing, coughing, or producing sputum. Tissues are flushed down the toilet, placed in a BIOHAZARD bag, or placed in a paper bag and burned. Hand washing after contact with sputum is essential.

DIGESTIVE DISORDERS
Vomiting
- These measures are needed:
  - Follow Standard Precautions and the Bloodborne Pathogen Standard.
  - Turn the person's head well to one side. This prevents aspiration.
  - Place a kidney basin under the person's chin.
  - Move vomitus away from the person.
  - Provide oral hygiene.
  - Observe vomitus for color, odor, and undigested food. If it looks like coffee grounds, it contains undigested blood. This signals bleeding. Report your observations.
  - Measure, report, and record the amount of vomitus. Also record the amount on the I&O record.
  - Save a specimen for laboratory study.
  - Dispose of vomitus after the nurse observes it.
  - Eliminate odors.
  - Provide for comfort.

Hepatitis
- Hepatitis is an inflammation of the liver. It can be mild or cause death. Signs and symptoms are listed in Box 26-14 in the textbook. Some people do not have symptoms.
- Protect yourself and others. Follow Standard Precautions and the Bloodborne Pathogen Standard. Isolation Precautions are ordered as necessary. Assist the person with hygiene and hand washing as needed.

URINARY SYSTEM DISORDERS
Urinary Tract Infections (UTIs)
- UTIs are common. Catheters, poor perineal hygiene, immobility, and poor fluid intake are common causes.

Prostate Enlargement
- The prostate grows larger as a man grows older. This is called benign prostatic hyperplasia (BPH). The enlarged prostate presses against the urethra. This obstructs urine flow through the urethra. Bladder function is gradually lost. Most men in their 60s and older have some symptoms of BPH.

REPRODUCTIVE DISORDERS
Sexually Transmitted Diseases
- A sexually transmitted disease (STD) is spread by oral, vaginal, or anal sex. Some people do not have signs and symptoms or are not aware of an infection. Others know but do not seek treatment because of embarrassment. Standard Precautions and the Bloodborne Pathogen Standard are followed.

ENDOCRINE DISORDERS
Diabetes
- In this disorder the body cannot produce or use insulin properly. Insulin is needed for glucose to move from the blood into the cells. Sugar builds up in the blood. Cells do not have enough sugar for energy and cannot function.
- Diabetes must be controlled to prevent complications. Complications include blindness, renal failure, nerve damage, and damage to the gums and teeth. Heart and blood vessel diseases are other problems. They can lead to stroke, heart attack, and slow healing. Foot and leg wounds and ulcers are very serious.
- Good foot care is needed. Corns, blisters, calluses, and other foot problems can lead to an infection and amputation.
- Blood glucose is monitored for:
  - *Hypoglycemia*—low sugar in the blood.
  - *Hyperglycemia*—high sugar in the blood.
- Review Table 26-1 in the textbook for the causes, signs, and symptoms of hypoglycemia and hyperglycemia. Both can lead to death if not corrected. You must call for the nurse at once.

IMMUNE SYSTEM DISORDERS
Acquired Immunodeficiency Syndrome
- Acquired immunodeficiency syndrome (AIDS) is caused by a virus. The virus is spread through body fluids—blood, semen, vaginal secretions, and breast milk. HIV is not spread by saliva, tears, sweat, sneezing, coughing, insects, or casual contact.
- Persons with AIDS are at risk for pneumonia, tuberculosis, Kaposi's sarcoma (a cancer), and nervous system damage.
- To protect yourself and others from the virus, follow Standard Precautions and the Bloodborne Pathogen Standard.
- Review Box 26-17, Caring for the Person With AIDS, in the textbook.
- Older persons also get AIDS. They get and spread HIV through sexual contact and IV drug use. Aging and some diseases can mask the signs and symptoms of AIDS. Older persons are less likely to be tested for HIV/AIDS.

CHAPTER 26 REVIEW QUESTIONS
Circle the BEST answer.
1. A person with cancer may need all the following *except*
   a. Pain relief or control
   b. Avoidance from you
   c. Fluids and nutrition
   d. Psychological support
2. The person had a stroke. Care includes all the following *except*
   a. Place the signal light on the person's strong side
   b. Reposition the person every 2 hours
   c. Perform ROM exercises as ordered
   d. Place objects on the affected side
3. The person with hemiplegia
   a. Is paralyzed on one side of the body
   b. Has both arms paralyzed
   c. Has both legs paralyzed
   d. Has all extremities paralyzed
4. The person with multiple sclerosis should be kept active as long as possible.
   a. True
   b. False
5. The person has paralysis in the legs and lower trunk. This is called
   a. Quadriplegia
   b. Paraplegia
   c. Hemiplegia
   d. Tetraplegia
6. A person is hard-of-hearing. You do the following *except*
   a. Face the person when speaking
   b. Speak clearly, distinctly, and slowly
   c. Use facial expressions and gestures to give clues
   d. Use long sentences

7. A person has taken his hearing aid out for the evening. You do the following *except*
   a. Make sure the hearing aid is turned off
   b. Keep the battery in the hearing aid
   c. Place the hearing aid in a safe place
   d. Handle the hearing aid carefully

8. A person is blind. You do the following *except*
   a. Identify yourself when you enter his room
   b. Describe people, places, and things thoroughly
   c. Rearrange his furniture without telling him
   d. Encourage him to do as much for himself as possible

9. Which statement about angina is *false?*
   a. Angina is chest pain.
   b. The person may be pale and perspire.
   c. Rest often relieves the symptoms.
   d. You do not report angina to the nurse.

10. A person has heart failure. You do all the following *except*
    a. Measure intake and output
    b. Measure weight daily
    c. Promote a diet that is high in salt
    d. Restrict fluids as ordered

11. Which position is usually best for the person with pneumonia?
    a. Semi-Fowler's
    b. Prone
    c. Supine
    d. Trendelenburg's

12. A person is vomiting. You should do all the following *except*
    a. Follow Standard Precautions and the Bloodborne Pathogen Standard
    b. Keep the person supine
    c. Provide oral hygiene
    d. Observe vomitus for color, odor, and undigested food

13. Which statement is *false?*
    a. Older persons are at high risk for urinary tract infections.
    b. Skin irritation and infection can occur if urine leaks onto the skin
    c. Benign prostatic hypertrophy may cause urinary problems in women.
    d. Some people may not be aware of having a sexually transmitted disease.

14. A person with diabetes is trembling, sweating, and feels faint. You
    a. Tell the nurse immediately
    b. Tell the nurse at the end of the shift
    c. Tell another nursing assistant
    d. Ignore the symptoms

15. Which statement about HIV is *false?*
    a. HIV is spread through body fluids.
    b. Standard Precautions and the Bloodborne Pathogen Standard are followed.
    c. Older persons cannot get and spread HIV.
    d. Older persons are less likely to be tested for HIV/AIDS.

Answers to these questions are on p. 425.

CHAPTER 27 CARING FOR PERSONS WITH MENTAL HEALTH PROBLEMS

- The whole person has physical, social, psychological, and spiritual parts. Each part affects the other.
- **Mental health** means the person copes with and adjusts to everyday stresses in ways accepted by society.
- **Mental illness** is a disturbance in the ability to cope with or adjust to stress. Behavior and function are impaired. Mental disorder, emotional illness, and psychiatric disorder also mean mental illness.

ANXIETY DISORDERS

- **Anxiety** is a vague, uneasy feeling in response to stress. The person may not know why or the cause. The person senses danger or harm—real or imagined. Some anxiety is normal. Review Box 27-1, Signs and Symptoms of Anxiety, in the textbook.
- Coping and defense mechanisms are used to relieve anxiety. Review Box 27-2, Defense Mechanisms, in the textbook.
- Some common anxiety disorders include panic disorder, phobias, obsessive-compulsive disorder, and post-traumatic stress disorder.
- *Panic disorder.* **Panic** is an intense and sudden feeling of fear, anxiety, terror, or dread. Onset is sudden with no obvious reason. The person cannot function. Signs and symptoms of anxiety are severe.
- *Phobias.* **Phobia** means an intense fear. The person has an intense fear of an object, situation, or activity that has little or no actual danger. The person avoids what is feared. When faced with the fear, the person has high anxiety and cannot function.
- *Obsessive-compulsive disorder (OCD).* An **obsession** is a recurrent, unwanted thought, idea, or image. **Compulsion** is repeating an act over and over again. The act may not make sense, but the person has much anxiety if the act is not done. Some persons with OCD also have depression, eating disorders, substance abuse, and other anxiety disorders.
- *Post-traumatic stress disorder (PTSD).* PTSD occurs after a terrifying ordeal. The ordeal involved physical harm or the threat of physical harm. Review Box 27-3, Signs and Symptoms of Post-Traumatic Stress Disorder, in the textbook.

Flashbacks are common. A **flashback** is reliving the trauma in thoughts during the day and in nightmares during sleep. During a flashback, the person may lose touch with reality. He or she may believe that the trauma is happening all over again. Signs and symptoms usually develop about 3 months after the harmful event. Or they may emerge years later. PTSD can develop at any age.

SCHIZOPHRENIA

- *Schizophrenia* means split mind. It is a severe, chronic, disabling brain disorder that involves:
  - **Psychosis**—a state of severe mental impairment. The person does not view the real or unreal correctly.
  - **Delusion**—a false belief.
  - **Hallucination**—seeing, hearing, smelling, or feeling something that is not real.
  - **Paranoia**—a disorder of the mind. The person has false beliefs (delusions). He or she is suspicious about a person or situation.
  - **Delusion of grandeur**—an exaggerated belief about one's importance, wealth, power, or talents.
  - **Delusion of persecution**—the false belief that one is being mistreated, abused, or harassed.
- The person with schizophrenia has problems relating to others. He or she may be paranoid. The person may have difficulty organizing thoughts. Responses are inappropriate. Communication is disturbed. The person may withdraw. Some people regress to an earlier time or condition. Some persons with schizophrenia attempt suicide.

MOOD DISORDERS

- Mood disorders involve feelings, emotions, and moods.

Bipolar Disorder

- The person with bipolar disorder has severe extremes in mood, energy, and ability to function. There are emotional lows (depression) and emotional highs (mania). This disorder is also called manic-depressive illness. This disorder must be managed throughout life. Review Box 27-4, Signs and Symptoms of Bipolar Disorder, in the textbook. Bipolar disorder can damage relationships and affect school or work performance. Some people are suicidal.

Major Depression

- Depression involves the body, mood, and thoughts. Symptoms affect work, study, sleep, eating, and other activities. The person is very sad.
- Depression is common in older persons. They have many losses—death of family and friends, loss of health, loss of body functions, loss of independence. Loneliness and the side effects of some drugs also are causes. Review Box 27-5, Signs and Symptoms of Depression in Older Persons, in the textbook. Depression in older persons is often overlooked or a wrong diagnosis is made.

SUBSTANCE ABUSE AND ADDICTION

Alcoholism

- Alcohol affects alertness, judgment, coordination, and reaction time. Over time, heavy drinking damages the brain, central nervous system, liver, heart, kidneys, and stomach. It causes changes in the heart and blood vessels. It also can cause forgetfulness and confusion. Alcoholism is a chronic disease. There is no cure. However, alcoholism can be treated. Counseling and drugs are used to help the person stop drinking. The person must avoid all alcohol to avoid a relapse.
- Alcohol effects vary with age. Even small amounts can make older persons feel "high." Older persons are at risk for falls, vehicle crashes, and other injuries from drinking. Mixing alcohol with some drugs can be harmful or fatal. Alcohol also makes some health problems worse.

SUICIDE

- **Suicide** means to kill oneself.
- People think about suicide when they feel hopeless or when they cannot see solutions to their problems. Suicide is most often linked to depression, alcohol or substance abuse, or stressful events. Review Box 27-6, Risk Factors for Suicide, in the textbook.
- If a person mentions or talks about suicide, take the person seriously. Call for the nurse at once. Do not leave the person alone.

CARE AND TREATMENT

- Treatment of mental health problems involves having the person explore his or her thoughts and feelings. This is done through psychotherapy and behavior, group, occupational, art, and family therapies. Often drugs are ordered.
- The care plan reflects the person's needs. The physical, safety and security, and emotional needs of the person must be met.
- Communication is important. Be alert to nonverbal communication.

CHAPTER 27 REVIEW QUESTIONS
Circle the BEST answer.
1. A person may not know why anxiety occurs.
   a. True
   b. False

2. Panic is an intense and sudden feeling of fear, anxiety, terror, or dread.
   a. True
   b. False
3. A person with an obsessive-compulsive disorder has a ritual that is repeated over and over again.
   a. True
   b. False
4. A person talks about suicide. You must do the following *except*
   a. Call the nurse at once
   b. Stay with the person
   c. Leave the person alone
   d. Take the person seriously
5. Which statement about depression in older persons is *false?*
   a. Depression is often overlooked in older persons.
   b. Depression rarely occurs in older persons.
   c. Loneliness may be a cause of depression in older persons.
   d. Side effects of some drugs may cause depression in older persons.
6. Which statement is *false?*
   a. Communication is important when caring for a person with a mental health problem.
   b. You should be alert to nonverbal communication when caring for a person with a mental health problem.
   c. The care plan reflects the needs of the person.
   d. The focus is only on the person's emotional needs.

Answers to these questions are on p. 426.

CHAPTER 28 CARING FOR PERSONS WITH CONFUSION AND DEMENTIA

- Changes in the brain and nervous system occur with aging. Review Box 28-1, Changes in the Nervous System From Aging, in the textbook.
- Changes in the brain can affect **cognitive function**—memory, thinking, reasoning, ability to understand, judgment, and behavior.

CONFUSION

- Confusion has many causes. Diseases, infections, hearing and vision loss, brain injury, and drug side effects are some causes.
- When caring for the confused person:
  - Follow the person's care plan.
  - Provide for safety.
  - Face the person and speak clearly.
  - Call the person by name every time you are in contact with him or her.
  - State your name. Show your name tag.

- Give the date and time each morning. Repeat as needed during the day and evening.
- Explain what you are going to do and why.
- Give clear, simple directions and answers to questions.
- Ask clear, simple questions. Give the person time to respond.
- Keep calendars and clocks with large numbers in the person's room.
- Have the person wear eyeglasses and hearing aids as needed.
- Use touch to communicate.
- Place familiar objects and pictures within the person's view.
- Provide newspapers, magazines, TV, and radio. Read to the person if appropriate.
- Discuss current events with the person.
- Maintain the day-night cycle.
- Provide a calm, relaxed, and peaceful setting.
- Follow the person's routine.
- Break tasks into small steps when helping the person.
- Do not rearrange furniture or the person's belongings.
- Encourage the person to take part in self-care.
- Be consistent.

DEMENTIA

- **Dementia** is the loss of cognitive function that interferes with routine personal, social, and occupational activities.
- Dementia is not a normal part of aging. Most older people do not have dementia.
- Some early warning signs include problems with dressing, cooking, and driving as well as getting lost in familiar places and misplacing items.
- Alzheimer's disease is the most common type of permanent dementia.

ALZHEIMER'S DISEASE

- Alzheimer's disease (AD) is a brain disease. Memory, thinking, reasoning, judgment, language, behavior, mood, and personality are affected.

Signs of AD

- The classic sign of AD is gradual loss of short-term memory. Warning signs include:
  - Asking the same questions over and over again.
  - Repeating the same story—word for word, again and again.
  - The person forgets activities that were once done regularly with ease.
  - Losing the ability to pay bills or balance a checkbook.
  - Getting lost in familiar places. Or misplacing household objects.

- Neglecting to bathe or wearing the same clothes over and over again. Meanwhile, the person insists that a bath was taken or that clothes were changed.
- Relying on someone else to make decisions or answer questions that he or she would have handled.
- Review Box 28-4, Signs of Alzheimer's Disease, in the textbook for other signs of AD.

Behaviors

- The following behaviors are common with AD:
  - *Wandering.* Persons with AD are not oriented to person, place, and time. They may wander away from home and not find their way back. The person cannot tell what is safe or dangerous.
  - *Sundowning.* With sundowning, signs, symptoms, and behaviors of AD increase during hours of darkness. As daylight ends, confusion, restlessness, anxiety, agitation, and other symptoms increase.
  - *Hallucinations.* The person with AD may see, hear, or feel things that are not real.
  - *Delusions.* People with AD may think they are some other person. A person may believe that the caregiver is someone else.
  - *Catastrophic Reactions.* The person reacts as if there is a disaster or tragedy.
  - *Agitation and Restlessness.* The person may pace, hit, or yell.
  - *Aggression and Combativeness.* These behaviors include hitting, pinching, grabbing, biting, or swearing.
  - *Screaming.* Persons with AD may scream to communicate.
  - *Abnormal Sexual Behaviors.* Sexual behaviors may involve the wrong person, the wrong time, and the wrong place. Persons with AD cannot control behavior.
  - *Repetitive Behaviors.* Persons with AD repeat the same motions over and over again.

CARE OF PERSONS WITH AD AND OTHER DEMENTIAS

- People with AD do not choose to be forgetful, incontinent, agitated, or rude. Nor do they choose to have other behaviors, signs, and symptoms of the disease. The disease causes the behaviors.
- Safety, hygiene, nutrition and fluids, elimination, and activity needs must be met. So must comfort and sleep needs. Review Box 28-6, Care of Persons With AD and Other Dementias, in the textbook.
- The person can have other health problems and injuries. However, the person may not recognize

pain, fever, constipation, incontinence, or other signs and symptoms. Carefully observe the person. Report any change in the person's usual behavior to the nurse.
- Infection is a risk. Provide good skin care, oral hygiene, and perineal care after bowel and bladder elimination.
- Supervised activities meet the person's needs and cognitive abilities.
- Impaired communication is a common problem. Avoid giving orders, wanting the truth, and correcting the person's errors.
- Always look for dangers in the person's room and in the hallways, lounges, dining areas, and other areas on the nursing unit. Remove the danger if you can.
- Every staff member must be alert to persons who wander. Such persons are allowed to wander in safe areas.

The Family

- The family may have physical, emotional, social, and financial stresses. The family often feels hopeless. No matter what is done, the person only gets worse. Anger and resentment may result. Guilt feelings are common.
- The family is an important part of the health team. They may help plan the person's care. For many persons, family members provide comfort. The family also needs support and understanding from the health team.

CHAPTER 28 REVIEW QUESTIONS
Circle the BEST answer.

1. Cognitive function involves all of the following *except*
   a. Memory and thinking
   b. Reasoning and understanding
   c. Personality and mood
   d. Judgment and behavior
2. When caring for a confused person, you do the following *except*
   a. Provide for safety
   b. Maintain the day-night schedule
   c. Keep calendars and clocks in the person's room
   d. Ask difficult-to-understand questions and give complex directions
3. Which statement about dementia is *false?*
   a. Dementia is a normal part of aging.
   b. The person may have changes in personality.
   c. Alzheimer's disease is the most common type of dementia.
   d. The person may have changes in behavior.

4. When caring for persons with AD, you do the following *except*
   a. Provide good skin care
   b. Talk to them in a calm voice
   c. Observe them closely for unusual behavior
   d. Allow personal choice in wandering

Answers to these questions are on p. 426.

CHAPTER 29 ASSISTING WITH EMERGENCY CARE
EMERGENCY CARE
- Rules for emergency care include:
  - Know your limits. Do not do more than you are able.
  - Stay calm.
  - Know where to find emergency supplies.
  - Follow Standard Precautions and the Bloodborne Pathogen Standard to the extent possible.
  - Check for life-threatening problems. Check for breathing, a pulse, and bleeding.
  - Keep the person lying down or as you found him or her.
  - Move the person only if the setting is unsafe. If the scene is not safe enough for you to approach, wait for help to arrive.
  - Perform necessary emergency measures.
  - Call for help.
  - Do not remove clothes unless necessary.
  - Keep the person warm. Cover the person with a blanket, coat, or sweater.
  - Reassure the person. Explain what is happening and that help was called.
  - Do not give the person food or fluids.
  - Keep onlookers away. They invade privacy.
- Review Box 29-1, Rules of Emergency Care, in the textbook for more information.

BASIC LIFE SUPPORT FOR ADULTS
- Cardiopulmonary resuscitation (CPR) supports breathing and circulation. It provides blood and oxygen to the heart, brain, and other organs until advanced emergency care is given. CPR is done if the person does not respond, is not breathing, and has no pulse.
- CPR involves four parts—the ABCDs of CPR:
  - *Airway*—the airway must be open and clear of obstructions. The head tilt-chin lift method opens the airway.
  - *Breathing*—the person must get oxygen. The rescuer looks, listens, and feels for adequate breathing. He or she *looks* to see if the chest rises and falls, *listens* for the escape of air, and *feels*

for the flow of air. If the person is not breathing adequately, the person is given breaths.
  - *Circulation*—the heart, brain, and other organs must receive blood. Chest compressions force blood through the circulatory system.
  - *Defibrillation*—ventricular fibrillation (VF, V-fib) is an abnormal heart rhythm. Rather than beating in a regular rhythm, the heart shakes and quivers. The heart does not pump blood. The heart, brain, and other organs do not receive blood and oxygen. A *defibrillator* is used to deliver a shock to the heart. This allows the return of a regular heart rhythm. Defibrillation as soon as possible after the onset of VF (V-fib) increases the person's chance of survival.

SEIZURES
- You cannot stop a seizure. However, you can protect the person from injury:
  - Follow the rules in Box 29-1 in the textbook.
  - Do not leave the person alone.
  - Lower the person to the floor.
  - Note the time the seizure started.
  - Place something soft under the person's head.
  - Loosen tight jewelry and clothing around the person's neck.
  - Turn the person onto his or her side. Make sure the head is turned to the side.
  - Do not put any object or your fingers between the person's teeth.
  - Do not try to stop the seizure or control the person's movements.
  - Move furniture, equipment, and sharp objects away from the person.
  - Note the time when the seizure ends.
  - Make sure the mouth is clear of food, fluids, and saliva after the seizure.
  - Provide basic life support if the person is not breathing after the seizure.

FAINTING
- **Fainting** is the sudden loss of consciousness from an inadequate blood supply to the brain.
- Warning signals are dizziness, perspiration, and blackness before the eyes. The person looks pale. The pulse is weak. Respirations are shallow if consciousness is lost. Emergency care includes:
  - Have the person sit or lie down before fainting occurs.
  - If sitting, the person bends forward and places the head between the knees.
  - If the person is lying down, raise the legs.
  - Loosen tight clothing.

- Keep the person lying down if fainting has occurred. Raise the legs.
- Do not let the person get up until symptoms have subsided for about 5 minutes.
- Help the person to a sitting position after recovery from fainting.

CHAPTER 29 REVIEW QUESTIONS
Circle the BEST answer.
1. During an emergency, you do all of the following *except*
   a. Perform only procedures you have been trained to do
   b. Keep the person lying down or as you found him or her
   c. Let the person become cold
   d. Reassure the person and explain what is happening
2. During an emergency, you keep onlookers away.
   a. True
   b. False
3. During a seizure, you do the following *except*
   a. Turn the person's body to the side
   b. Place your fingers in the person's mouth
   c. Note the time the seizure started and ended
   d. Turn the person's head to the side
4. Which statement about fainting is *false*?
   a. If standing, have the person sit down before fainting.
   b. If sitting, have the person bend forward and place his head between his knees before fainting occurs.
   c. Tighten the person's clothing.
   d. Raise the legs if the person is lying down.
Answers to these questions are on p. 426.

CHAPTER 30 CARING FOR THE DYING PERSON
ATTITUDES ABOUT DEATH
- Attitudes about death often change as a person grows older and with changing circumstances.

Culture and Religion
- Practices and attitudes about death differ among cultures. Also, attitudes about death are closely related to religion.

Age
- Adults fear pain and suffering, dying alone, and the invasion of privacy. They also fear loneliness and separation from loved ones. Adults often resent death because it affects plans, hopes, dreams, and ambitions.

- Older persons usually have fewer fears than younger adults. Some welcome death as freedom from pain, suffering, and disability. Death also means reunion with those who have died. Like younger adults, they often fear dying alone.

THE STAGES OF DYING
- Dr. Kubler-Ross described five stages of dying. They are:
  - *Stage 1: Denial.* The person refuses to believe he or she is going to die.
  - *Stage 2: Anger.* There is anger and rage, often at family, friends, and the health team.
  - *Stage 3: Bargaining.* Often the person bargains with God for more time.
  - *Stage 4: Depression.* The person is sad and mourns things that were lost.
  - *Stage 5: Acceptance.* The person is calm and at peace. The person accepts death.
- Dying persons do not always pass through all five stages. A person may never get beyond a certain stage. Some move back and forth between stages.

THE PERSON'S NEEDS
- Dying people have psychological, social, and spiritual needs. You need to listen and use touch.
  - *Listening.* Let the person express feelings and emotions in his or her own way. Do not worry about saying the wrong thing or finding the right words. You do not need to say anything.
  - *Touch.* Touch shows caring and concern. Sometimes the person does not want to talk but needs you nearby. Silence, along with touch, is a meaningful way to communicate.
- Some people may want to see a spiritual leader. Or they may want to take part in religious practices.

Vision, Hearing, and Speech
- Vision blurs and gradually fails. Explain what you are doing to the person or in the room. Provide good eye care.
- Hearing is one of the last functions lost. Always assume that the person can hear.
- Speech becomes difficult. Anticipate the person's needs. Do not ask questions that need long answers.

Mouth, Nose, and Skin
- Frequent oral hygiene is given as death nears.
- Crusting and irritation of the nostrils can occur. Carefully clean the nose.
- Skin care, bathing, and preventing pressure ulcers are necessary. Change linens and gowns whenever needed.

Elimination
- Urinary and fecal incontinence may occur. Give perineal care as needed.

Comfort and Positioning
- Skin care, personal hygiene, back massages, oral hygiene, and good alignment promote comfort.
- Frequent position changes and supportive devices promote comfort.
- Semi-Fowler's position is usually best for breathing problems.

The Person's Room
- The person's room should be comfortable and pleasant. It should be well lit and well ventilated. Remove unnecessary equipment.
- Mementos, pictures, cards, flowers, and religious items provide comfort. The person and family arrange the room as they wish.

THE FAMILY
- This is a hard time for family. The family goes through stages like the dying person. Be available, courteous, and considerate.
- The person and family need time together. However, you cannot neglect care because the family is present. Most agencies let family members help give care.

LEGAL ISSUES
- *Living wills.* A living will is a document about measures that support or maintain life when death is likely. A living will may instruct doctors not to start measures that promote dying or to remove measures that prolong dying.
- *Durable power of attorney for health care.* This gives the power to make health care decisions to another person. When a person cannot make health care decisions, the person with durable power of attorney can do so.
- *"Do Not Resuscitate" (DNR) order.* This means the person will not be resuscitated. The person is allowed to die with peace and dignity. The orders are written after consulting with the person and family.
- You may not agree with care and resuscitation decisions. However, you must follow the person's or family's wishes and the doctor's orders. These may be against your personal, religious, and cultural values. If so, discuss the matter with the nurse. An assignment change may be needed.

SIGNS OF DEATH
- There are signs that death is near:
  - Movement, muscle tone, and sensation are lost.
  - Abdominal distention, fecal incontinence, nausea, and vomiting are common.

- Body temperature rises. The person feels cool, looks pale, and perspires heavily.
- The pulse is fast, weak, and irregular. Blood pressure starts to fall.
- Slow or rapid respirations are observed. Mucus collects in the airway. This causes the death rattle that is heard.
- Pain decreases as the person loses consciousness. Some people are conscious until the moment of death.
- The signs of death include no pulse, no respirations, and no blood pressure. The pupils are dilated and fixed.

CARE OF THE BODY AFTER DEATH
- Post-mortem care is done to maintain a good appearance of the body.
- Moving the body when giving post-mortem care can cause remaining air in the lungs, stomach, and intestines to be expelled. When air is expelled, sounds are produced.
- When giving post-mortem care, follow Standard Precautions and the Bloodborne Pathogen Standard.

CHAPTER 30 REVIEW QUESTIONS
Circle the BEST answer.
1. Which statement is *false?*
   a. Adults fear dying alone.
   b. Older persons usually have fewer fears about dying than younger adults.
   c. Adults often resent death.
   d. All adults welcome death.
2. Persons in the denial stage of dying
   a. Are angry
   b. Bargain with God
   c. Refuse to believe that they are dying
   d. Are calm and at peace
3. When caring for a person who is dying, you should do the following *except*
   a. Listen to the person
   b. Talk about your feelings about death
   c. Provide privacy during spiritual moments
   d. Use touch to show care and concern
4. When caring for a dying person, you provide all of the following *except*
   a. Eye care
   b. Oral hygiene
   c. Good skin care
   d. Physical exercise
5. When giving post-mortem care, you should wear gloves.
   a. True
   b. False
Answers to these questions are on p. 426.

PRACTICE EXAMINATION 1

This test contains 75 questions. For each question, circle the BEST answer.

1. A nurse asks you to give a person his drug when he is done in the bathroom. Your response to the nurse is
   A. "I will give the drug for you."
   B. "I will ask the other nursing assistant to give the drug."
   C. "I am sorry, but I cannot give that drug. I will let you know when he is out of the bathroom."
   D. "I refuse to give that drug."

2. An ethical person
   A. Does not judge others
   B. Avoids persons whose standards and values are different from his or hers
   C. Is prejudiced and biased
   D. Causes harm to another person

3. You smell alcohol on the breath of a co-worker. You
   A. Ignore the situation
   B. Tell the co-worker to get counseling
   C. Take a break and drink some alcohol too
   D. Tell the nurse at once

4. A person's signal light goes unanswered. He gets out of bed and falls. His leg is broken. This is
   A. Neglect
   B. Emotional abuse
   C. Physical abuse
   D. Malpractice

5. Your mom asks you about a person on your unit. How should you respond?
   A. "She is walking better now that she is receiving physical therapy."
   B. "I'm sorry, but I cannot talk about her. It is unprofessional, and violates her privacy and confidentiality."
   C. "Don't tell anyone I told you, but she is getting worse."
   D. "She has been very sad recently and needs visitors."

6. You are going off duty. The nursing assistant coming on duty is on the unit with you. A person puts her light on. Your response is
   A. "I'm ready to go. I will let you answer that light."
   B. "I've been here all day so I am not answering that light."
   C. "No one helped me answer lights when I came on duty."
   D. "I will answer that light so you can get organized for the shift."

7. When recording in the medical record, you
   A. Write in pencil
   B. Spell words incorrectly
   C. Use only center-approved abbreviations
   D. Record what your co-worker did

8. You are answering the phone in the nurses' station. You
   A. Answer in a rushed manner
   B. Give a courteous greeting
   C. End the conversation and hang-up without saying good-bye
   D. Give confidential information about a resident to the caller

9. A person who was admitted to the nursing center yesterday does not feel safe. You
   A. Are rude as you care for the person
   B. Ignore the person's requests for information
   C. Show the person around the nursing center
   D. Act rushed as you care for the person

10. A person is angry and is shouting at you. You should
    A. Yell back at the person
    B. Stay calm and professional
    C. Put the person in a room away from others
    D. Call the family

11. When speaking with another person, you
    A. Use medical terms that may not be familiar to the person
    B. Mumble your words as you talk
    C. Ask several questions at a time
    D. Speak clearly and distinctly

12. To use a transfer or gait belt safely, you should
    A. Ignore the manufacturer's instructions
    B. Leave the excess strap dangling
    C. Apply the belt over bare skin
    D. Apply the belt under the breasts
13. When you are listening to a person, you
    A. Look around the room
    B. Sit with your arms crossed
    C. Act rushed and not interested in what the person is saying
    D. Have good eye contact with the person
14. When caring for a person who is comatose, you
    A. Make jokes about how sick the person is
    B. Care for the person without talking to him or her
    C. Explain what you are doing to him or her
    D. Discuss your problems with the other nursing assistant in the room with you
15. You need to give care to a person when a visitor is present. You
    A. Politely ask the visitor to leave the room
    B. Do the care in the presence of the visitor
    C. Expose the person's body in front of the visitor
    D. Rudely tell the visitor where to wait while you care for the person
16. A person tells you he wants to talk with a minister. You
    A. Ignore the request
    B. Tell the nurse
    C. Ask what the person wants to discuss with the minister
    D. Tell the person there is no need to talk with a minister
17. When you care for a person who has a restraint, you
    A. Observe the person every 15 minutes
    B. Remove the restraint and reposition the person every 4 hours
    C. Apply the restraint tightly
    D. Apply the restraint incorrectly
18. As a person ages
    A. The skin becomes less dry
    B. Muscle strength increases
    C. Reflexes are faster
    D. Bladder muscles weaken
19. A person you are caring for touches your buttocks several times. You
    A. Tell the person you like being touched
    B. Ask the person not to touch you again
    C. Tell the person's daughter
    D. Tell the person's girlfriend

20. You see a person sliding out of a wheelchair. You
    A. Ignore the person
    B. Tell the nursing assistant assigned to the person
    C. Position the person correctly in the wheelchair
    D. Tell the nurse the person needs repositioning
21. You cannot read the person's name on the ID bracelet. You
    A. Tell the nurse so a new bracelet can be made
    B. Ignore the fact that you cannot read the name
    C. Ask another nursing assistant to identify the person
    D. Tell the family the person needs a new ID bracelet
22. The universal sign of choking is
    A. Holding your breath
    B. Clutching at the throat
    C. Having difficulty breathing
    D. Coughing
23. A person is on a diabetic diet. You
    A. Serve the person's meals late
    B. Let the person eat whenever he or she is hungry
    C. Sometimes check the tray to see what was eaten
    D. Tell the nurse about changes in the person's eating habits
24. With mild airway obstruction
    A. The person is usually unconscious
    B. The person cannot speak
    C. Forceful coughing often does not remove the object
    D. Forceful coughing often can remove the object
25. To relieve severe airway obstruction in a conscious adult, you do
    A. Abdominal thrusts
    B. Back thrusts
    C. Chest compressions
    D. A finger sweep
26. Faulty electrical equipment
    A. Can be used in a nursing center
    B. Should be given to the nurse
    C. Should be taken home by you for repair
    D. Should be used only with alert persons
27. A warning label has been removed from a hazardous substance container. You
    A. May use the substance if you know what is in the container
    B. Leave the container where it is
    C. Take the container to the nurse and explain the problem
    D. Tell another nursing assistant about the missing label

28. A person's beliefs and values are different from your views. What should you do?
    A. Refuse to care for the person.
    B. Delegate care to another nursing assistant.
    C. Tell the nurse about your concerns.
    D. Tell the person how you feel.
29. You find a person smoking in the nursing center. You should
    A. Ignore the situation
    B. Tell the person to leave
    C. Tell another nursing assistant
    D. Ask the person to put the cigarette out and show him or her where smoking is permitted
30. During a fire, the first thing you do is
    A. Rescue persons in immediate danger
    B. Sound the nearest fire alarm
    C. Close doors and windows to confine the fire
    D. Extinguish the fire
31. A person with Alzheimer's disease has increased restlessness and confusion as daylight ends. You
    A. Try to reason with the person
    B. Ask the person to tell you what is bothering him or her
    C. Provide a calm, quiet setting late in the day
    D. Complete his or her treatments and activities late in the day
32. To prevent suffocation, you should
    A. Make sure dentures fit loosely
    B. Cut food into large pieces
    C. Make sure the person can chew and swallow the food served
    D. Ignore loose teeth or dentures
33. When using a wheelchair, you should
    A. Lock both wheels before you transfer a person to and from the wheelchair
    B. Lock only one wheel before you transfer a person to and from the wheelchair
    C. Let the person's feet touch the floor when the chair is moving
    D. Let the person stand on the footplates
34. A person begins to fall while you are walking him or her. You should
    A. Try to prevent the fall
    B. Ease the person to the floor
    C. Yell at the person for falling
    D. Tell the nurse at the end of the shift
35. A person has a restraint on. You know that
    A. Restraints are used for staff convenience
    B. Death from strangulation is a risk factor to using a restraint
    C. Restraints may be used to punish a person
    D. A written nurse's order is required for a restraint

36. Before feeding a person, you
    A. Tell the other nursing assistant
    B. Go to the restroom
    C. Wash your hands
    D. Tell the nurse
37. When wearing gloves, you remember to
    A. Wear them several times before discarding them
    B. Wear the same ones from room to room
    C. Wear gloves with a tear or puncture
    D. Change gloves when they become contaminated with urine
38. When washing your hands, you
    A. Use hot water
    B. Let your uniform touch the sink
    C. Keep your watch at your wrist
    D. Keep your hands and forearms lower than your elbows
39. You need to move a box from the floor to the counter in the utility room. You
    A. Bend from your waist to pick up the box
    B. Hold the box away from your body as you pick it up
    C. Bend your knees and squat to lift the box
    D. Stand with your feet close together as you pick up the box
40. The nurse asks you to place a person in Fowler's position. You
    A. Put the bed flat
    B. Raise the head of the bed between 45 and 60 degrees
    C. Raise the head of the bed between 80 and 90 degrees
    D. Raise the head of the bed 15 degrees
41. You accidentally scratch a person. This is
    A. Neglect
    B. Negligence
    C. Malpractice
    D. Physical abuse
42. You positioned a person in a chair. For good body alignment, you
    A. Have the person's back and buttocks against the back of the chair
    B. Leave the person's feet unsupported
    C. Have the backs of the person's knees touch the edge of the chair
    D. Have the person sit on the edge of the chair
43. You need to transfer a person with a weak left leg from the bed to the wheelchair. You
    A. Get the person out of bed on the left side
    B. Get the person out of bed on the right side
    C. Keep the person in bed
    D. Ask the person what side moves first

44. A person tries to scratch and kick you. You should
    A. Protect yourself from harm
    B. Argue with the person
    C. Become angry with the person
    D. Ignore the person
45. When moving a person up in bed
    A. Window coverings may be left open so people can look in
    B. Body parts may be exposed
    C. Ask the person to help
    D. Ask the person to lie still
46. For comfort, most older persons prefer
    A. Rooms that are cold
    B. Restrooms that smell of urine
    C. Loud talking and laughter in the nurses' station
    D. Lighting that meets their needs
47. Signal lights are
    A. Placed on the person's strong side
    B. Answered when time permits
    C. Kept on the bedside table
    D. Kept on the person's weak side
48. A nurse asks you to inspect a person's closet. You
    A. Tell the nurse you cannot do this
    B. Inspect the closet when the person is in the dining room
    C. Ask the person if you can inspect his or her closet
    D. Tell the nurse to inspect the closet
49. When changing bed linens, you
    A. Hold the linen close to your uniform
    B. Shake the sheet when putting it on the bed
    C. Take only needed linen into the person's room
    D. Put dirty linen on the floor
50. To use a fire extinguisher, you
    A. Keep the safety pin in the extinguisher
    B. Direct the hose or nozzle at the top of the fire
    C. Squeeze the lever to start the stream
    D. Sweep the stream at the top of the fire
51. When doing mouth care for an unconscious person, you
    A. Do not need to wear gloves
    B. Give mouth care at least every 2 hours
    C. Place the person in a supine position
    D. Keep the mouth open with your fingers

52. A person is angry because he did not get to the activity room on time because a co-worker did not come to work. How should you respond to him?
    A. "It's not my fault. A co-worker called off today and we are short-staffed."
    B. "I'm sorry you were late for activities. I will try to plan better."
    C. "I am doing the best I can."
    D. "I'm just too busy."
53. You are asked to clean a person's dentures. You
    A. Use hot water
    B. Hold the dentures firmly and line the basin with a towel
    C. Wrap the dentures in tissues after cleaning
    D. Store the dentures in a denture cup with the person's room number on it
54. When bathing a person, you notice a rash that was not there before. You
    A. Do nothing
    B. Tell the person
    C. Tell the nurse and record it in the medical record
    D. Tell the person's daughter
55. When washing a person's eyes, you
    A. Use soap
    B. Clean the eye near you first
    C. Wipe from the inner to the outer aspect of the eye
    D. Wipe from the outer aspect to the inner aspect of the eye
56. When giving a back massage, you
    A. Use cold lotion
    B. Use light strokes
    C. Massage reddened bony areas
    D. Look for bruises and breaks in the skin
57. You need to give perineal care to a female. You
    A. Separate the labia and clean downward from front to back
    B. Separate the labia and clean upward from back to front
    C. Wear gloves only if there is drainage
    D. Only use water
58. When giving a person a tub bath or shower, you
    A. Do not give the person a signal light
    B. Turn the hot water on first, then the cold water
    C. Stay within hearing distance if the person can be left alone
    D. Direct water toward the person while adjusting the water temperature
59. A person is on an anticoagulant. You
    A. Use a safety razor
    B. Use an electric razor
    C. Let him grow a beard
    D. Let him choose which type of razor to use

60. A person with a weak left arm wants to remove his or her sweater. You
    A. Let the person do it without any assistance
    B. Help the person remove the sweater from his or her right arm first
    C. Help the person remove the sweater from his or her left arm first
    D. Tell the person to keep the sweater on
61. When talking with a person, you should call the person
    A. "Honey"
    B. By his or her first name
    C. By his or her title—Mr. or Mrs. or Miss
    D. "Grandpa" or "Grandma"
62. A person has an indwelling catheter. You
    A. Let the person lie on the tubing
    B. Disconnect the catheter from the drainage tubing every 8 hours
    C. Secure the catheter to the lower leg
    D. Measure and record the amount of urine in the drainage bag
63. A person needs to eat a diet that contains carbohydrates. Carbohydrates
    A. Are needed for tissue repair and growth
    B. Provide energy and fiber for bowel elimination
    C. Add flavor to food and help the body use certain vitamins
    D. Are needed for nerve and muscle function
64. You are taking a rectal temperature with a glass thermometer. You
    A. Insert the thermometer before lubricating it
    B. Leave the privacy curtain open
    C. Leave the thermometer in place for 10 minutes
    D. Hold the thermometer in place
65. A person has a blood pressure of 86/58. You
    A. Report the BP to the nurse at once
    B. Record the BP but do not tell the nurse
    C. Ask the unit secretary to tell the nurse
    D. Retake the BP in 30 minutes before telling the nurse
66. On which person would you take an oral temperature?
    A. An unconscious person
    B. The person receiving oxygen
    C. The person who breathes through his or her mouth
    D. A conscious person
67. When caring for a person who is blind or visually impaired, you
    A. Offer the person your arm and have the person walk a half step behind you
    B. Do as much for the person as possible
    C. Shout at the person when talking with him or her
    D. Touch the person before indicating your presence

68. You are caring for a person with dementia. You
    A. Misplace the person's clothes
    B. Choose the activities the person attends
    C. Send personal items home
    D. Let the family make choices if the person cannot
69. When caring for a person with a disability, you
    A. Can shout or scream at the person
    B. Can hit or strike the person
    C. Can call the person names
    D. Discuss your anger with the nurse
70. While bathing a person, you
    A. Keep doors and windows open
    B. Wash from the dirtiest areas to cleanest areas
    C. Encourage the person to help as much as possible
    D. Rub the skin dry
71. When a person is dying
    A. Assume that the person can hear you
    B. Oral care is done every 5 hours
    C. Skin care is done weekly
    D. Reposition the person every 3 hours
72. A person is on intake and output. You
    A. Measure only liquids such as water and juice
    B. Measure ice cream and gelatin as part of intake
    C. Measure IV fluids
    D. Measure tube feedings
73. A person has been on bedrest. You need to have the person walk. What will you do first?
    A. Help the person move quickly.
    B. Have the person dangle before getting out of bed.
    C. Have the person sit in a chair.
    D. Walk with the person as soon as he or she gets out of bed.
74. Your ring accidentally causes a skin tear on an elderly person. You
    A. Tell yourself to be more careful the next time
    B. Tell the nurse at once
    C. Do nothing
    D. Hope no one finds out
75. To protect a person's privacy, you should
    A. Keep all information about the person confidential
    B. Discuss the person's treatment with another nursing assistant in the lunch room
    C. Open the person's mail
    D. Keep the privacy curtain open when providing care to the person

PRACTICE EXAMINATION 2

This test contains 75 questions. For each question, circle the BEST answer.

1. You can refuse to do a delegated task when
   A. You are too busy
   B. You do not like the task
   C. The task is not in your job description
   D. It is the end of the shift

2. Mr. Smith does not want life-saving measures. You
   A. Explain to Mr. Smith why he should have life-saving measures
   B. Respect his decision
   C. Explain to Mr. Smith's family why life-saving measures are needed
   D. Tell your friend about Mr. Smith's decision

3. You are walking by a resident's room. You hear a nurse shouting at a person. This is
   A. Battery
   B. Malpractice
   C. Verbal abuse
   D. Neglect

4. When communicating with a foreign-speaking person, you
   A. Speak loudly or shout
   B. Use medical terms the person may not understand
   C. Use words the person seems to understand
   D. Speak quickly and mumble

5. To protect a person from getting burned, you
   A. Allow smoking in bed
   B. Turn hot water on first, then cold water
   C. Assist the person with drinking or eating hot food
   D. Let the person sleep with a heating pad

6. To prevent equipment accidents, you should
   A. Use two-pronged plugs on all electrical devices
   B. Follow the manufacturer's instructions
   C. Wipe up spills when you have time
   D. Use unfamiliar equipment without training

7. To prevent a person from falling, you should
   A. Ignore signal lights
   B. Use throw rugs on the floor
   C. Keep the bed in a high position
   D. Use grab bars in showers

8. You need to wash your hands
   A. Before you document a procedure
   B. After you remove gloves
   C. After you talk with a person
   D. After you talk with a co-worker

9. You need to turn a heavy person in bed. You
   A. Do the procedure alone
   B. Keep the privacy curtain open
   C. Ask the person to lie still
   D. Use good body mechanics

10. When transferring a person from a bed to a wheelchair, you never
    A. Ask a co-worker to help you
    B. Use a transfer or gait belt
    C. Have the person put his or her arms around your neck
    D. Lock the wheels on the wheelchair

11. When making a bed, you
    A. Keep the bed in the low position
    B. Wear gloves when removing linen
    C. Raise the head of the bed
    D. Raise the foot of the bed

12. To give perineal care to a male, you
    A. Use a circular motion and work toward the meatus
    B. Use a circular motion and start at the meatus and work outward
    C. Wear gloves only if there is drainage
    D. Use only water

13. A person with a weak left arm wants to put his or her sweater on. You
    A. Let the person do it without any assistance
    B. Help the person put the sweater on his or her right arm first
    C. Help the person put the sweater on his or her left arm first
    D. Tell the person to keep the sweater off

14. A person has an indwelling catheter. You
    A. Let the drainage bag touch the floor
    B. Keep the drainage bag higher than the bladder
    C. Hang the drainage bag on a bed rail
    D. Have the drainage bag hang from the bed frame or chair

15. A person needs to eat a diet that contains protein. Protein
    A. Is needed for tissue repair and growth
    B. Provides energy and fiber for bowel elimination
    C. Adds flavor to food and helps the body use certain vitamins
    D. Is needed for nerve and muscle function

16. Older persons
    A. Have an increased sense of thirst
    B. Need less water than younger persons
    C. May not feel thirsty
    D. Seldom need to have water offered to them

17. A person is NPO. You
    A. Post a sign in the bathroom
    B. Keep the water pitcher filled at the bedside
    C. Remove the water pitcher and glass from the room
    D. Provide oral hygiene every day

18. A person drank 3 oz of milk at lunch. He or she drank
    A. 30 mL
    B. 60 mL
    C. 90 mL
    D. 120 mL

19. When feeding a person, you
    A. Offer fluids at the end of the meal
    B. Use forks
    C. Do not talk to the person
    D. Allow time for chewing and swallowing

20. You need to do ROM to a person's right shoulder. You
    A. Force the joint beyond its present ROM
    B. Move the joint quickly
    C. Force the joint to the point of pain
    D. Support the part being exercised

21. A person has a weak left leg. The person should
    A. Hold the cane in his or her left hand
    B. Hold the cane in his or her right hand
    C. Hold the cane in either hand
    D. Use a walker

22. To promote comfort and relieve pain, you
    A. Keep wrinkles in the bed linens
    B. Position the person in good alignment
    C. Talk loudly to the person
    D. Use sudden and jarring movements of the bed or chair

23. A person is receiving oxygen through a nasal cannula. You
    A. Turn the oxygen higher when he or she is short of breath
    B. Fill the humidifier when it is not bubbling
    C. Check behind the ears and under the nose for signs of irritation
    D. Remove the cannula when the person goes to the dining room

24. You accidentally dropped a mercury glass thermometer. You
    A. Tell the nurse at once
    B. Put the mercury in your pocket
    C. Pick up the pieces of glass with your hands
    D. Touch the mercury

25. When taking a person's pulse, you
    A. Use the brachial pulse
    B. Take the pulse for 30 seconds if it is irregular
    C. Tell the nurse if the pulse is less than 60
    D. Use your thumb to take a pulse

26. You are counting respirations on a person. You
    A. Tell the person you are counting his or her respirations
    B. Count for 1 minute if an abnormal breathing pattern is noted
    C. Report a rate of 16 to the nurse at once
    D. Count for 30 seconds if an abnormal breathing pattern is noted

27. You are taking blood pressures on people assigned to you. An older person has a blood pressure of 188/96. You
    A. Report the BP to the nurse at once
    B. Finish taking all the blood pressures before telling the nurse
    C. Retake the BP in 30 minutes before telling the nurse
    D. Ask the unit secretary to tell the nurse about the BP

28. When would you take a rectal temperature?
    A. The person has diarrhea
    B. The person is confused
    C. The person is unconscious
    D. The person is agitated

29. A person has been admitted to the nursing center recently. You
    A. Look through his or her belongings
    B. Ignore his or her questions
    C. Speak in a gentle, calm voice
    D. Enter the person's room without knocking

30. When taking a person's height and weight, you
    A. Let the person wear shoes
    B. Have the person void before being weighed
    C. Weigh the person at different times of the day
    D. Balance the scale every 6 months

31. A person is bedfast. To prevent pressure ulcers, you
    A. Reposition the person at least every 3 hours
    B. Massage reddened areas
    C. Let heels and ankles touch the bed
    D. Keep the skin free of moisture from urine, stools, or perspiration

32. A person has a hearing problem. When talking with the person, you
    A. Keep the TV or radio on
    B. Shout
    C. Face the person
    D. Speak quickly

33. When caring for a person who is blind or visually impaired, you
    A. Place furniture and equipment where the person walks
    B. Keep the lights off
    C. Explain the location of food and beverages
    D. Rearrange furniture and equipment

34. You are caring for a person with dementia. You
    A. Share information about the person's care
    B. Share information about the person's condition
    C. Protect confidential information
    D. Expose the person's body when you provide care

35. When caring for a confused person, you
    A. Call the person "Honey"
    B. Do not need to explain what you are doing
    C. Ask clear, simple questions
    D. Remove the calendar from the person's room

36. A person with Alzheimer's disease likes to wander. You
    A. Keep the person in his or her room
    B. Restrain the person
    C. Argue with the person who wants to leave
    D. Exercise the person as ordered

37. Restorative nursing programs
    A. Help maintain the lowest level of function
    B. Promote self-care measures
    C. Focus on the disability, not the person
    D. Help the person lose strength and independence

38. When caring for a person with a disability, you
    A. Focus on his or her limitations
    B. Expect progress in a rehabilitation program to be fast
    C. Remind the person of his or her progress in the rehabilitation program
    D. Deny the disability

39. After a person dies, you
    A. Can expose his or her body unnecessarily
    B. Can discuss the person's diagnosis with your family
    C. Can talk about the family's reactions to your friends
    D. Respect the person's right to privacy

40. You enter a person's room and find a fire in the wastebasket. Your first action is to
    A. Remove the person from the room
    B. Close the door
    C. Call for help
    D. Activate the fire alarm

41. You leave a person lying in urine and he or she develops a bedsore. This is
    A. Fraud
    B. Neglect
    C. Assault
    D. Battery

42. A nurse asks you to place a drug and a sterile dressing on a small foot wound. You
    A. Agree to do the task
    B. Ask another nursing assistant to do the task
    C. Politely tell the nurse you cannot do that task
    D. Report the nurse to the director of nursing

43. You observe a person's urine is foul-smelling and dark amber. Your first action is to
    A. Tell the other nursing assistant
    B. Tell the person
    C. Tell the nurse
    D. Record the observation

44. A daughter asks you for water for her mom. Your response is
    A. "I am not caring for your mom. I will get her nursing assistant for you."
    B. "I do not have time to do that."
    C. "That's not my job."
    D. "I will be happy to do that."

45. A person has a restraint on. You
    A. Observe the person for breathing and circulation complications every 30 minutes
    B. Know that unnecessary restraint is false imprisonment
    C. Use the most restrictive type of restraint
    D. Know that restraints decrease confusion and agitation

46. The nurse asks you to place a person in the supine position. You
    A. Elevate the head of the bed 45 degrees
    B. Elevate the foot of the bed 15 degrees
    C. Place the person on his or her back with the bed flat
    D. Place the person on his or her abdomen

47. The most important way to prevent or avoid spreading infection is to
    A. Wash hands
    B. Cover your nose when coughing
    C. Use disposable gloves
    D. Wear a mask
48. You are eating lunch and a nursing assistant begins to gossip about another person. You
    A. Join the conversation and talk about the person
    B. Remove yourself from the group
    C. Tell your roommate about the gossip you heard at lunch
    D. Tell another nursing assistant about the gossip you heard
49. When moving a person up in bed, you should
    A. Raise the head of the bed
    B. Ask the person to keep his or her legs straight
    C. Cause friction and shearing
    D. Ask a co-worker to help you
50. A person is on a sodium-controlled diet. This means
    A. Canned vegetables are omitted from his or her diet
    B. Salt may be added to food at the table
    C. Large amounts of salt are used in cooking
    D. Ham is eaten regularly
51. Elastic stockings
    A. Are applied after a person gets out of bed
    B. Should not have wrinkles or creases after being applied
    C. Come in one size only
    D. Are forced on the person
52. While walking, the person begins to fall. You
    A. Call for help
    B. Reach for a chair
    C. Ease the person to the floor
    D. Ask a visitor to help
53. Before bathing a person, you should
    A. Offer the bedpan or urinal
    B. Partially undress the person
    C. Raise the head of the bed
    D. Open the privacy curtain
54. When taking a rectal temperature, you insert the thermometer
    A. 1 inch
    B. 1.5 inches
    C. 2 inches
    D. 2.5 inches
55. Touch
    A. Is a form of nonverbal communication
    B. Is a form of verbal communication
    C. Means the same thing to everyone
    D. Should be used for all persons

56. You may share information about a person's care and condition to
    A. The staff caring for the person
    B. The person's daughter
    C. Your family members
    D. The volunteer in the gift shop
57. A person tells you he or she has pain upon urination. You
    A. Tell the nurse
    B. Let the nurse document this information
    C. Ask the person to tell you if it happens again
    D. Tell the person's son
58. A person's culture and religion are different from yours. You
    A. Laugh about the person's customs
    B. Tell your family about the person's customs
    C. Ask the person to explain his or her beliefs and practices to you
    D. Tell the person his or her beliefs and customs are silly
59. You need to wear gloves when you
    A. Do range-of-motion exercises
    B. Feed a person
    C. Give perineal care
    D. Walk a person
60. An older person is normally alert. Today he or she is confused. What should you do?
    A. Ask the person why he or she is confused
    B. Ignore the confusion
    C. Check to see if the person is confused later in the day
    D. Tell the nurse
61. While walking with a person, he tells you he feels faint. What do you do first?
    A. Have the person sit down.
    B. Call for the nurse.
    C. Open the window.
    D. Ask the person to take a deep breath.
62. You are asked to encourage fluids for a person. You
    A. Increase the person's fluid intake
    B. Decrease the person's fluid intake
    C. Limit fluids to mealtimes
    D. Keep fluids where the person cannot reach them
63. Communication fails when you
    A. Use words the other person understands
    B. Talk too much
    C. Let others express their feelings and concerns
    D. Talk about a topic that is uncomfortable
64. During bathing, a person may
    A. Decide what products to use
    B. Be exposed in the shower room
    C. Have visitors present without his or her permission
    D. Have no personal choices

65. People in late adulthood need to
    A. Adjust to increased income
    B. Adjust to their health being better
    C. Develop new friends and relationships
    D. Adjust to increased strength
66. When measuring blood pressure, you should do the following except
    A. Apply the cuff to a bare upper arm
    B. Turn off the TV
    C. Locate the brachial artery
    D. Use the arm with an IV infusion
67. You find clean linen on the floor in a person's room. You
    A. Use the linen to make the bed
    B. Return the linen to the linen cart
    C. Put the linen in the laundry
    D. Tell the nurse
68. When doing mouth care on an unconscious person, you
    A. Use a large amount of fluid
    B. Position the person on his or her side
    C. Do the task without telling the person what you are doing
    D. Insert his or her dentures when done
69. When brushing or combing a person's hair, you
    A. Cut matted or tangled hair
    B. Encourage the person to do as much as possible
    C. Style the hair as you want
    D. Perform the task weekly
70. When providing nail and foot care, you
    A. Cut fingernails with scissors
    B. Trim toenails for a diabetic person
    C. Trim toenails for a person with poor circulation
    D. Check between the toes for cracks and sores

71. An indwelling catheter becomes disconnected from the drainage system. You
    A. Reconnect the tubing to the catheter quickly without gloves
    B. Tell the nurse at once
    C. Get a new drainage system
    D. Touch the ends of the catheter
72. Urinary drainage bags are
    A. Hung on the bed rail
    B. Emptied and measured at the end of each shift
    C. Kept on the floor
    D. Kept higher than the person's bladder
73. A person needs a condom catheter applied. You remember to
    A. Apply it to a penis that is red and irritated
    B. Use adhesive tape to secure the catheter
    C. Use elastic tape to secure the catheter
    D. Act in an unprofessional manner
74. For comfort during bowel elimination
    A. Have the person use the bedpan rather than the bathroom or commode if possible
    B. Permit visitors to stay
    C. Keep the door and privacy curtain open
    D. Leave the person alone if possible
75. You are transferring a person with a weak right side from the wheelchair to the bed. You
    A. Place the wheelchair on the left side of the bed
    B. Place the wheelchair on the right side of the bed
    C. Keep the person in the wheelchair
    D. Ask the person what side moves first

SKILLS EVALUATION REVIEW

Each state has its own policies and procedures for the skills test. The following information is an overview of what to expect:

- To pass the skills evaluation, you will need to perform all 5 skills correctly.
- A nurse evaluates your performance of certain skills. Having someone watch as you work is not a new experience. Your instructor evaluated your performance during your training program. While you are working, your supervisor evaluates your skills.
- Mannequins and people are used as "patients" or "residents," depending on the skills you are performing.
- If you make a mistake, tell the evaluator what you did wrong. Then perform the skill correctly. Do not panic.
- Take whatever equipment you normally take or use at work. Wear a watch with a second hand. You may need it to measure vital signs and check how much time you have left.

BEFORE AND DURING THE PROCEDURE

- Hand washing is evaluated at the beginning of the skills test. You are expected to know when to wash your hands. Therefore you may not be told to do so. Follow the rules for hand hygiene during the test.
- Before entering a person's room, knock on the door. Greet the person by name and introduce yourself before beginning a procedure. Check the ID or the photo ID to make certain you are giving care to the right person.
- Explain what you are going to do before beginning the procedure and as needed throughout the procedure.
- Always follow the rules of medical asepsis. For example, remove gloves and dispose of them properly. Keep clean linen separated from dirty linen.
- Always protect the person's rights throughout the skills test.
- Communicate with the person as you give care. Focus on the person's needs and interests. Always

treat the person with respect. Do not talk about yourself or your personal problems.

- Provide privacy. This involves pulling the privacy curtain around the bed, closing doors, and asking visitors to leave the room.
- Promote safety for the person. For example, lock the wheelchair when you transfer a person to and from it. Place the bed in the lowest horizontal position when the person must get out of bed or when you are done giving care.
- Make sure the signal light is within the person's reach. Attaching it to the bed or bed rail does not mean the person can reach it.
- Use good body mechanics. Raise the bed and overbed table to a good working height.
- Provide for comfort:
  - Make sure the person and linens are clean and dry. The person may have become incontinent during the procedure.
  - Change or straighten bed linens as needed.
  - Position the person for comfort and in good alignment.
  - Provide pillows as directed by the nurse and the care plan.
  - Raise the head of the bed as the person prefers and allowed by the nurse and the care plan.
  - Provide for warmth. The person may need an extra blanket, a lap blanket, a sweater, socks, and so on.
  - Adjust lighting to meet the person's needs.
  - Make sure eyeglasses and hearing aids are in place as needed.
  - Ask the person if he or she is comfortable.
  - Ask the person if there is anything else you can do for him or her.
  - Make sure the person is covered for warmth and privacy.

SKILLS

Ask your instructor to tell you which of the following skills are tested in your state. Place a checkmark in the box in front of each tested skill so it will be easy for you to reference. The skills marked with an asterisk (*) are used with permission of Pearson VUE. These skills are offered as a study guide to you. The word "client" refers to the resident or person receiving care. You are responsible for following the most current standards, practices, and guidelines of your state.

The steps in boldface type are critical element steps. Critical element steps must be done correctly to pass the skill. If you miss a critical element step, you will not pass the skills evaluation. For example, you are to transfer a client from the bed to a wheelchair. You will fail if you do not lock the wheels on the wheelchair before transferring the person. An automatic failure is one that could potentially cause harm to a person. Your state may mark critical element steps in another way—underline or italics. If your state has one, review the candidate's handbook.

❏ *WASHES HANDS (CHAPTER 11)

1. Addresses client by name and introduces self to client by name
2. Turns on water at sink
3. Wets hands and wrists thoroughly
4. Applies skin cleanser or soap to hands
5. **Lathers all surfaces of hands, wrists, and fingers, producing friction for at least 15 (fifteen) seconds**
6. Cleans fingernails by rubbing fingertips against palms of the opposite hand
7. Rinses all surfaces of wrists, hands, and fingers, keeping hands lower than the elbows and the fingertips down
8. Uses clean, dry paper towel to dry all surfaces of hands, wrists, and fingers
9. Uses clean, dry paper towel to turn off faucet or uses knee or foot control to turn off faucet
10. Does not touch inside of sink at any time
11. Disposes of used paper towel(s) in wastebasket immediately after shutting off faucet

❏ *APPLIES ONE KNEE-HIGH ELASTIC STOCKING (CHAPTER 23)

1. Explains procedure to client, speaking clearly, slowly, and directly, maintaining face-to-face contact whenever possible
2. Provides for client's privacy during procedure with curtain, screen, or door
3. Ensures client is in supine position (lying down in bed) while stocking is applied
4. Turns stocking inside out at least to heel area
5. Places foot of stocking over toes, foot, and heel
6. Pulls top of stocking over foot, heel, and leg

7. Moves client's foot and leg gently and naturally, avoiding force and over-extension of limb and joints throughout the procedure
8. **Finishes procedures with no twists or wrinkles and heel of stocking (if present) is over heel opening and opening in the toe area (if present) is under or over toe area**
9. Places signaling device within client's reach
10. Leaves bed in low position
11. Washes hands

❏ *ASSISTS CLIENT TO AMBULATE USING A TRANSFER BELT (CHAPTER 22)

1. Explains procedure to client, speaking clearly, slowly, and directly, maintaining face-to-face contact whenever possible
2. **Before assisting to stand, ensures client is wearing non-skid footwear**
3. Before assisting to stand, places bed at a safe and appropriate level for the client
4. Before assisting to stand, checks and locks bed wheels
5. Before assisting to stand, client is assisted to a sitting position with feet flat on the floor
6. Before assisting to stand, provides instructions to enable client to assist in standing, including prearranged signal to alert client to begin standing
7. Stands in front of and facing client
9. Braces client's lower extremities
10. Places transfer belt around client's waist and grasps the belt, counts to three (or says other prearranged signal), and gradually assists client to stand while grasping transfer belt on both sides with an upward grasp
11. Walks slightly behind and to one side of client for the full distance, while holding on to the belt
12. After ambulation, assists client to a position of comfort and safety in bed and removes transfer belt
13. Places signaling device within client's reach
14. Leaves bed in low position
15. Washes hands

❏ ASSISTS CLIENT WITH USE OF BEDPAN (CHAPTER 17)

1. Explains procedure to client, speaking clearly, slowly, and directly, maintaining face-to-face contact whenever possible
2. Provides for client's privacy during procedure with curtain, screen, or door

---

*From the candidate handbook and the Pearson VUE website. Used with the permission of Pearson VUE, Inc.

3. Before placing bedpan, lowers head of bed
4. Puts on clean gloves before handling bedpan
5. **Places bedpan correctly under client's buttocks (Standard bedpan: Position bedpan so wider end of pan is aligned with client's buttocks; Fracture pan: Position bedpan with handle toward foot of bed)**
6. Removes and disposes of gloves (without contaminating self) into waste container and washes hands
7. Raises head of bed
8. Puts toilet tissue within client's reach
9. Supplies for hand washing or hand wipes are placed within the client's reach and the client is instructed to clean hands when finished
10. Leaves signaling device within client's reach while client is using bedpan
11. Asks client to signal when finished (candidate remains outside curtain until called by client)
12. Puts on clean gloves before removing bedpan
13. Lowers head of bed before removing bedpan
14. Avoids completely exposing client
15. Removes bedpan
16. Empties and rinses bedpan, and pours rinse into toilet
17. Returns bedpan to proper storage
18. Removes and disposes of gloves into wastebasket and washes hands
19. Places signaling device within client's reach
20. Leaves bed in low position

❑ *CLEANS AND STORES DENTURES (CHAPTER 15)

1. Puts on clean gloves before handling dentures
2. Before handling dentures, protects dentures from possible breakage (e.g., by lining sink/basin with a towel/washcloth or by filling it with water)
3. Rinses dentures in moderate temperature running water before brushing them
4. Applies toothpaste or denture cleanser to toothbrush
5. Brushes dentures on all surfaces
6. Rinses all surfaces of dentures under moderate temperature running water
7. Rinses denture cup before placing clean dentures in it
8. Places dentures in clean denture cup with moderate temperature water/solution and places lid on cup
9. Returns denture cup to proper storage (e.g., bedside stand)
10. Cleans and returns implements to proper storage

11. Maintains clean technique with placement of dentures and toothbrush throughout procedure
12. Disposes of sink liner in appropriate container or drains sink/basin
13. Removes and disposes of gloves into wastebasket
14. Washes hands

❑ *COUNTS AND RECORDS RADIAL PULSE (CHAPTER 20)

1. Explains procedure to client, speaking clearly, slowly, and directly, maintaining face-to-face contact whenever possible
2. Places fingertips on thumb side of client's wrist to locate pulse
3. Counts beats for 1 full minute
4. Places signaling device within client's reach
5. Washes hands
6. **Records pulse rate within plus or minus 4 beats of evaluator's reading**

❑ *COUNTS AND RECORDS RESPIRATIONS (CHAPTER 20)

1. Explains procedure to client (for testing purposes), speaking clearly, slowly, and directly, maintaining face-to-face contact whenever possible
2. Counts respirations for 1 full minute
3. Places signaling device within client's reach
4. Washes hands
5. **Records respiration rate within plus or minus 2 breaths of evaluator's reading**

❑ *DRESSES CLIENT WITH AFFECTED (WEAK) RIGHT ARM (CHAPTER 16)

1. Explains procedure to client, speaking clearly, slowly, and directly, maintaining face-to-face contact whenever possible
2. Provides for client's privacy during procedure with curtain, screen, or door
3. Asks client which top he/she would like to wear and dresses him/her in top of choice
4. Removes client's gown without completely exposing client. Removes garments from the unaffected side first, then removes garments from the affected side
5. **Assists client to put the right (affected/weak) arm through the right sleeve of the top before placing garment on left (unaffected) arm**

*From the candidate handbook and the Pearson VUE website. Used with the permission of Pearson VUE, Inc.

6. While putting on items, moves client's body gently and naturally, avoiding force and over-extension of limbs and joints
7. Finishes with client dressed appropriately (e.g., clothing right side out, zippers/buttons fastened, and so on)
8. Places gown in soiled linen container
9. Places signaling device within client's reach
10. Leaves bed in low position
11. Washes hands

❑ *FEEDS CLIENT WHO CANNOT FEED SELF (CHAPTER 19)

1. Explains procedure to client, speaking clearly, slowly, and directly, maintaining face-to-face contact whenever possible
2. Before feeding, picks up name card and verifies that client has received the tray prepared for him/her
3. **Before feeding client, ensures client is in an upright sitting position (45 to 90 degrees)**
4. Places tray where it can be easily seen by client
5. Cleans client's hands before beginning feeding
6. Sits facing client
7. Tells client what foods are on tray and asks what client would like to eat first, allowing for personal choice
8. Offers the food in bite-size pieces
9. Makes sure client's mouth is empty before next bite of food or sip of beverage
10. Offers beverage to client throughout the meal
11. Wipes food from client's mouth and hands as necessary during the meal
12. At end of meal, wipes client's mouth and cleans client's hands
13. Removes food tray and places tray in proper area
14. Places signaling device within client's reach
15. Washes hands

❑ *GIVES MODIFIED BED BATH (FACE AND ONE ARM, HAND, AND UNDERARM) (CHAPTER 15)

1. Explains procedure to client, speaking clearly, slowly, and directly, maintaining face-to-face contact whenever possible
2. Provides for client's privacy during procedure with curtain, screen, or door
3. Removes or folds back top bedding, keeping client covered with bath blanket
4. Removes client's gown while keeping client covered

5. Tests water temperature and ensures it is safe and comfortable before bathing client, and adjusts if necessary
6. Beginning with eyes, washes eyes with wet washcloth (no soap), using a different area of the washcloth for each eye, washing inner aspect to outer aspect, then proceeds to wash face
7. Dries face with towel, using a blotting motion
8. Exposes one arm and places towel underneath arm
9. Using soapy washcloth, washes arm, hand, and underarm
10. Rinses and dries arm, hand, and underarm
11. Moves client's body gently and naturally, avoiding force and over-extension of limbs and joints throughout the procedure
12. Puts clean gown on client
13. Pulls up bedcovers and removes bath blanket
14. Empties, rinses, and dries bath basin and returns to proper storage
15. Places soiled clothing and linen in soiled linen container
16. Avoids contact between candidate clothing and soiled linens/pads throughout procedure
17. Places signaling device within client's reach
18. Leaves bed in low position
19. Washes hands

❑ *MAKES AN OCCUPIED BED (CHAPTER 14)

1. Explains procedure to client, speaking clearly, slowly, and directly, maintaining face-to-face contact whenever possible
2. Places clean linen on clean surface within candidate's reach (e.g., bedside stand, overbed table, or chair)
3. Provides for client's privacy throughout procedure with curtain, screen, or door
4. Covers client while linens are changed
5. Lowers head of bed before moving client
6. Loosens top linen from the end of the bed on working side
7. Unfolds bath blanket over the top sheet and removes top sheet
8. Raises side rail on side to which client will move, goes to other side, and then slowly rolls client onto side toward raised side rail
9. Loosens bottom soiled linen on working side and moves bottom soiled linen toward center of bed
10. Places and tucks in clean bottom linen or fitted bottom sheet on working side (if flat sheet is used, tucks in at top and working side), then raises side rail

11. Goes to other side of bed, lowers side rail, and then assists client to turn onto clean bottom sheet
12. Removes soiled bottom linen
13. Pulls and tucks in clean bottom linen, finishing with bottom sheet free of wrinkles
14. Covers client with clean top sheet and removes bath blanket
15. Changes pillowcase
16. Linen is centered and tucked at foot of bed
17. Avoids contact between candidate's clothing and soiled linen throughout procedure
18. Disposes of soiled linen in soiled linen container
19. Places signaling device within client's reach
20. Leaves bed in low position
21. Washes hands

❏ *MEASURES AND RECORDS BLOOD PRESSURE (ONE-STEP PROCEDURE) (CHAPTER 20)

1. Explains procedure to client, speaking clearly, slowly, and directly, maintaining face-to-face contact whenever possible
2. Before using stethoscope, wipes diaphragm and earpieces of stethoscope with alcohol
3. Exposes client's upper arm and positions arm with palm up
4. Locates brachial artery with fingertips
5. Places blood pressure cuff snugly on client's upper arm with sensor/arrow over brachial artery site
6. Places earpieces of stethoscope in ears and bell/diaphragm over brachial artery site
7. Candidate does one of the following:
   a. Inflates cuff between 160 mm Hg and 180 mm Hg (if beat heard immediately upon cuff deflation, completely deflate cuff). Re-inflates cuff to no more than 200 mm Hg OR
   b. Locates radial or brachial pulse; inflates cuff 30 mm Hg beyond where pulse was last heard or felt
8. Deflates cuff slowly and notes the first sound (systolic reading), and last sound (diastolic reading) (If rounding needed, measurements are rounded up to the nearest 2 mm Hg)
9. Removes cuff
10. Places signaling device within client's reach
11. Washes hands
12. **Records both systolic and diastolic pressures, each within plus or minus 8 mm Hg of evaluator's reading**

❏ *MEASURES AND RECORDS URINARY OUTPUT (CHAPTER 20)

1. Puts on clean gloves before handling bedpan
2. Pours the contents of the bedpan into measuring container without spilling or splashing any of the urine
3. Measures the amount of urine at eye level
4. After measuring urine, empties contents of measuring container into toilet without splashing
5. Rinses measuring container and pours rinse water into toilet
6. Rinses bedpan and pours rinse water into toilet
7. Returns bedpan and measuring container to proper storage
8. Removes and disposes of gloves into wastebasket
9. Washes hands before recording output
10. **Records contents of container within plus or minus 25 mL of evaluator's reading**

❏ *MEASURES AND RECORDS WEIGHT OF AMBULATORY CLIENT (CHAPTER 20)

1. Explains procedure to client, speaking clearly, slowly, and directly, maintaining face-to-face contact whenever possible
2. Candidate ensures client has shoes on before walking to scale
3. Starts with scale balanced at zero before weighing client
4. Assists client to step up onto center of the scale
5. Determines client's weight
6. Assists client off scale before recording weight
7. **Records weight within plus or minus 2 pounds of evaluator's reading (If weight recorded in kg, weight is within plus or minus 0.9 kg of evaluator's reading)**
8. Leaves client in position of comfort
9. Places signaling device within client's reach
10. Washes hands

❏ *POSITIONS CLIENT ON SIDE (CHAPTER 13)

1. Explains procedure to client, speaking clearly, slowly, and directly, maintaining face-to-face contact whenever possible
2. Provides for client's privacy during procedure with curtain, screen, or door

---

*From the candidate handbook and the Pearson VUE website. Used with the permission of Pearson VUE, Inc.

3. Before turning client, lowers head of bed
4. Raises side rail on side to which client's body will be turned
5. Slowly rolls client onto side as one unit toward raised side rail
6. Places or adjusts pillow under client's head for support
7. Adjusts shoulder so client is not lying on arm
8. Supports top arm with body or supportive device
9. Places supportive device behind client's back
10. Places supportive device between legs with top knee flexed; knee and ankle supported
11. Covers client with top linen
12. Places signaling device within client's reach
13. Leaves bed in low position
14. Washes hands

❏ *PROVIDES CATHETER CARE (CHAPTER 17)

1. Explains procedure to client, speaking clearly, slowly, and directly, maintaining face-to-face contact whenever possible
2. Provides for client's privacy during procedure with curtain, screen, or door
3. Tests water temperature in basin to determine if it is safe and comfortable before washing, and adjusts if necessary
4. Puts on clean gloves before washing
5. Places towel or linen protector under client's buttocks before washing
6. Covers client with bath blanket and moves top linens to foot of bed
7. Exposes only area surrounding catheter
8. Applies soap to wet washcloth and cleans area around urinary meatus using a clean area of washcloth for each stroke
9. **Holds catheter near meatus without tugging and cleans at least 4 inches of catheter nearest meatus, moving in only one direction (i.e., away from meatus) using a clean area of the cloth for each stroke**
10. **Holds catheter near meatus without tugging and rinses at least 4 inches of catheter nearest meatus, moving only in one direction (i.e., away from meatus) using a clean area of the cloth for each stroke**
11. Holds the catheter near meatus without tugging and dries 4 inches of catheter moving away from meatus
12. Replaces top covers and removes bath blanket

13. Disposes of linen in soiled linen container
14. Avoids contact between candidate clothing and soiled linen/pads throughout procedure
15. Empties, rinses, and dries basin and returns to proper storage
16. Removes and disposes of gloves into wastebasket
17. Places signaling device within client's reach
18. Leaves bed in low position
19. Washes hands

❏ *PROVIDES FINGERNAIL CARE ON ONE HAND (CHAPTER 16)

1. Explains procedure to client, speaking clearly, slowly, and directly, maintaining face-to-face contact whenever possible
2. Provides for client's privacy during procedure with curtain, screen, or door
3. Tests water temperature and ensures it is safe and comfortable before immersing client's fingers in water and adjusts if necessary
4. Places basin in a comfortable position for client
5. Soaks client's fingers (fingernails) in basin of water
6. Puts on clean gloves before cleaning under fingernails
7. Cleans under each fingernail with orangewood stick
8. Wipes orangewood stick on towel after each nail
9. Dries client's hand/fingers, including between fingers
10. Grooms nails with file or emery board
11. Finishes with nails smooth and free of rough edges
12. Disposes of orangewood stick and emery board into wastebasket (for testing purposes)
13. Empties, rinses, and dries basin, and returns to proper storage
14. Disposes of soiled linen in soiled linen container
15. Removes and disposes of gloves in wastebasket
16. Places signaling device within client's reach
17. Washes hands

❏ *PROVIDES FOOT CARE ON ONE FOOT (CHAPTER 16)

1. Explains procedure to client, speaking clearly, slowly, and directly, maintaining face-to-face contact whenever possible

2. Provides for client's privacy during procedure with curtain, screen, or door
3. Tests water temperature and ensures it is safe and comfortable before placing client's foot in water and adjusts if necessary
4. Places basin in comfortable position on protective barrier
5. Completely submerges and soaks foot in water
6. Puts on clean gloves before washing foot
7. Washes entire foot, including between the toes, with soapy washcloth
8. Rinses entire foot, including between the toes
9. Dries entire foot, including between the toes
10. Applies lotion to top and bottom of foot, removing excess (if any) with a towel
11. Supports foot and ankle properly throughout procedure
12. Empties, rinses, and dries bath basin, and returns to proper storage
13. Disposes of soiled linen in soiled linen container
14. Removes and disposes of gloves in wastebasket
15. Places signaling device within client's reach
16. Washes hands

❏ ***PROVIDES MOUTH CARE (CHAPTER 15)**
1. Explains procedure to client, speaking clearly, slowly, and directly, maintaining face-to-face contact whenever possible
2. Provides for client's privacy throughout procedure with curtain, screen, or door
3. Before providing mouth care, ensures client is in an upright sitting position (45 to 90 degrees)
4. Puts on clean gloves before cleaning client's mouth
5. Places towel across client's chest before providing mouth care
6. Moistens toothbrush or toothette
7. Applies toothpaste to toothbrush or toothette
8. **Cleans entire mouth (including tongue and all surfaces of teeth) using gentle motions**
9. Holds emesis basin to client's chin and assists client to rinse his or her mouth
10. Wipes client's mouth and removes towel
11. Disposes of soiled linen in soiled linen container
12. Maintains clean technique with placement of toothbrush or toothette throughout the procedure
13. Empties, rinses, and dries basin; rinses toothbrush (if used); and returns to proper storage

14. Removes and disposes of gloves into wastebasket
15. Places signaling device within client's reach
16. Leaves bed in low position
17. Washes hands

❏ ***PROVIDES PERINEAL CARE (PERI-CARE) FOR FEMALE (CHAPTER 15)**
1. Explains procedure to client, speaking clearly, slowly, and directly, maintaining face-to-face contact whenever possible
2. Provides for client's privacy during procedure with curtain, screen, or door
3. Tests water temperature and ensures it is safe and comfortable before washing and adjusts if necessary
4. Puts on clean gloves before washing perineal area
5. Covers client with bath blanket and moves top linens to foot of bed
6. Places a pad or linen protector under perineal area before washing
7. Exposes only perineal area
8. Applies soap to wet washcloth
9. **Washes perineal area with soapy washcloth, moving from front to back, while using a clean area of the washcloth or clean washcloth for each stroke**
10. **Using a clean washcloth, rinses perineal area, moving from front to back, while using a clean area of the washcloth or clean washcloth for each stroke**
11. Dries perineal area moving from front to back, using a blotting motion with towel
12. Turns client on to side
13. Washes and rinses rectal area moving from front to back using a clean area of washcloth or a clean washcloth for each stroke; then dries with towel
14. Removes pad or linen protector
15. Repositions client
16. Replaces top covers and removes bath blanket
17. Disposes of soiled linen and pad/linen protector in proper container
18. Avoids contact between candidate clothing and soiled linens/pads throughout procedure
19. Empties, rinses, and wipes basin and returns to proper storage
20. Removes and disposes of gloves into wastebasket
21. Places signaling device within client's reach
22. Leaves bed in low position
23. Washes hands

❏ ***TRANSFERS CLIENT FROM BED TO WHEELCHAIR USING TRANSFER BELT (CHAPTER 13)**

1. Explains procedure to client, speaking clearly, slowly, and directly, maintaining face-to-face contact whenever possible
2. Provides for client's privacy during procedure with curtain, screen, or door
3. Positions wheelchair along side of bed, at head of bed, and facing the foot of the bed
4. Before assisting client to stand, folds up footplates
5. Before assisting client to stand, places bed at a safe and appropriate level for the client
6. **Before assisting client to stand, locks wheels on wheelchair**
7. Before assisting client to stand, checks and/or locks bed wheels
8. Before assisting client to stand, supports client's back and hips and assists client to sitting position with feet flat on the floor
9. Before assisting client to stand, puts non-skid footwear on client, making sure they are securely fastened
10. Before assisting client to stand, applies transfer belt securely over clothing or gown
11. Before assisting client to stand, provides instructions to enable client to assist in transfer, including prearranged signal to alert client when to begin standing
12. Stands facing client, positioning self to ensure safety of candidate and client during transfer (e.g., knees bent, feet apart, back straight); counts to three (or says prearranged signal) to alert client to begin standing
13. On signal, gradually assists client to stand by grasping transfer belt on both sides with an upward grasp and maintaining stability of client's legs
14. Assists client to turn to stand in front of wheelchair with back of client's legs against wheelchair
15. Lowers client into wheelchair
16. Positions client with hips touching back of wheelchair and removes transfer belt
17. Positions client's feet on footplates
18. Places signaling device within client's reach
19. Washes hands

❏ ***PERFORMS PASSIVE RANGE-OF-MOTION (ROM) FOR ONE KNEE AND ONE ANKLE (CHAPTER 22)**

1. Explains procedure to client, speaking clearly, slowly, and directly, maintaining face-to-face contact whenever possible

2. Provides for client's privacy during procedure with curtain, screen, or door
3. Instructs client to inform candidate if pain is felt during exercise
4. Supports client's leg at knee and ankle while performing range-of-motion for knee
5. Bends the knee to the point of resistance and then returns leg to client's normal position (extension/flexion) (Performs AT LEAST 3 TIMES unless pain occurs)
6. Supports foot and ankle close to the bed while performing range-of-motion for ankle
7. Pushes/pulls foot toward head (dorsiflexion), and pushes/pulls foot down, toes point down (plantar flexion) (Performs AT LEAST 3 TIMES unless pain occurs)
8. **While supporting the limb, moves joints gently, slowly, and smoothly through the range-of-motion to the point of resistance, discontinuing exercise if pain occurs**
9. Places signaling device within client's reach
10. Leaves bed in low position
11. Washes hands

❏ ***PERFORMS PASSIVE RANGE-OF-MOTION (ROM) FOR ONE SHOULDER (CHAPTER 22)**

1. Explains procedure to client, speaking clearly, slowly, and directly, maintaining face-to-face contact whenever possible
2. Provides for client's privacy during procedure with curtain, screen, or door
3. Instructs client to inform candidate if pain is felt during exercise
4. Supports client's arm at elbow and wrist while performing range-of-motion for shoulder
5. Raises client's straightened arm from side position forward above head and returns arm to side of body (flexion/extension) (Performs AT LEAST 3 TIMES unless pain occurs)
6. Raises client's straightened arm away from the side of body to shoulder level and returns arm to side of body (abduction/adduction) (Performs AT LEAST 3 TIMES unless pain occurs)
7. **While supporting the limb, moves joint gently, slowly, and smoothly through the range-of-motion to the point of resistance, discontinuing exercise if client reports pain**
8. Places signaling device within client's reach
9. Leaves bed in low position
10. Washes hands

*From the candidate handbook and the Pearson VUE website. Used with the permission of Pearson VUE, Inc.

❏ PASSIVE RANGE-OF-MOTION OF LOWER EXTREMITY (HIP, KNEE, ANKLE) (CHAPTER 22)

1. Washes hands before contact with client
2. Identifies self to client by name and addresses client by name
3. Explains procedure to client, speaking clearly, slowly, and directly, maintaining face-to-face contact whenever possible
4. Provides for client's privacy during procedure with curtain, screen, or door
5. Positions client supine and in good body alignment
6. Supports client's leg by placing one hand under knee and other hand under heel
7. Moves entire leg away from body (Performs AT LEAST 3 TIMES unless pain occurs)
8. Moves entire leg toward body (Performs AT LEAST 3 TIMES unless pain occurs)
9. Bends client's knee and hip toward client's trunk (Performs AT LEAST 3 TIMES unless pain occurs)
10. Straightens knee and hip (Performs AT LEAST 3 TIMES unless pain occurs)
11. Flexes and extends ankle through range-of-motion exercises (Performs AT LEAST 3 TIMES unless pain occurs)
12. Rotates ankle through range-of-motion exercises (Performs AT LEAST 3 TIMES unless pain occurs)
13. **While supporting limb, moves joints gently, slowly, and smoothly through range-of-motion to point of resistance, discontinuing exercise if pain occurs**
14. Provides for comfort
15. Before leaving client, places signaling device within client's reach
16. Washes hands

❏ PASSIVE RANGE-OF-MOTION OF UPPER EXTREMITY (SHOULDER, ELBOW, WRIST, FINGER) (CHAPTER 22)

1. Washes hands before contact with client
2. Identifies self to client by name and addresses client by name
3. Explains procedure to client, speaking clearly, slowly, and directly, maintaining face-to-face contact whenever possible
4. Provides for client's privacy during procedure with curtain, screen, or door
5. Supports client's extremity above and below joints while performing range-of-motion

6. Raises client's straightened arm toward ceiling and back toward head of bed and returns to flat position (flexion/extension) (Performs AT LEAST 3 TIMES unless pain occurs)
7. Moves client's straightened arm away from client's side of body toward head of bed, and returns client's straightened arm to midline of client's body (abduction/adduction) (Performs AT LEAST 3 TIMES unless pain occurs)
8. Moves client's shoulder through rotation range-of-motion exercises (Performs AT LEAST 3 TIMES unless pain occurs)
9. Flexes and extends elbow through range-of-motion exercises (Performs AT LEAST 3 TIMES unless pain occurs)
10. Provides range-of-motion exercises to wrist (Performs AT LEAST 3 TIMES unless pain occurs)
11. Moves finger and thumb joints through range-of-motion exercises (Performs AT LEAST 3 TIMES unless pain occurs)
12. **While supporting body part, moves joint gently, slowly, and smoothly through range-of-motion to point of resistance, discontinuing exercise if pain occurs**
13. Before leaving client, places signaling device within client's reach
14. Washes hands

❏ MAKES AN UNOCCUPIED BED (CHAPTER 14)

1. Washes hands
2. Collects clean linen
3. Places clean linen on a clean surface
4. Raises the bed for good body mechanics
5. Puts on gloves
6. Removes linen without contaminating uniform. Rolls each piece away from self
7. Discards linen into laundry bag
8. Moves the mattress to the head of the bed
9. Applies mattress pad
10. Applies bottom sheet, keeping it smooth and free of wrinkles
11. Places the top sheet and bedspread on the bed, keeping them smooth and free of wrinkles
12. Tucks in top linens at the foot of the bed. Makes mitered corners
13. Applies clean pillowcase with zippers and/or tags to inside of pillowcase
14. Lowers the bed to its lowest position. Locks the bed wheels
15. Washes hands

❑ *DONS AND REMOVES GOWN AND GLOVES (CHAPTER 11)

1. Removes watch and all jewelry
2. Rolls up uniform sleeves
3. Washes hands
4. Holds a clean gown out in front and lets it unfold
5. Facing the back opening of gown, places hands and arms through the sleeves
6. Makes sure the gown covers all of the body from neck to knees and shoulders to wrists
7. Ties the strings at the back of the neck
8. Overlaps the back of the gown and ties the waist strings
9. Puts on the gloves, making sure gloves overlap gown at the wrists
10. With one gloved hand, grasps the other glove at the palm, pulls glove off
11. Slips fingers from ungloved hand underneath cuff of remaining glove at wrist; removes glove turning it inside out as it is removed
12. Disposes of gloves in appropriate container without contaminating self
13. After removing gloves, unties gown at neck and waist
14. Removes gown without touching outside of gown
15. While removing gown, holds gown away from body, turns gown inward, and keeps it inside out
16. Disposes of gown in appropriate container without contaminating self
17. Washes hands

❑ PERFORMS ABDOMINAL THRUSTS (CHAPTER 8)

1. Asks client if he or she is choking
2. Stands behind the client
3. Wraps arms around client's waist
4. Makes a fist with one hand
5. Places thumb side of fist against the client's abdomen
6. Positions fist in middle above navel and below sternum (breastbone)
7. Grasps fist with other hand
8. Presses fist and other hand into client's abdomen with quick upward thrusts
9. Repeats thrusts until object is expelled or client becomes unresponsive

❑ AMBULATION WITH CANE OR WALKER (CHAPTER 22)

1. Explains procedure to client, speaking clearly, slowly, and directly, maintaining face-to-face contact whenever possible
2. Locks bed wheels or wheelchair brakes
3. Assists client to a sitting position
4. **Before ambulating, puts on and properly fastens non-skid footwear**
5. Positions cane or walker correctly. Cane is on the client's strong side
6. Assists client to stand, using correct body mechanics
7. Stabilizes cane or walker and ensures client stabilizes cane or walker
8. Stands behind and slightly to the side of client
9. Ambulates client
10. Assists client to pivot and sit, using correct body mechanics
11. Before leaving client, places signaling device within client's reach
12. Washes hands

❑ FLUID INTAKE (CHAPTER 20)

1. Observes dinner tray
2. Determines, in milliliters (mL), the amount of fluid consumed from each container
3. Determines total fluid consumed in mL
4. Records total fluid consumed on I&O sheet
5. Calculated total is within required range of evaluator's reading

❑ BRUSHES OR COMBS CLIENT'S HAIR (CHAPTER 16)

1. Explains procedure to client, speaking clearly, slowly, and directly, maintaining face-to-face contact whenever possible
2. Collects brush or comb and bath towel
3. Places towel across the person's back and shoulders or across the pillow
4. Asks client how he or she wants his or her hair styled
5. Combs/brushes hair gently and completely
6. Leaves hair neatly brushed, combed, and/or styled
7. Removes towel
8. Removes hair from comb or brush
9. Before leaving client, places signaling device within client's reach
10. Washes hands

*From the candidate handbook and the Pearson VUE website. Used with the permission of Pearson VUE, Inc.

❑ TRANSFERS A CLIENT USING A MECHANICAL LIFT (CHAPTER 13)

1. Assembles required equipment; performs safety check of slings, straps, hooks, and chains
2. Checks client's weight to ensure it does not exceed the lift's capacity
3. Asks a co-worker to help
4. Explains procedure to client, speaking clearly, slowly, and directly, maintaining face-to-face contact whenever possible
5. Provides for privacy during procedure with curtain, screen, or door
6. Locks the bed wheels
7. Raises the bed for proper body mechanics
8. Lowers the head of the bed to a level appropriate for the client
9. Stands on one side of the bed; co-worker stands on the other side
10. Lowers the bed rails if up
11. Centers the sling under the client following the manufacturer's instructions
12. Ensures that the sling is smooth
13. Positions the client in semi-Fowler's position
14. Positions a chair to lower the client into it
15. Lowers the bed to its lowest position
16. Raises the lift to position it over the client
17. Positions the lift over the client
18. Attaches the sling to the swivel bar; checks fasteners for security
19. Crosses the client's arms over the chest
20. Raises the lift high enough until the client and sling are free of the bed
21. Instructs co-worker to support the client's legs as candidate moves the lift and the client away from the bed
22. Positions the lift so the client's back is toward the chair
23. Slowly lowers the client into the chair
24. Places client in comfortable position, in correct body alignment
25. Lowers the swivel bar and unhooks the sling
26. Removes the sling from under the client unless otherwise indicated. Moves lift away from client
27. Puts footwear on the client
28. Covers the client's lap and legs with a lap blanket
29. Positions the chair as the client prefers
30. Places signaling device within client's reach
31. Washes hands

❑ PROVIDES MOUTH CARE FOR AN UNCONSCIOUS CLIENT (CHAPTER 15)

1. Explains procedure to client, speaking clearly, slowly, and directly, maintaining face-to-face contact whenever possible
2. Provides for privacy during procedure with curtain, screen, or door
3. Washes hands
4. Positions client on side with head turned well to one side
5. Puts on gloves
6. Places the towel under the client's face
7. Places the kidney basin under the chin
8. Uses swabs or toothbrush and toothpaste or other cleaning solution
9. Cleans inside of mouth including the gums, tongue, and teeth
10. Cleans and dries face
11. Removes the towel, kidney basin
12. Applies lubricant to the lips
13. Positions client for comfort and safety
14. Removes and discards the gloves
15. Places signal light within the client's reach
16. Washes hands

❑ PASSING FRESH WATER (CHAPTER 19)

1. Washes hands
2. Assembles equipment—ice, scoop, pitcher
3. Explains procedure to client, speaking clearly, slowly, and directly, maintaining face-to-face contact whenever possible
4. Uses the scoop to fill the pitcher with ice; does not let the scoop touch the rim or inside of the pitcher
5. Places scoop in appropriate receptacle after each use
6. Adds water to pitcher
7. Places the pitcher, disposable cup, and straw (if used) on the overbed table, within the person's reach
8. Before leaving, places signaling device within client's reach
9. Washes hands

❑ PROVIDES PERINEAL CARE FOR UNCIRCUMCISED MALE (CHAPTER 15)

1. Explains procedure to client, speaking clearly, slowly, and directly, maintaining face-to-face contact whenever possible
2. Provides for privacy during procedure with curtain, screen, or door

3. Washes hands
4. Fills basin with comfortably warm water
5. Puts on gloves
6. Elevates bed to working height
7. Places waterproof pad under buttocks
8. Gently grasps penis
9. Retracts the foreskin
10. Using a circular motion, cleans the tip by starting at the meatus of the urethra and working outward
11. Rinses the area with another washcloth
12. Returns the foreskin to its natural position
13. Cleans the shaft of the penis with firm, downward strokes and rinses the area
14. Cleans the scrotum
15. Pats dry the penis and the scrotum
16. Cleans the rectal area
17. Removes the waterproof pad
18. Lowers the bed
19. Removes and discards the gloves
20. Washes hands
21. Before leaving, places signaling device within client's reach

❏ EMPTIES AND RECORDS CONTENT OF URINARY DRAINAGE BAG (CHAPTER 17)

1. Explains procedure to client, speaking clearly, slowly, and directly, maintaining face-to-face contact whenever possible
2. Washes hands
3. Puts on gloves
4. Places a paper towel on the floor
5. Places the graduate on the paper towel
6. Places the graduate under the collection bag
7. Ensures the bag is below the bladder and the drainage tube is not kinked
8. Opens the clamp on the drain
9. Lets all urine drain into the graduate—does not let the drain touch the graduate
10. Closes and positions the clamp
11. Measures urine
12. Removes and discards the paper towel
13. Empties the contents of the graduate into the toilet and flushes
14. Rinses the graduate
15. Returns the graduate to its proper place
16. Removes the gloves
17. Washes hands
18. Records the time and amount on the intake and output (I&O) record
19. Provides for client comfort
20. Places the signal light within reach of client

❏ APPLYING A VEST RESTRAINT (CHAPTER 10)

1. Obtains the correct type and size of restraint
2. Checks straps for tears or frays
3. Washes hands
4. Explains procedure to client, speaking clearly, slowly, and directly, maintaining face-to-face contact whenever possible
5. Provides for privacy during procedure with curtain, screen, or door
6. Makes sure the client is comfortable and in good alignment
7. Assists the person to a sitting position
8. Applies the restraint following the manufacturer's instructions—the "V" part of the vest crosses in front
9. Makes sure the vest is free of wrinkles in the front and back
10. Brings the straps through the slots
11. Makes sure the client is comfortable and in good alignment
12. Secures the straps to the chair or to the movable part of the bed frame
13. Uses a secure knot that can be released with one pull
14. Makes sure the vest is snug—slide an open hand between the restraint and the client
15. Places the signal light within the client's reach
16. Washes hands

❏ PERFORMS A BACK RUB (MASSAGE) (CHAPTER 15)

1. Washes hands
2. Explains procedure to client, speaking clearly, slowly, and directly, maintaining face-to-face contact whenever possible
3. Provides for privacy during procedure with curtain, screen, or door
4. Raises the bed for good body mechanics
5. Lowers the bed rail near the candidate, if up
6. Positions the person in the prone or side-lying position
7. Exposes the back, shoulders, upper arms, and buttocks
8. Warms the lotion
9. Rubs entire back in upward, outward motion for approximately 2 to 3 minutes; does not massage reddened bony areas
10. Straightens and secures clothing or sleepwear

11. Returns client to comfortable and safe position
12. Places the signal light within reach
13. Lowers the bed to its lowest position
14. Washes hands

❑ POSITION FOLEY CATHETER (CHAPTER 17)

1. Explains procedure to client, speaking clearly, slowly, and directly, maintaining face-to-face contact whenever possible
2. Washes hands
3. Puts on gloves
4. Secures catheter and drainage tubing according to facility procedure
5. Places tubing over leg
6. Positions drainage tubing so urine flows freely into drainage bag and has no kinks
7. Attaches bag to bed frame, below level of bladder
8. Washes hands

❑ APPLY COLD PACK OR WARM COMPRESS (CHAPTER 23)

1. Washes hands
2. Collects needed equipment
3. Explains procedure to client, speaking clearly, slowly, and directly, maintaining face-to-face contact whenever possible
4. Provides for privacy during procedure with curtain, screen, or door
5. Positions the client for the procedure
6. Covers cold pack or warm compress with towel or other protective cover
7. Properly places cold pack or warm compress on site
8. Checks the client for complications every 5 minutes
9. Checks the cold pack or warm compress every 5 minutes
10. Removes the application at the specified time—usually after 15 to 20 minutes
11. Provides for comfort
12. Places the signal light within reach
13. Washes hands

❑ POSITION FOR AN ENEMA (CHAPTER 18)

1. Washes hands
2. Explains procedure to client, speaking clearly, slowly, and directly, maintaining face-to-face contact whenever possible
3. Provides for privacy

4. Positions the client in Sims' position or in a left side-lying position
5. Covers client appropriately
6. Provides for comfort
7. Places the signal light within reach
8. Washes hands

❑ POSITION CLIENT FOR MEALS (CHAPTER 19)

1. Washes hands
2. Explains procedure to client, speaking clearly, slowly, and directly, maintaining face-to-face contact whenever possible
3. If the person will eat in bed:
   a. Raises the head of the bed to a comfortable position—usually Fowler's or high Fowler's position is preferred
   b. Removes items from the overbed table and cleans the overbed table
   c. Adjusts the overbed table in front of the person
   d. Places the client in proper body alignment
4. If the person will sit in a chair:
   a. Positions the person in a chair or wheelchair
   b. Provides support for the client's feet
   c. Removes items from the overbed table and cleans the table
   d. Adjusts the overbed table in front of the person
   e. Places the client in proper body alignment
5. Places the signal light within reach
6. Washes hands

❑ TAKES AND RECORDS AXILLARY TEMPERATURE, PULSE, AND RESPIRATIONS (CHAPTER 20)

1. Washes hands before contact with client
2. Identifies self to client by name and addresses client by name
3. Explains procedure to client, speaking clearly, slowly, and directly, maintaining face-to-face contact whenever possible
4. Provides for client's privacy during procedure with curtain, screen, or door
5. Turns on digital oral thermometer
6. Dries axilla and places thermometer in the center of the axilla
7. Holds thermometer in place for appropriate length of time
8. Removes and reads thermometer
9. Records temperature on pad of paper
10. **Recorded temperature is within required range**

11. Discards sheath from thermometer
12. Places fingertips on thumb side of client's wrist to locate radial pulse
13. Counts beats for 1 full minute
14. Records pulse rate on pad of paper
15. **Recorded pulse is within required range**
16. Counts respirations for 1 full minute
17. Records respirations on pad of paper
18. **Recorded respirations are within required range**
19. Before leaving client, places signaling device within client's reach
20. Washes hands

❑ TRANSFERS CLIENT FROM WHEELCHAIR TO BED (CHAPTER 13)

1. Washes hands before contact with client
2. Identifies self to client by name and addresses client by name
3. Explains procedure to client, speaking clearly, slowly, and directly, maintaining face-to-face contact whenever possible
4. Provides for client's privacy during procedure with curtain, screen, or door
5. Positions wheelchair close to bed with arm of wheelchair almost touching bed
6. Before transferring client, ensures client is wearing non-skid footwear
7. Before transferring client, folds up footplates
8. Before transferring client, places bed at safe and appropriate level for client
9. **Before transferring client, locks wheels on wheelchair and locks bed brakes**
10. With transfer (gait) belt: Stands in front of client, positioning self to ensure safety of candidate and client during transfer (for example, knees bent, feet apart, back straight), places belt around client's waist, and grasps belt. Tightens belt so that fingers of candidate's hand can be slipped between transfer/gait belt and client

    Without transfer belt: Stands in front of client, positioning self to ensure safety of candidate and client during transfer (for example, knees bent, feet apart, back straight, arms around client's torso under arms)
11. Provides instructions to enable client to assist in transfer, including prearranged signal to alert client to begin standing
12. Braces client's lower extremities to prevent slipping
13. Counts to three (or says other prearranged signal) to alert client to begin transfer

14. On signal, gradually assists client to stand
15. Assists client to pivot and sit on bed in manner that ensures safety
16. Removes transfer belt, if used
17. Assists client to remove non-skid footwear
18. Assists client to move to center of bed
19. Provides for comfort and good body alignment
20. Before leaving client, places signaling device within client's reach
21. Washes hands

❑ WEIGHING AND MEASURING HEIGHT OF AN AMBULATORY CLIENT (CHAPTER 20)

1. Washes hands before contact with client
2. Identifies self to client by name and addresses client by name
3. Explains procedure to client, speaking clearly, slowly, and directly, maintaining face-to-face contact whenever possible
4. Starts with scale balanced at zero before weighing client
5. Assists client to step up onto center of scale
6. Determines client's weight and height
7. Assists client off scale before recording weight and height
8. Before leaving client, places signaling device within client's reach
9. Records weight and height within required range
10. Washes hands

❑ AFTER A PROCEDURE

After you demonstrate a skill, complete a safety check of the room:

- The person is wearing eyeglasses and hearing aids as needed.
- The signal light is plugged in and within reach.
- Bed rails are up or down according to the care plan.
- The bed is in the lowest horizontal position.
- The bed position is locked if needed.
- Manual bed cranks are in the down position.
- Bed wheels are locked.
- Assistive devices are within reach. Walker, cane, and wheelchair are examples.
- The overbed table, filled water pitcher and cup, tissues, phone, TV controls, and other needed items are within reach.
- Unneeded equipment is unplugged or turned off.

- Harmful substances are stored properly. Lotion, mouthwash, shampoo, after-shave, and other personal care products are examples.
- Food and other items brought by the family and visitors are safe for the person.
- Floors are free of spills and clutter.

❏ AFTER THE TEST

- Celebrate—you have completed the competency evaluation! The length of time for you to get your test results varies with each state. In the meantime, try to relax. Continue your daily routine, and be the best nursing assistant you can be.

ANSWERS TO REVIEW QUESTIONS IN TEXTBOOK CHAPTERS REVIEW

Chapter 1
1. c
2. b
3. a
4. a
5. d

Chapter 2
1. b
2. d
3. a
4. b
5. b
6. c
7. c
8. b
9. a
10. d
11. b
12. c
13. a

Chapter 3
1. c
2. c
3. a
4. d
5. d
6. b

Chapter 4
1. a
2. d
3. a
4. d
5. c

Chapter 5
1. b
2. d
3. d
4. c
5. d
6. b
7. a

8. c
9. d
10. c
11. c
12. d
13. a
14. b

Chapter 7
1. b
2. d
3. c
4. c
5. d
6. c
7. d

Chapter 8
1. b
2. d
3. a
4. d
5. c
6. c
7. b
8. c
9. b
10. c
11. b

Chapter 9
1. a
2. d
3. b
4. c
5. c
6. c

Chapter 10
1. a
2. c
3. a
4. a
5. b
6. b

Chapter 11
1. b
2. d
3. d
4. a
5. a
6. c

Chapter 12
1. c
2. b
3. c
4. c

Chapter 13
1. c
2. a
3. c
4. b
5. a
6. d

Chapter 14
1. T
2. T
3. T
4. F
5. T
6. T
7. c
8. b
9. c
10. d
11. d
12. c
13. a
14. d

Chapter 15
1. c
2. d
3. b
4. d
5. c
6. b

7. a
8. c
9. d
10. a
11. a

Chapter 16
1. T
2. F
3. T
4. T
5. F
6. T
7. T
8. T
9. F
10. b
11. d

Chapter 17
1. b
2. d
3. c
4. a
5. b
6. c
7. c

Chapter 18
1. b
2. d
3. d
4. a

Chapter 19
1. d
2. a
3. b
4. a
5. d
6. d

Chapter 20
1. b
2. a
3. b
4. b
5. a
6. c
7. c
8. d

Chapter 22
1. c
2. a
3. b
4. a

Chapter 23
1. d
2. c
3. a
4. c
5. d
6. d
7. c

Chapter 24
1. c
2. b
3. a
4. c
5. d

Chapter 25
1. a
2. a
3. d
4. a
5. b

Chapter 26
1. b
2. d
3. a
4. a
5. b

6. d
7. b
8. c
9. d
10. c
11. a
12. b
13. c
14. a
15. c

Chapter 27

1. a
2. a
3. a
4. c
5. b
6. d

Chapter 28

1. c
2. d
3. a
4. d

Chapter 29

1. c
2. a
3. b
4. c

Chapter 30

1. d
2. c
3. b
4. d
5. a

ANSWERS TO PRACTICE EXAMINATION 1

1. **C** You never give drugs. You may politely refuse to do a task that you have not been trained to do. However, you need to tell the nurse. Do not ignore a request to do something. Pages 16 and 23, Chapter 2.
2. **A** An ethical person does not judge others or cause harm to another person. Ethical behavior involves not being prejudiced or biased. Ethical behavior also involves not avoiding persons whose standards and values are different from your own. Page 24, Chapter 2.
3. **D** An ethical person is knowledgeable of what is right conduct and wrong conduct. Health care workers do not drink alcohol before coming to work and do not drink alcohol while working. Page 33, Chapter 3.
4. **A** Neglect is failure to provide a person with the goods or services needed to avoid physical harm, mental anguish, or mental illness. Page 28, Chapter 2.
5. **B** The person's information is confidential. Information about the patient or resident is shared only among health team members involved in his or her care. Page 39, Chapter 3.
6. **D** End-of-shift is a time for good teamwork. Continue to do your job. Your attitude is important. Page 62, Chapter 4.
7. **C** Write in ink, spell words correctly, and use only center-approved abbreviations. Page 55, Chapter 4.
8. **B** Give a courteous greeting. End the conversation politely and say good-bye. Confidential information about a resident or employee is not given to any caller. Page 60, Chapter 4.
9. **C** Safety and security needs relate to feeling safe from harm, danger, and fear. Health care agencies are strange places with strange routines and equipment. People feel safer if they know what to expect. Be kind and understanding. Show the person the nursing center, listen to his or her concerns, explain routines and procedures. Page 66, Chapter 5.
10. **B** When a person is angry or hostile, stay calm and professional. The person is usually not angry with you. He or she may be angry at another person or situation. Page 67, Chapter 5.
11. **D** Use words that are familiar to the person. Speak clearly, slowly, and distinctly. Also, ask one question at a time and wait for an answer. Page 68, Chapter 5.
12. **D** Follow the manufacturer's instructions. The excess strap should be tucked under the belt. The belt is applied over clothing and under the breasts. Page 126, Chapter 9.
13. **D** Listening requires that you care and have interest in the other person. Have good eye contact with the person. Focus on what the person is saying. Page 70, Chapter 5.
14. **C** Assume that a comatose person hears and understands you. Talk to the person and tell him or her what you are going to do. Page 73, Chapter 5.
15. **A** Protect a person's right to privacy when giving care. Politely ask visitors to leave the room. Do not expose the person's body in front of them. Show visitors where to wait. Page 73, Chapter 5.
16. **B** If a person wants to talk with a minister or spiritual leader, tell the nurse. Many people find comfort and strength from prayer and religious practices. Page 67, Chapter 5.
17. **A** Observe the person with a restraint at least every 15 minutes. Remove the restraint and reposition the person every 2 hours. Apply a restraint so it is snug and firm, but not tight. You could be negligent if the restraint is not applied properly. Page 137, Chapter 10.
18. **D** The skin becomes more dry, muscle strength decreases, reflexes are slower, and bladder muscles weaken. Page 98, Chapter 7.
19. **B** Always act in a professional manner. Page 101, Chapter 7.
20. **C** If you see something unsafe, correct the matter right away. Page 118, Chapter 8.
21. **A** Tell the nurse at once. It is important to do the correct procedure on the right person. You have to be able to read the person's name on the ID bracelet or use the photo ID to identify the person. Page 106, Chapter 8.
22. **B** Clutching at the throat is the "universal sign of choking." Page 108, Chapter 8.

23. **D** When a person is on a diabetic diet, tell the nurse about changes in the person's eating habits. The person's meals and snacks need to be served on time. The person needs to eat at regular intervals to maintain a certain blood sugar. Always check the tray to see what was eaten. Page 331, Chapter 19.

24. **D** With mild airway obstruction, the person is conscious and can speak. Often forceful coughing can remove the object. Page 107, Chapter 8.

25. **A** Abdominal thrusts are used to relieve severe airway obstruction. Page 108, Chapter 8.

26. **B** Do not use faulty electrical equipment in nursing centers. Take the item to the nurse. Page 110, Chapter 8.

27. **C** If a warning label is removed or damaged, do not use the substance. Take the container to the nurse and explain the problem. Page 112, Chapter 8.

28. **C** An ethical person realizes a person's values and standards may be different from his or hers. Page 24, Chapter 2.

29. **D** Remind a person not to smoke inside the center. Page 113, Chapter 8.

30. **A** During a fire, remember the word RACE. Page 114, Chapter 8.

31. **C** If a person with Alzheimer's disease has sundowning (increased restlessness and confusion as daylight ends), provide a calm, quiet setting late in the day. Do not try to reason with the person because he or she cannot understand what you are saying. Do not ask the person to tell you what is bothering him or her. Communication is impaired. Complete treatments and activities early in the day. Page 496, Chapter 28.

32. **C** Make sure dentures fit properly. Cut food into small pieces, and make sure the person can chew and swallow the food served. Report loose teeth or dentures to the nurse. Page 107, Chapter 8.

33. **A** Lock both wheels before you transfer a person to and from the wheelchair. The person's feet are on the footplates before moving the chair. Do not let the person stand on the footplates. Page 200, Chapter 13.

34. **B** Ease the person to the floor. Do not try to prevent the fall or yell at the person. The person should not get up before the nurse checks for injuries. Therefore the nurse needs to be told as soon as the fall occurs. Page 127, Chapter 9.

35. **B** Death from strangulation is the most serious risk factor to using a restraint. Restraints are not used for staff convenience or to punish a person. A written doctor's order is required before a restraint can be applied. Page 135, Chapter 10.

36. **C** Wash your hands before and after giving care to a person. Page 153, Chapter 11.

37. **D** Gloves need to be changed when they become contaminated with blood, body fluids, secretions, and excretions. Page 163, Chapter 11.

38. **D** When washing your hands, keep your hands and forearms lower than your elbows. Do not use hot water or let your uniform touch the sink. Push your watch up your arm so you can wash past your wrist. Page 153, Chapter 11.

39. **C** Bend your knees and squat to lift a heavy object. Hold items close to your body when lifting a heavy object. For a wider base of support and more balance, stand with your feet apart. Do not bend from your waist when lifting objects. Page 173, Chapter 12.

40. **B** The head of the bed is raised between 45 and 60 degrees for Fowler's position. Page 177, Chapter 12.

41. **B** Negligence—an unintentional wrong in which a person did not act in a reasonable and careful manner and causes harm to a person or the person's property. Page 26, Chapter 2.

42. **A** Have the person's back and buttocks against the back of the chair. Feet are flat on the floor or on the wheelchair footplates. Backs of the person's knees and calves are slightly away from the edge of the seat. Page 179, Chapter 12.

43. **B** Help the person out of bed on his or her strong side. In transferring, the strong side moves first. It pulls the weaker side along. Page 200, Chapter 13.

44. **A** When a person tries to bite, scratch, pinch, or kick you, you need to protect the person, others, and yourself from harm. Page 67, Chapter 5.

45. **C** Protect the person's right to privacy at all times. Screen the person properly, and do not expose body parts. Page 183, Chapter 13.

46. **D** For comfort, adjust lighting to meet the person's changing needs. Nursing centers maintain a temperature range of 71° F to 81° F. Unpleasant odors may be offensive or embarrassing to people. Many older persons are sensitive to noise. Page 214, Chapter 14.

47. **A** Signal lights are placed on the person's strong side and kept within the person's reach. Signal lights are answered promptly. Page 219, Chapter 14.

48. **C** You must have the person's permission to open or search closets or drawers. Page 220, Chapter 14.

49. **C** When handling linens, do not take unneeded linen to a person's room. Once in the room, extra linen is considered contaminated. Because your uniform is considered dirty, always hold linen away from your body. To prevent the spread of microbes, never shake linen. Never put clean or dirty linens on the floor. Page 223, Chapter 14.

50. **C** To use a fire extinguisher, remember the word PASS. P—pull the safety pin, A—aim low, S—squeeze the lever, S—sweep back and forth. Page 114, Chapter 8.

51. **B** Mouth care is given at least every 2 hours for an unconscious person. To prevent aspiration, you position the person on one side with the head turned well to the side. Use a padded tongue blade to keep the person's mouth open. Wear gloves. Page 243, Chapter 15.

52. **B** A good attitude is needed at work. Be willing to help others. Be pleasant and respectful of others. Page 42, Chapter 3.

53. **B** During cleaning, firmly hold dentures over a basin of water lined with a towel. This prevents them from falling onto a hard surface and breaking. Clean and store dentures in cool water. Hot water causes dentures to lose their shape. To prevent losing dentures, label the denture cup with the person's name. Page 245, Chapter 15.

54. **C** Report and record the location and description of the rash. Page 248, Chapter 15.

55. **C** Gently wipe the eye from the inner aspect to the outer aspect of the eye. Clean the far eye first. Do not use soap. Page 250, Chapter 15.

56. **D** When giving a back massage, wear gloves if the person's skin has open areas. Warm the lotion before applying it to the person. Use firm strokes. Do not massage reddened bony areas. This can lead to more tissue damage. Page 258, Chapter 15.

57. **A** Separate the labia and clean downward from front to back. Wear gloves and use soap. Page 262, Chapter 15.

58. **C** Stay within hearing distance if the person can be left alone. Place the signal light within the person's reach. Cold water is turned on first, then hot water. Direct water away from the person while adjusting the water temperature. Page 254, Chapter 15.

59. **B** Electric razors are used when a person is on an anticoagulant. An anticoagulant prevents or slows down blood clotting. Bleeding occurs easily. A nick or cut from a safety razor can cause bleeding. Page 274, Chapter 16.

60. **B** Remove clothing from the strong or "good" (unaffected) side first. Page 279, Chapter 16.

61. **C** Address a person with dignity and respect. Call the person by his or her title—Mr., or Mrs., or Miss. Address a person by his or her first name, or another name, if the person asks you to do so. Page 65, Chapter 5.

62. **D** Measure and record the amount of urine in the drainage bag. The catheter is secured to the person's thigh or abdomen. Do not disconnect the catheter from the drainage tubing. Do not let the person lie on the tubing. Page 299, Chapter 17.

63. **B** Carbohydrates provide energy and fiber for bowel elimination. Page 327, Chapter 19.

64. **D** When taking a rectal temperature, the thermometer is held in place so it is not lost into the rectum or broken. Lubricate the bulb end of the thermometer for easy insertion and to prevent tissue damage. Provide for privacy. A glass thermometer remains in place for 2 minutes or as required by policy. Page 352, Chapter 20.

65. **A** Report any systolic pressure below 90 mm Hg and any diastolic pressure below 60 mm Hg at once. Record the BP. If the nurse tells you, retake the BP in 30 minutes. It is your responsibility to tell the nurse, not the unit secretary. Page 363, Chapter 20.

66. **D** Oral temperatures are not taken on unconscious persons, persons receiving oxygen, or persons who breathe through their mouth. Page 350, Chapter 20.

67. **A** To assist with walking, offer the person your arm and have the person walk a half step behind you. When caring for a person who is blind or visually impaired, let the person do as much for himself or herself as possible. Use a normal voice tone. Do not shout at the person. Identify yourself when you enter the room. Do not touch the person until you have indicated your presence. Page 465, Chapter 26.

68. **D** The person with confusion and dementia has the right to personal choice. He or she also has the right to keep and use personal items. The family makes choices if the person cannot. Page 496, Chapter 28.

69. **D** No one can shout, scream, or hit the person. Nor can they call the person names. The person did not choose loss of function. Discuss your feelings with the nurse. Page 444, Chapter 25.

70. **C** Encourage the person to help as much as possible. Doors and windows are closed to reduce drafts. You wash from the cleanest areas to the dirtiest areas. Pat the skin dry to avoid irritating or breaking the skin. Page 247, Chapter 15.

71. **A** When a person is dying, always assume that the person can hear you. Reposition the person every 2 hours to promote comfort. Skin care, personal hygiene, back massages, oral hygiene, and good body alignment promote comfort. Page 520, Chapter 30.

72. **B** Foods that melt at room temperature (ice cream, sherbet, custard, pudding, gelatin,and Popsicles) are measured and recorded as intake. The nurse measures and records IV fluids and tube feedings. Page 367, Chapter 20.

73. **B** After bedrest, activity increases slowly and in steps. First the person dangles. Sitting in a chair follows. Next the person walks in the room and then in the hallway. Page 197, Chapter 13.

74. **B** Tell the nurse at once if you find or cause a skin tear. Page 410, Chapter 23.

75. **A** Treat the resident with respect and ensure privacy. The resident has a right not to have his or her private affairs exposed or made public without giving consent. Only staff involved in the resident's care should see, handle, or examine his or her body. Page 8, Chapter 1.

ANSWERS TO PRACTICE EXAMINATION 2

1. **C** You may politely refuse to do a task that is not in your job description. Page 23, Chapter 2.
2. **B** An ethical person realizes a person's values and standards may be different from his or hers. You may not agree with advance directive or resuscitation decisions. However, you must respect the person's wishes. Page 24, Chapter 2 and Page 524, Chapter 30.
3. **C** Verbal abuse is using oral or written words or statements that speak badly of, sneer at, criticize, or condemn a person. Page 28, Chapter 2.
4. **C** Speak in a normal tone. Use words the person seems to understand, and speak slowly and distinctly. Page 72, Chapter 5.
5. **C** Do not allow smoking in bed. Turn cold water on first, then hot water. Assist the person with drinking or eating hot food. Do not let the person sleep with a heating pad. Page 107, Chapter 8.
6. **B** Use three-pronged plugs on all electrical devices, and follow the manufacturer's instructions on equipment. Wipe up spills right away. Do not use unfamiliar equipment. Ask for training if you are unfamiliar with something. Page 110, Chapter 8.
7. **D** Answer signal lights promptly. Throw rugs, scatter rugs, and area rugs are not used. The person's bed should be in the lowest horizontal position, except when giving care. Grab bars should be used when the person showers. Page 122, Chapter 9.
8. **B** Decontaminate your hands after removing gloves. Page 153, Chapter 11.
9. **D** Use good body mechanics, provide for privacy, and use pillows as directed by the nurse. The signal light should be placed within the person's reach after positioning. Page 183, Chapter 13.
10. **C** A person must not put his or her arms around your neck. He or she can pull you forward or cause you to lose your balance. Neck, back, and other injuries from falls are possible. Ask a co-worker to help you, and you should use a transfer or gait belt. Lock the wheels on the wheelchair. Page 201, Chapter 13.
11. **B** Wear gloves when removing linen. Linens may contain blood, body fluids, secretions, or excretions. Raise the bed for good body

mechanics. The bed is flat when you place clean linens on it. Page 224, Chapter 14.
12. **B** Use a circular motion, start at the meatus, and work outward. Gloves are worn. Soap is used. Page 264, Chapter 15.
13. **C** Put clothing on the weak (affected) side first. Page 279, Chapter 16.
14. **D** The drainage bag hangs from the bed frame or chair. It must not touch the floor. The bag is always kept lower than the person's bladder. The drainage bag does not hang on the bed rail. Page 299, Chapter 17.
15. **A** Protein is needed for tissue repair and growth. Page 327, Chapter 19.
16. **C** Older persons may not feel thirsty (decreased sense of thirst). Offer water often. Page 334, Chapter 19.
17. **C** NPO means nothing by mouth. An NPO sign is posted above the bed. The water pitcher and glass are removed from the room. Oral hygiene is performed frequently. Page 334, Chapter 19.
18. **C** 1 oz equals 30 mL. 3 oz equals 90 mL. Page 367, Chapter 20.
19. **D** Allow time for chewing and swallowing. Fluids are offered during the meal. A teaspoon, rather than a fork, is used for feeding. Sit and talk with the person. Page 338, Chapter 19.
20. **D** Support the part being exercised. Do not force a joint beyond its present ROM. Move the joint slowly, smoothly, and gently. Do not force the joint to the point of pain. Page 393, Chapter 22.
21. **B** A cane is held on the strong side of the body. If the left leg is weak, the cane is held in the right hand. Page 400, Chapter 22.
22. **B** Position the person in good alignment. Bed linens are kept tight and wrinkle-free. Talk softly and gently. Avoid sudden and jarring movements of the bed or chair. Page 233, Chapter 14.
23. **C** Check behind the ears and under the nose for signs of irritation. Never remove an oxygen device. Do not adjust the oxygen flow rate. Do not fill the humidifier. Page 436, Chapter 24.
24. **A** Tell the nurse at once. Mercury is a hazardous substance. Do not touch the mercury. Follow special procedures for handling hazardous materials. Page 351, Chapter 20.

25. **C** Record and report at once a pulse rate less than 60 or more than 100 beats per minute. The radial pulse is used for routine vital signs. If the pulse is irregular, count it for 1 minute. Do not use your thumb to take a pulse. Page 359, Chapter 20.

26. **B** Count the respirations for 1 minute if an abnormal breathing pattern is noted. People change their breathing patterns when they know respirations are being counted. Therefore the person should not know that you are counting respirations. The healthy adult has 12 to 20 respirations per minute. Page 361, Chapter 20.

27. **A** Report at once any systolic pressure above 140 mm Hg and any diastolic pressure above 80 mm Hg. Then continue to take blood pressures on other persons. Retake the BP in 30 minutes if the nurse asks you to. It is your responsibility to tell the nurse, not the unit secretary's responsibility. Page 363, Chapter 20.

28. **C** Rectal temperatures are not taken if a person has diarrhea, is confused, or is agitated. Page 350, Chapter 20.

29. **C** Residents must be cared for in a manner that promotes dignity and self-esteem. Use the right tone of voice. Respect private space and property. Listen to the person with interest. Knock on the door and wait to be asked in before entering. Page 10, Chapter 1.

30. **B** Have the person void before being weighed. A full bladder adds weight. No footwear is worn. Footwear adds to the weight and height measurements. Weigh the person at the same time of day, usually before breakfast. Balance the scale before weighing the person. Page 370, Chapter 20.

31. **D** Keep the skin free of moisture from urine, stools, or perspiration. Reposition the person at least every 2 hours. Do not massage reddened areas. Keep the heels and ankles off the bed. Page 408, Chapter 23.

32. **C** Face the person when speaking. Reduce or eliminate background noise. Speak in a normal voice tone. Speak clearly, distinctly, and slowly. Page 461, Chapter 26.

33. **C** Explain the location of food and beverages. Keep furniture and equipment out of areas where the person walks. Provide lighting as the person prefers. Do not rearrange furniture and equipment. Page 464, Chapter 26.

34. **C** The person with confusion and dementia has the right to privacy and confidentiality. Information about the person's care and condition is shared only with those involved in providing the care. Protect the person from exposure. Page 500, Chapter 28.

35. **C** Ask clear, simple questions. Explain what you are going to do and why. Call the person by name every time you are in contact with him or her. Keep calendars and clocks in the person's room. Page 491, Chapter 28.

36. **D** Exercise the person as ordered. Adequate exercise often reduces wandering. Do not keep the person in his or her room. Involve the person in activities. Do not restrain the person or argue with the person who wants to leave. Page 496, Chapter 28.

37. **B** Restorative nursing programs promote self-care measures. They help maintain the person's highest level of function. The programs focus on the whole person. The care helps the person regain health, strength, and independence. Page 439, Chapter 25.

38. **C** Remind the person of his or her progress in the rehabilitation program. Focus on the person's abilities and strengths. Progress may be slow. Do not deny the disability. Page 443, Chapter 25.

39. **D** Respect the person's right to privacy. Do not expose the person's body unnecessarily. Only those involved in the person's care need to know the person's diagnosis. The final moments of death are kept confidential. So are family reactions. Page 525, Chapter 30.

40. **A** Remember the word RACE. Your first action is to Rescue the person in immediate danger. Then sound the Alarm, Confine the fire, and Extinguish the fire. Page 114, Chapter 8.

41. **B** Failure to provide a person with the goods or services needed to avoid physical harm or mental anguish is neglect. Page 28, Chapter 2.

42. **C** You have not been trained to give drugs or to perform sterile procedures. Do not perform tasks that are not in your job description. Page 16, Chapter 2.

43. **C** Ask the nurse to observe urine that looks or smells abnormal. Then record your observation. Page 290, Chapter 17.

44. **D** A good attitude is needed at work. People rely on you to give good care. You are expected to be pleasant and respectful. Always be willing to help others. Page 38, Chapter 3.

45. **B** Unnecessary restraint is false imprisonment. Observe the person for complications every 15 minutes. The least restrictive type of restraint is ordered by the doctor. Restraints

can increase confusion and agitation. Page 136, Chapter 10.

46. **C** The supine position is the back-lying position. For good alignment, the bed is flat and the head and shoulders are supported on a pillow. Place arms and hands at the sides. Page 177, Chapter 12.

47. **A** Hand washing is the most important way to prevent or avoid spreading infection. Page 153, Chapter 11.

48. **B** To gossip means to spread rumors or talk about the private matters of others. Gossiping is unprofessional and hurtful. If others are gossiping, you need to remove yourself from the group. Do not make or repeat any comment that can hurt another person. Page 38, Chapter 3.

49. **D** Ask a co-worker to help you. The head of the bed is lowered. The person flexes both knees. Friction and shearing cause skin tears and need to be prevented. Page 188, Chapter 13.

50. **A** On a sodium-controlled diet, high-sodium foods such as ham and canned vegetables are omitted. Salt is not added to food at the table. The amount of salt used in cooking is limited. Page 331, Chapter 19.

51. **B** Elastic stockings should not have wrinkles or creases after being applied. Wrinkles and creases can cause skin breakdown. Apply stockings before the person gets out of bed. Apply the correct size. Page 413, Chapter 23.

52. **C** When a person begins to fall, ease him or her to the floor. Also protect the person's head. Page 127, Chapter 9.

53. **A** Before bathing, allow the person to use the bathroom, bedpan, or urinal. Page 247, Chapter 15.

54. **A** Insert a rectal thermometer 1 inch into the rectum. Page 354, Chapter 20.

55. **A** Touch is a form of nonverbal communication. It conveys comfort and caring. Touch means different things to different people. Some people do not like to be touched. Page 68, Chapter 5.

56. **A** A person's information is confidential. The information is shared only among health team members involved in the person's care. Page 39, Chapter 3.

57. **A** Report and record complaints of urgency, burning, dysuria, or other urinary problems. Page 291, Chapter 17.

58. **C** Respect a person's culture and religion. Learn about his or her beliefs and practices. This helps you understand the person and give better care. Page 66, Chapter 5.

59. **C** Wear gloves when giving perineal care. Gloves are needed whenever contact with blood, body fluids, secretions, excretions, mucous membranes, and non-intact skin is likely. Page 163, Chapter 11.

60. **D** Report any changes from normal or changes in the person's condition to the nurse at once. Then record your observation. Page 54, Chapter 4.

61. **A** If a person is standing, have him or her sit before fainting occurs. Page 515, Chapter 29.

62. **A** The person drinks an increased amount of fluid. Keep fluids within the person's reach. Offer fluids regularly. Page 334, Chapter 19.

63. **B** Communication fails when you talk too much and fail to listen. Page 72, Chapter 5.

64. **A** During bathing, a person has the right to privacy and the right to personal choice. Page 247, Chapter 15.

65. **C** People in late adulthood need to develop new friends and relationships. They need to adjust to retirement and reduced income, decreased strength, and loss of health. They need to cope with a partner's death and prepare for their own death. Page 97, Chapter 7.

66. **D** Blood pressure is not taken on an arm with an IV (intravenous) infusion. When taking a blood pressure, apply the cuff to the bare upper arm. Make sure the room is quiet. Talking, TV, radio, and sounds from the hallway can affect an accurate measurement. Place the diaphragm of the stethoscope over the brachial artery. Page 364, Chapter 20.

67. **C** Never put clean or dirty linen on the floor. The floor is dirty. You cannot use the linen. Page 223, Chapter 14.

68. **B** To prevent aspiration, position the unconscious person on one side when you do mouth care. Use a small amount of fluid to clean the mouth. Tell the person what you are doing. Dentures are not worn when the person is unconscious. Page 243, Chapter 15.

69. **B** Encourage people to do their own hair care. Do not cut matted or tangled hair. The person chooses his or her hair style. Brushing and combing are done with morning care and whenever needed. Page 269, Chapter 16.

70. **D** Check between the toes for cracks and sores. These areas are often overlooked. If left untreated, a serious infection could occur. Fingernails are cut with nail clipper, not scissors. You do not trim or cut toenails if a person has diabetes or has poor circulation. Page 276, Chapter 16.

71. **B** If an indwelling catheter becomes disconnected from the drainage system, you tell the nurse at once. Page 302, Chapter 17.
72. **B** Urinary drainage bags are emptied and the contents measured at the end of each shift. Drainage bags must not touch the floor. The bag is always kept lower than the person's bladder. Page 302, Chapter 17.
73. **C** Use elastic tape to secure a condom catheter. Elastic tape expands when the penis changes size, and adhesive tape does not. Do not apply a condom catheter if the penis is red and irritated. Always act in a professional manner. Page 304, Chapter 17.
74. **D** For comfort during bowel elimination, leave the person alone if possible. Provide for privacy. Help the person to the toilet or commode if possible. Page 311, Chapter 18.
75. **A** Help the person from the wheelchair to the bed on his or her strong side. In transferring, the strong side moves first. It pulls the weaker side along. Page 204, Chapter 13.